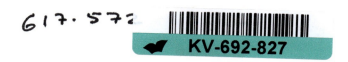

Complications of Shoulder Surgery

TREATMENT AND PREVENTION

Complications of Shoulder Surgery

TREATMENT AND PREVENTION

EDITED BY

▬ THOMAS J. GILL, MD

Associate Professor
Harvard Shoulder Service
Harvard Medical School
Department of Orthopaedic Surgery
Massachusetts General Hospital
Boston, Massachusetts

▬ RICHARD J. HAWKINS, MD

Clinical Professor of Orthopaedic Surgery
University of Colorado
Team Physician
Denver Broncos and Colorado Rockies,
Denver, Colorado
Consultant
Steadman Hawkins Clinic
Vail, Colorado
Steadman Hawkins Clinic of the Carolinas
Spartanburg, South Carolina

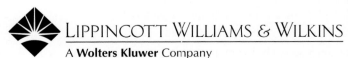

LIPPINCOTT WILLIAMS & WILKINS
A **Wolters Kluwer** Company
Philadelphia • Baltimore • New York • London
Buenos Aires • Hong Kong • Sydney • Tokyo

Acquisitions Editor: Robert A. Hurley
Managing Editor: Jenny Kim
Project Manager: Fran Gunning
Marketing Manager: Sharon Zinner
Manufacturing Manager: Ben Rivera
Design Coordinator: Doug Smock
Production Services: Maryland Composition Co., Inc.
Printer: Edwards Brothers

Library of Congress Cataloging-in-Publication Data

Complications of shoulder surgery : treatment and prevention / edited
  by Thomas J. Gill, Richard J. Hawkins.
     p. ; cm.
  Includes bibliographical references and index.
  ISBN 0-7817-5729-0
  1. Shoulder—Surgery—Complications.   I. Gill, Thomas J., 1964-
II. Hawkins, Richard J.
  [DNLM: 1. Postoperative Complications—therapy.   2. Shoulder Joint
—surgery.   3. Arthroscopy.   4. Orthopedic Procedures—adverse effects.
5. Shoulder—surgery.   WE 810 C7375 2006]
  RD557.5.C654 2006
  617.5′72059—dc22

                        2005026526

Care has been taken to confirm the accuracy of the information presented and to describe generally accepted practices. However, the authors, editors, and publisher are not responsible for errors or omissions or for any consequences from application of the information in this book and make no warranty, expressed or implied, with respect to the currency, completeness, or accuracy of the contents of the publication. Application of this information in a particular situation remains the professional responsibility of the practitioner.

The authors, editors, and publisher have exerted every effort to ensure that drug selection and dosage set forth in this text are in accordance with current recommendations and practice at the time of publication. However, in view of ongoing research, changes in government regulations, and the constant flow of information relating to drug therapy and drug reactions, the reader is urged to check the package insert for each drug for any change in indications and dosage and for added warnings and precautions. This is particularly important when the recommended agent is a new or infrequently employed drug.

Some drugs and medical devices presented in this publication have Food and Drug Administration (FDA) clearance for limited use in restricted research settings. It is the responsibility of the health care provider to ascertain the FDA status of each drug or device planned for use in their clinical practice.

To purchase additional copies of this book, call our customer service department at (800) 638-3030 or fax orders to (301) 223-2320. International customers should call (301) 223-2300.

Visit Lippincott Williams & Wilkins on the Internet at LWW.com. Lippincott Williams & Wilkins customer service representatives are available from 8:30 AM to 6 PM, EST.

10 9 8 7 6 5 4 3 2 1

Contents

SECTION I: OPEN SURGERY 1

1 Complications of Surgery for Anterior Shoulder Instability 3
Thomas J. Gill and Bertram Zarins

2 Complications of Surgery for Posterior/Multidirectional Instability 14
James D. O'Holleran and Russel F. Warren

3 Complications of Rotator Cuff Repair 31
Joseph Iannotti and Michael Codsi

4 Complications of Total Shoulder Arthroplasty 43
George F. Hatch, III, John G. Costouros, Peter J. Millett, and Jon J.P. Warner

5 Complications of Fracture Management 70
Theodore F. Schlegel, Patrick N. Siparsky, and Richard J. Hawkins

6 Complications of Surgery to the Acromioclavicular and Sternoclavicular Joints 77
Jonathan P. Braman and Evan L. Flatow

7 Neurologic Injury 85
Robert H. Cofield and Scott P. Steinmann

8 Frozen Shoulder 95
Laith M. Jazrawi, Andrew S. Rokito, and Joseph D. Zuckerman

9 Complications of Glenohumeral Arthrodesis 113
Gregory J. Gilot, David J. Clare, Bertrand Coulet, and Charles A. Rockwood, Jr.

10 Complications of Scapulothoracic Arthrodesis 118
Sumant G. Krishnan, Richard J. Hawkins, and Wayne Z. Burkhead

SECTION II: ARTHROSCOPY 123

11 General Complications of Arthroscopic Shoulder Surgery 125
Sumant G. Krishnan, Scott D. Pennington, Daniel E. Cooper, and Wayne Z. Burkhead

12 Arthroscopy: Complications of Surgery for Instability 132
Carlos A. Guanche and Stephen J. Snyder

13 Arthroscopy: Complications of Rotator Cuff Repair 144
Samer S. Hasan and Gary M. Gartsman

14 Complications of Arthroscopic Subacromial Decompression and Acromioclavicular Joint Resection 162
Ilya Voloshin, Kevin J. Setter, Sean F. Bak, and Louis U. Bigliani

15 Complications of Thermal Capsulorrhaphy 172
Charles L. Getz, Matthew L. Ramsey, David Glaser, and Gerald R. Williams, Jr.

Preface

Shoulder surgery, like many aspects of medicine, is fraught with potential complications. When they arise, it is helpful to consult with other shoulder surgeons and to collect opinions about preferred treatment approaches. Although doing a literature review on a topic can provide valuable information, some of the best advice and recommendations come from the invaluable experience of our colleagues. Many times no individual surgeon has collected enough cases of a specific complication to report a well-documented approach to resolving them. However, the contributors to this text have many years of experience in treating shoulder problems, and they have acquired valuable practical knowledge that can provide the basis for "pearls of wisdom."

The purpose of this book is different from other books in the field. Rather than simply relying on published reports and summarizing the literature, we have asked a well-recognized and highly respected group of shoulder experts to contribute a chapter that summarizes their own approaches to a given set of complications, i.e., to provide their own "pearls" about accurate diagnosis and treatment of a variety of shoulder complications. In essence, we have tried to create a portable consultation reference that can help the practicing surgeon to select a suitable approach to treating a variety of difficult complications of shoulder surgery. Thus, this book is similar to an "Ask the Experts" forum, and we hope that it can serve as a guide—a good second opinion—when the surgeon has to make difficult decisions.

There is a saying that success comes from experience, and that "experience" comes from failures. We would like to thank all of the authors who have made this important endeavor possible by sharing their own such successes and failures. We hope that this book will enable the reader to learn from their collective experience, thereby contributing to better care for our patients.

Thomas J. Gill, MD
Richard J. Hawkins, MD

Contributors

SEAN F. BAK, MD The Shoulder Service, New York Orthopaedic Hospital, Columbia-Presbyterian Medical Center, New York, New York

LOUIS U. BIGLIANI, MD Frank E. Stinchfield Professor and Chairman, Department of Orthopaedic Surgery, New York Presbyterian Hospital, Columbia-Presbyterian Medical Center, Columbia University, New York, New York

JONATHAN P. BRAMAN, MD Mount Sinai School of Medicine, New York, New York

WAYNE Z. BURKHEAD, MD Clinical Associate Professor, Department of Orthopaedec Surgery, University of Texas Southwestern Medical Center, Attending Orthopaedic Surgeon, Shoulder and Elbow Service, W.B. Carrell Memorial Clinic, Dallas, Texas

DAVID J. CLARE, MD Nebraska Orthopaedic & Sports Medicine, P.C., Lincoln, Nebraska

MICHAEL CODSI, MD Department of Orthopedic Surgery, The Cleveland Clinic, Cleveland, Ohio

ROBERT H. COFIELD, MD Professor, Mayo Medical School, Consultant, Department of Orthopedic Surgery, Mayo Clinic, Rochester, Minnesota

DANIEL E. COOPER, MD Attending Orthopaedic Surgeon W.B. Carrell Memorial Clinic, Dallas, Texas

JOHN G. COSTOUROS, MD Clinical Instructor, Harvard Shoulder Service, Department of Orthopaedic Surgery, Harvard Medical School, Massachusetts General Hospital, Boston, Massachusetts

BERTRAND COULET, MD Hand and Orthopaedics Surgery Department, Lapeyronie Hospital, Montpellier, France

EVAN L. FLATOW, MD Professor of Orthopedic Surgery, Chief of Shoulder Surgery, Mount Sinai School of Medicine, New York, New York

GARY M. GARTSMAN, MD Clinical Professor, University of Texas Health Science Center, Fondren Orthopaedic Group, Houston, Texas

CHARLES L. GETZ, MD Assistant Professor, Penn Presbyterian Medical Center, University of Pennsylvania, Philadelphia, Pennsylvania

THOMAS J. GILL, MD Associate Professor, Harvard Shoulder Service, Harvard Medical School, Department of Orthopedic Surgery, Massachusetts General Hospital, Boston, Massachusetts

GREGORY J. GILOT, MD Assistant Professor, Department of Orthopedics, Indiana University School of Medicine, Indianapolis, Indiana

DAVID L. GLASER, MD Assistant Professor of Orthopaedic Surgery, Shoulder and Elbow Service, Penn Presbyterian Medical Center, University of Pennsylvania, Philadelphia, Pennsylvania

CARLOS A. GUANCHE, MD Southern California Orthopedic Institute, Van Nuys, California

SAMER S. HASAN, MD, PhD Cincinnati Sports Medicine and Orthopaedic Center, Cincinnati, Ohio

GEORGE F. (RICK) HATCH, III, MD Assistant Professor of Orthopaedics, USC Sports Medicine, Shoulder & Elbow Service, Department of Orthopaedic Surgery, University of Southern California, Keck School of Medicine, Los Angeles, California

RICHARD J. HAWKINS, MD Clinical Professor of Orthopedic Surgery, University of Colorado, Team Physician, Denver Broncos and Colorado Rockies, Denver, Colorado, Consultant, Steadman Hawkins Clinic, Vail, Colorado, Steadman Hawkins Clinic of the Carolinas, Spartanburg, South Carolina

JOSEPH IANNOTTI, MD, PhD Professor and Chairman, Department of Orthopedic Surgery, The Cleveland Clinic, Cleveland, Ohio

LAITH M. JAZRAWI, MD Assistant Professor, New York University School of Medicine, New York University Hospital for Joint Diseases, New York, New York

SUMANT G. KRISHNAN, MD Clinical Assistant Professor, Department of Orthopaedec Surgery, University of Texas Southwestern Medical Center, Attending Orthopaedic Surgeon, Shoulder and Elbow Service, W.B. Carrell Memorial Clinic, Dallas, Texas

PETER J. MILLETT, MD, MSc   Associate Director, Harvard Shoulder Service, Assistant Professor of Orthopaedics, Harvard Medical School, Department of Orthopaedic Surgery, Brigham and Women's Hospital, Boston, Massachusetts

JAMES D. O'HOLLERAN, MD   Hospital for Special Surgery, New York, New York

SCOTT D. PENNINGTON, MD   Shoulder and Elbow Service, W.B. Carrell Memorial Clinic, Dallas, Texas

MATTHEW L. RAMSEY, MD   Associate Professor of Orthopaedic Surgery, Chief, Shoulder and Elbow Service, Department of Orthopaedic Surgery, Penn Presbyterian Medical Center, Philadelphia, Pennsylvania

CHARLES A. ROCKWOOD, JR., MD   Professor and Chairman Emeritus, The University of Texas Health Science Center, Department of Orthopedics, San Antonio, Texas

ANDREW S. ROKITO, MD   Chief, Shoulder and Elbow Service, New York University, Hospital for Joint Diseases, New York, New York

THEODORE F. SCHLEGEL, MD   Orthopedic Surgeon, Steadman Hawkins Clinic, Denver, Assistant Clinical Professor, Department of Orthopedics, University of Colorado, Medical Director, Denver Broncos Football Team, Assistant Team Physician, Colorado Rockies, Greenwood Village, Colorado

KEVIN J. SETTER, MD   The Shoulder Service, New York Orthopaedic Hospital, Columbia-Presbyterian Medical Center, New York, New York

PATRICK N. SIPARSKY, BS   University of Colorado School of Medicine, Denver, Colorado

STEPHEN J. SNYDER, MD   Orthopedic Surgeon, Southern California Orthopedic Institute, Van Nuys, California

SCOTT P. STEINMANN, MD   Assistant Professor, Mayo Medical School, Consultant, Department of Orthopedic Surgery, Mayo Clinic, Rochester, Minnesota

ILYA VOLOSHIN, MD   The Shoulder Service, New York Orthopaedic Hospital, Columbia-Presbyterian Medical Center, New York, New York

JON J.P. WARNER, MD   Chief, Harvard Shoulder Service, Professor of Orthopaedics, Harvard Medical School, Massachusetts General Hospital Yawkey Center for Outpatient Care, Boston, Massachusetts

RUSSELL F. WARREN, MD   Professor of Orthopedic Surgery, Weill Medical College of Cornell University, Hospital for Special Surgery, New York, New York

GERALD R. WILLIAMS, JR., MD   Professor of Orthopaedic Surgery, Shoulder and Elbow Service, Chief of Orthopaedic Surgery, Penn Presbyterian Medical Center, Philadelphia, Pennsylvania

BERTRAM ZARINS, MD   Chief, Sports Medicine Service, Department of Orthopedic Surgery, Massachusetts General Hospital, Boston, Massachusetts

JOSEPH D. ZUCKERMAN, MD   Chairman, Department of Orthopaedic Surgery, New York University Hospital for Joint Diseases, Walter A.L. Thompson Professor of Orthopaedic Surgery, New York University School of Medicine, New York, New York

Complications of Shoulder Surgery

TREATMENT AND PREVENTION

Open Surgery

Complications of Surgery for Anterior Shoulder Instability

Thomas J. Gill   *Bertram Zarins*

The goals of surgery for shoulder instability are to restore stability while maintaining a pain-free, maximal range of motion. In the past, surgeons have performed operations that restored glenohumeral stability, but often at the price of decreased mobility or stiffness (1). Examples of these procedures are the Putti-Platt and Magnuson-Stack procedures. Recent outcome studies have reported that patients' priorities are full mobility and function, even to the exclusion of absolute stability (2).

When complications do arise, the problems generally fall into one of several categories. These categories include recurrent instability, loss of motion without arthrosis, loss of motion with arthrosis, subscapularis ruptures, neurologic injuries, and hardware-related problems. In order to treat these complications successfully, there are several principles of treatment that are helpful to consider.

PRINCIPLES

Perhaps the most important principle of treatment when evaluating a complication of open instability surgery is to diagnose the exact reason for failure of the prior surgery (3). It is not enough to simply assume that a revision Bankart operation can be used to treat the recurrent instability. A precise anatomic explanation for the instability should be determined whenever possible.

It is helpful to start the patient interview by obtaining a history about the events that led up to the first instability procedure. What kind of symptoms was the patient having that led to the surgical intervention? Was it instability or pain only? If a trauma was involved, did the shoulder actually dislocate and require a formal reduction? In what position was the arm when the trauma occurred, and what position of the arm exacerbated the symptoms? These types of questions help to confirm that an accurate diagnosis of anterior instability was made prior to performing an anterior stabilization procedure.

If the patient had an initial Bankart procedure, but upon questioning had symptoms more consistent with posterior instability, then the reason for the patient's instability complaints may not be due to a failed primary surgery, but rather that the wrong procedure was performed for the wrong diagnosis. It should also be remembered that not all cases of anterior instability are due to Bankart lesions alone. Anterior-inferior labral tears are present in 65% to 90% of shoulders (2,4–7). Other pathology includes Hill-Sachs lesions in 77%, injury to the glenoid rim (including fracture) in 73% (6,8), and glenoid avulsion fractures in 4% of shoulders. Rotator cuff tears are identified in up to 13%, and posterior glenoid labral tears in 10% of shoulders (9). A redundant capsule and deficient subscapularis muscle can also contribute to shoulder instability (5).

If it is determined that the initial diagnosis and treatment were more than likely appropriate, the next step is to diagnose the current cause for symptoms. It is helpful to determine whether the complaints are acute and the result of a recent significant trauma, or whether the shoulder has never felt quite right since the initial surgery. Complaints of pain versus instability are important to differentiate. Instability symptoms may be due to failure of the initial repair, whereas pain may be due to arthrosis or concomitant rotator cuff pathology. Differentiating these conditions can typically be accomplished through a careful physical examination and appropriate radiographs. The single most important finding for recurrent instability on examination is the presence of the apprehension sign.

Once the diagnosis of recurrent anterior instability has been made, it is essential to obtain the previous operative report whenever possible before deciding upon revision treatment. It cannot be assumed that a revision Bankart operation is indicated for every case. For example, a Bankart alone may not be successful if the initial procedure was a Latarjet or Bristow done in the presence of a large bony Bankart lesion. Choosing a revision Bankart operation will also not be successful if the cause of recurrent instability is a subscapularis rupture or insufficiency. Therefore, it is useful to know whether the subscapularis was divided during the initial surgery or split along its fibers, which would be less likely to cause this complication.

The initial postoperative course can also provide useful information regarding the patient's current condition. Questions should be asked about the rehabilitation program that was performed. An overly aggressive program may be an indication that the surgical repair has been disrupted. Failure to do appropriate range-of-motion exercises in a timely fashion may have more to do with loss of motion in a patient than an overly tight surgical repair. Asking whether the patient ever experienced an abrupt change in his or her status during the course of the rehabilitation program, and what exercises they were doing at the time, can also yield helpful information. Issues related to voluntary instability are also pertinent (10).

NONANATOMIC AND HISTORICAL REPAIRS

The surgeon should be familiar with a variety of historical instability procedures and nonanatomic repairs (11). Specific complications are inherent to specific nonanatomic repairs. This knowledge will allow a better understanding of the pathology that might be encountered at revision surgery and allow appropriate preoperative planning to be performed. In rare cases, some of these operations may be used as the revision procedure itself to salvage a specific earlier repair.

For example, the Bristow procedure scars the subscapularis tendon and muscle. This typically causes a loss of exter-

nal rotation up to 23 degrees (12) and decreases internal rotation of the shoulder. Athletes who require overhead use of their arms are frequently unable to return to high-performance levels due to the alteration of normal anatomy (13,14). The typical complications following the Bristow procedure include recurrent painful anterior instability, articular cartilage damage, nonunion of the coracoid bone block, loosening and migration of hardware (15), neurovascular injury (especially musculocutaneous nerve), and posterior instability (16). Revision of a failed Bristow procedure is very difficult due to the significant scarring that occurs. Consider the need for bone grafting, hardware removal, and soft tissue repair, if necessary.

In the Putti-Platt procedure, a vertical incision is made in the subscapularis tendon and capsule. The tendon and capsule are then shortened by overlapping them in a "pants-over-vest" fashion. Intra-articular pathology (such as labral tears) is not repaired. The Putti-Platt procedure can result in complications such as limitation of external rotation and degenerative arthritis (17). Patients are typically unable to return to competitive throwing. Common revision issues include the need for soft-tissue release, tendon lengthening, or the treatment of various stages of arthritis.

The Magnuson-Stack procedure (18) involves lateral transfer of the subscapularis tendon from its insertion on the lesser tuberosity to the greater tuberosity. The procedure, like the Putti-Platt, is designed to restrict external rotation without addressing any underlying pathology that causes shoulder instability. Recurrence rates range from 2% (19) to 17% (20), whereas loss of external rotation ranges from 10 to 30 degrees (19,20). Glenohumeral arthritis and muscle weakness are reported as well (21,22).

RECURRENT INSTABILITY

Recurrent instability following an anterior shoulder stabilization procedure must be assessed carefully and systematically. For example, following a previous Bankart operation, a new trauma can cause a disruption of a well-performed capsulo-labral repair done for correctly diagnosed anterior instability. Alternatively, the new trauma may not disrupt the prior repair but rather result in a new cause for instability, such as a subscapularis rupture or bony Bankart injury. If the previous repair was not performed adequately, a relatively minor trauma can also lead to recurrent instability. While interviewing the patient, it may become clear that preoperative symptoms were never eliminated. This is an indication that either an incorrect diagnosis was made initially or the correct procedure was not performed. Lastly, a strong repair may have been done for the wrong initial diagnosis, such as an anterior Bankart repair done in the presence of a missed posterior instability.

Recurrent instability following anterior stabilization of

the shoulder occurs in 0% to 11% of patients (4,23,24). The most common causes for failure are: (a) an avulsed anterior capsulo-labral complex from the glenoid rim (unrepaired Bankart lesion or failed initial repair), (b) excessive capular laxity, (c) an enlarged "rotator interval," and (d) failure to diagnose the correct direction(s) of instability. Other causes include large osseous defects that are not treated at the time of the initial stabilization (25), the presence of a Hill-Sachs lesion, reduced humeral head retroversion (26), excessive glenoid cavity retroversion, avulsion of the anterior capsule from its lateral humeral attachment (HAGL lesion) (27), un-recognized scapular winging, and a ruptured, scarred, or weakened subscapularis muscle or tendon.

Specific guidelines for treatment to correct recurrent anterior shoulder instability after prior treatment have previously been reported by Zarins and Kolettis (28) and Gill et al. (29). The critical element is to make an anatomic diagnosis of the etiology for recurrent instability and then choose a revision procedure that directly addresses the pathology. Often, this diagnosis can be made on history and physical examination, in conjunction with appropriate imaging. Missed instability patterns, especially posterior instability or multidirectional instability, should be specifically investigated on examination. Increased passive external rotation, a positive belly press test, or positive liftoff test suggests disruption of the subscapularis tendon.

Judicious use of imaging can also elucidate the etiology of recurrent instability. Appropriate use of plain radiographs is very useful to rule out any osseous defects. In particular, the axillary view can give an assessment of the anterior and posterior glenoid rims, the West Point view gives good visualization of the anterior-inferior glenoid rim to better assess the presence of a bony Bankart lesion, and the Stryker notch view can be used to delineate the size of a Hill-Sachs lesion. If bony lesions are suspected, computed tomography (CT) imaging should be performed to quantify the degree of bone loss. Postsurgical changes may make standard magnetic resonance imaging (MRI) difficult to interpret, although subscapularis tendon ruptures can be confirmed. The use of magnetic resonance arthrography increases the sensitivity of detecting recurrent labral tears. Even if an open approach to revision surgery is preferred, as is often the case, an initial arthroscopic examination can be very useful to make or confirm a diagnosis of a failed prior labral repair or to rule out an associated posterior labral tear, which may indicate an undiagnosed posterior component of the instability. In addition, arthroscopy allows for a dynamic assessment of whether a Hill-Sachs lesion engages the anterior glenoid rim with external rotation, indicating the possible need for either osseous reconstruction, or intentionally preventing the degree of external rotation necessary to engage the defect (Fig. 1-1).

SURGICAL OPTIONS

Some of the etiologies of recurrent instability are relatively straightforward to address. If the diagnosis is made of a

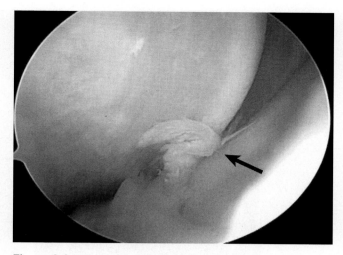

Figure 1-1 Arthroscopic view of a large Hill-Sachs deformity about to engage the anterior rim of the glenoid. The potential contribution of the bony humeral head deformity to recurrent instability can be dynamically assessed under direct arthroscopic visualization with the arm is varying positions of abduction and external rotation.

recurrent Bankart lesion, then a revision Bankart procedure (either open or arthroscopic) can be performed. However, other etiologies offer more complex challenges.

Osseous defects of either the glenoid or humeral head are often overlooked or undiagnosed. Patients are suspected to have this lesion if they have failed prior instability surgery and/or have had many instability episodes with decreasing force necessary for each episode. Historically, Rowe's qualitative assessment of one-third glenoid bone loss as a basis for deciding about soft-tissue repair was the surgeon's best method (6). This might be expected to underestimate the degree of glenoid loss and cause the surgeon to err on the side of a biomechanically weak soft-tissue reconstruction using a conventional Bankart repair technique (30). Burkhart and DeBeer (31,32) observed a failure rate greater than 80% in athletically active individuals who had anterior glenoid erosion treated with arthroscopic Bankart repair. Gerber and Nyffler (33) described a criterion to determine the need for glenoid bone grafting. The authors recommend a bone graft if the length of the glenoid defect is longer than the maximum radius of the glenoid (Fig. 1-2). Other studies have supported this concept (30,34–38). Preoperative CT imaging of patients suspected of severe glenoid bone loss can identify candidates for glenoid reconstruction preoperatively.

In one study, a 4% (11/262) incidence of severe glenoid insufficiency in the setting of recurrent anterior instability after trauma was reported (25), which was thought to be directly responsible for the patient's instability. Most of these patients (9/11) had recurrent instability following conventional Bankart repair. Several options are available to address a deficient glenoid rim. The Bristow-Helfet and the Laterjet procedures involve transfer of the coracoid process and conjoined tendon through the subscapularis and onto

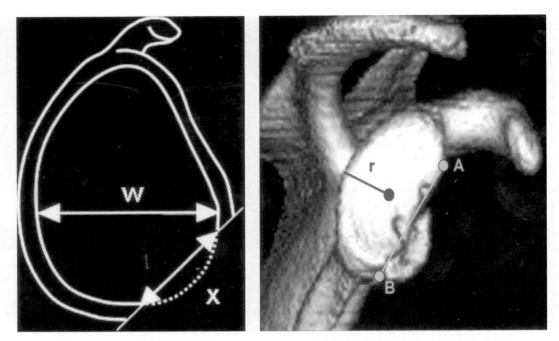

Figure 1-2 If the length of the glenoid defect is longer than one-half the greatest diameter of the glenoid concavity, the force needed to dislocate the shoulder is markedly reduced and the osseous defect bone grafted.

the anterior scapular neck (23,39–46). The mechanism of stability is through creation of an anterior bone block, as well as both the passive sling effect and active stabilizing effect of the conjoined tendon. Although these series have reported very satisfactory outcomes with this technique, some have observed significant problems including loss of motion, hardware impingement and loosening, nonunion of the bone graft, and arthritis. Furthermore, revision surgery can be very challenging due to scarring and distortion of the anatomy around the subscapularis muscle and brachial plexus (16). We prefer an anatomic reconstruction of the anterior glenoid rim using tricortical iliac crest bone graft (Fig. 1-3). Excellent results have been reported with this technique, with very few complications (25).

Although they are more rare, large Hill-Sachs deformities can also contribute to recurrent instability. A CT scan with three-dimensional reconstruction is very useful to assess the size of the bony defect. A rough guideline for reconstructing the humeral head is a defect larger than 30% (6,47). We find it useful to perform a dynamic arthroscopic examination to directly visualize whether the head engages the glenoid rim with passive external rotation if we think this is a possibility (Fig. 1-1). Miniaci has presented excellent results following allograft humeral head reconstruction of large Hill-Sachs lesion (47), which is our preferred approach. Simple overtightening of the anterior capsule to prevent external rotation can also be performed. However, this carries the risk of causing posterior humeral subluxation. Another alternative is transfer of the greater tuberosity and attached infraspinatus into the humeral head defect

(Connolly procedure) (48). This procedure is effective in restoring stability, but causes loss of motion. A rotational proximal humeral osteotomy or Eden-Hybinette-type anterior bone block technique can also be used.

Revision Bankart procedures are usually successful in restoring shoulder stability. Rowe and Zarins (6) reported successful results in 22 of 24 shoulders (92%) that were treated using revision Bankart procedures. No degenerative changes were noted intraoperatively at the time of revision surgery (49). The prognosis following reoperation for involuntary instability is much better than the prognosis for instability that can be reproduced voluntarily by the patient. The ultimate treatment for failed instability surgery is arthrodesis (28).

If scapular winging is identified, there are several therapeutic options. An electromyelogram (EMG) is helpful to identify a neurologic injury that may be contributing to the winging. During the physical examination, compress the scapula manually against the thoracic cage to limit scapular mobility. If the patient's motion is improved and symptoms alleviated, treatment of the winging is indicated. If rehabilitation of the periscapular muscles alone is not successful, either scapulothoracic fusion or pectoralis major transfer can be considered. We prefer pectoralis major transfer using a fascia lata autograft. The fascia lata autograft lengthens the effective distance of the pectoralis major tendon, minimizing tension at the attachment site at the inferior angle of the scapula. Good results have been reported using this technique (50).

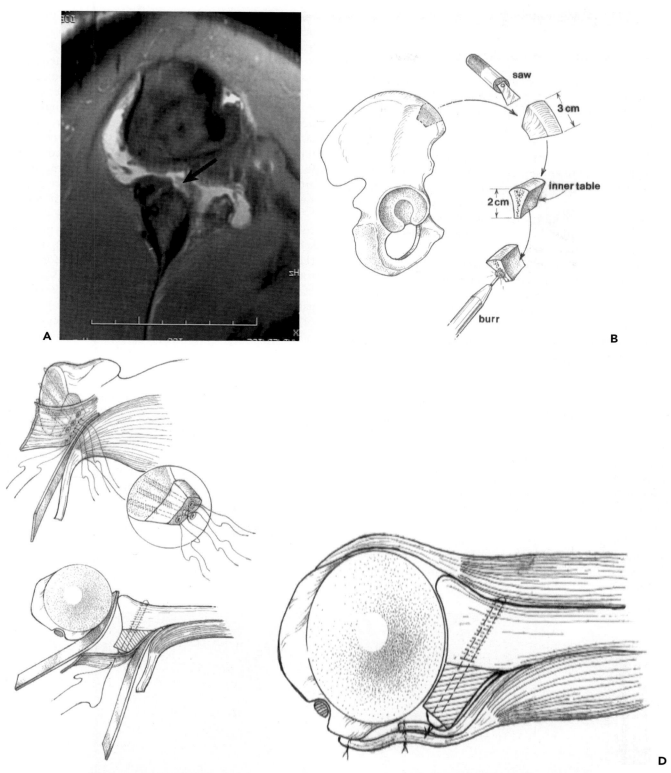

Figure 1-3 **A:** MRI view of a large bony Bankart lesion. **B:** Technique for harvesting a tricortical bone block from the anterior superior iliac spine. The graft is then contoured with a high-speed burr to match the actual glenoid defect. **C:** Diagram depicting the intra-articular placement of the graft and attachment of the capsule to the fixation screws and graft. **D:** Anatomical reconstruction of the glenoid rim. Due to paradoxical shortening of the capsule, it is typically sutured to the overlying subscapularis at the muscle-tendon junction.

ILLUSTRATIVE CASES

Loss of Motion without Arthrosis

A 24-year-old man had a Bankart repair for anterior instability of his shoulder. Six months postoperatively, he still has some pain with only 0 degrees of external rotation despite rigorous rehabilitation. His radiographs are normal, but he is not happy with the functional outcome.

Loss of external rotation is perhaps the most common complication of open surgery for the treatment of anterior instability. The risks of leaving a patient with a significant loss of motion (e.g., >30 degrees) not only include an impaired ability to perform recreational, occupational, and daily living activities, but also the potential development of future pain and arthrosis.

As with patients who have recurrent instability, the anatomic basis of the limited motion must be identified if the proper corrective revision surgery is to be performed. Etiologies of the restricted motion include overtightening of the capsule during a Bankart repair (i.e., capsulotomy made too far laterally), excessive shortening of the subscapularis after tenotomy and subsequent reattachment, or subdeltoid adhesions with or without a capsular contracture.

Clues to the anatomic basis of the motion loss can be found on physical examination. A loss of external rotation in adduction that improves at 90 degrees of abduction implies that the limitation in external rotation rests with the subscapularis, which moves above the center of joint rotation at 90 degrees of abduction. Loss of external rotation at both 0 and 90 degrees of abduction indicates that the capsule is tight as well. Significant impingement signs and subacromial crepitus on motion testing also suggest the possibility of subdeltoid adhesions.

Deciding how to correct the loss of motion depends on the procedure that was done previously. If the patient still cannot externally rotate past 0 degrees after 6 months of

rehabilitation following a Bankart-type repair with capsular or rotator interval tightening, an arthroscopic capsular release and subacromial debridement should be performed. Releasing the inferior capsule arthroscopically helps to improve forward elevation, as well as external rotation in abduction. It does risk injury to the axillary nerve, although by staying sufficiently lateral in the pouch, an injury to this nerve is rare. If needed, the articular side of the subscapularis can also be progressively released arthroscopically until the desired amount of rotation is restored. Waiting for a longer period of time risks the onset of glenohumeral arthrosis from increased glenohumeral contact pressure, sometimes with the head being subluxated posteriorly.

An open Z-lengthening of the subscapularis should be considered if rotation is still restricted following the arthroscopic release, or if the surgeon prefers an open approach (Fig. 1-4). The open approach is also preferred for external rotation contractures following Putti-Platt or Magnuson-Stack procedures. In general, 20 degrees of rotation is gained for every 1 cm of lengthening. At least 30 degrees of external rotation and 50 degrees of elevation can typically be gained using this approach. If there is still not adequate restoration of motion following the Z-lengthening, the subdeltoid and subcoracoid spaces should be released as well. Leaving the patient with an internal rotation contracture will increase the joint compressive forces with attempted rotation while causing the humeral head to translate posteriorly over time. The sequelae of such situations include degenerative arthrosis in the posterior aspect of the joint or occasionally posterior instability. The goals of performing a capsular release as early as 6 months postoperatively are relief of pain, improved function, and prevention of developing osteoarthrosis.

Loss of Motion with Arthrosis

A 48-year-old man had a repair for anterior instability at age 38 years. He presents 10 years postoperatively with a significant

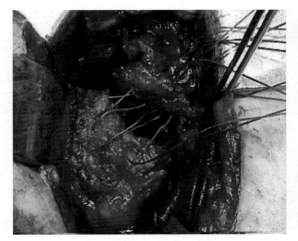
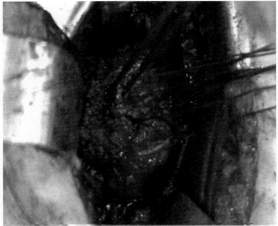

Figure 1-4 Intra-operative photo of a Z-plasty lengthening of the subscapularis. An oblique tenotomy is performed from lateral to medial. (Courtesy of Dr. J.P. Warner.)

internal rotation deformity of his arm. His other motions are acceptable but he has pain. His radiographs show osteoarthritis.

Late degenerative arthrosis has been documented following Bankart reconstruction (2,51). In one study (51), 14 of 33 shoulders had minimal changes, three had moderate changes, and one had severe changes at 15 years follow-up. There was a relationship between degenerative radiographic changes, length of follow-up, and restriction of external rotation with the arm abducted 90 degrees. The most common cause of glenohumeral arthrosis following surgery for anterior instability is an excessively tight reconstruction. The actual severity of arthrosis can be directly correlated to the degree of limitation in external rotation (52). Other etiologies of arthrosis include transfer of the coracoid process to the anterior glenoid rim, which causes impingement of the humeral head on the coracoid tip (16,21), as well as corrective osteotomies of the glenoid, which enter the joint. Misplacement and loosening of hardware around the joint are also causative factors of arthrosis (15,51–54).

Osteoarthrosis of the glenohumeral joint is particularly common after procedures that are designed to limit external rotation of the joint. The osteoarthrosis that results from this limited rotation is likely the result of increased joint contact pressures and shear forces with continued attempts at rotation. Such procedures include the Putti-Platt capsulorraphy (55), Magnuson-Stack, and duToit (21). Following a Putti-Platt procedure, disabling pain is typically seen 10–13 years postoperatively in association with substantial limitation of motion (17,21,55). The limitation of motion is frequently disabling, and is often as much as a 30- to 40-degree internal-rotation contracture. The Bristow procedure has also been associated with loss of motion due to scarring of the subscapularis and subsequent arthrosis (16). In essence, arthrosis may result from any procedure that makes the shoulder too tight and limits motion.

Treatment of this complication depends on the degree of functional limitation, the amount of pain, and the extent of the arthrosis. Mild symptoms and mild arthrosis are treated with an alteration in activities, physiotherapy and anti-inflammatory medications. Symptoms and arthrosis that are moderately severe can often be successfully treated by an arthroscopic anterior release or open Z-plasty lengthening of the subscapularis and capsule (Fig. 1-4) (17,55,56). An arthroscopic release is most successful when there is still a concentric joint space with intact sphericity of the humeral head. Once the sphericity is lost, the reduction in symptoms is far less predictable. The goal of a capsular release for the treatment of the loss of motion with arthrosis is to restore a more pain-free range of motion while reducing contact pressures in the joint. By doing so, an arthroscopic release can help to diminish overall pain, increase function, and hopefully slow the progression of the arthrosis.

In patients who have more severe joint degeneration, or whose joint concentricity and sphericity are lost, a prosthetic replacement should be considered. A soft-tissue procedure to increase rotation should be performed at the same time as the arthroplasty. Options include an anterior Z-plasty lengthening, a 360-degree capsular release, and/or an anterior interval release. The use of a smaller prosthetic humeral head and more medial reattachment of the subscapularis and capsule can also improve motion. Anteroposterior radiographs alone frequently underestimate the extent of joint-space narrowing.

Debate remains as to whether to resurface both sides of the glenohumeral joint or only the humeral head. Hemiarthroplasty is indicated if the glenoid cavity is concentric, still has the majority of its articular cartilage in tact, and the humeral head is centered on the axillary radiographic view. This is especially true in a younger population. If the glenoid fossa is flattened and posteriorly eroded, a total shoulder arthroplasty is much more likely to relieve pain and restore function. When performing the arthroplasty with a posterior glenoid erosion, the humeral prosthesis should be implanted with less retroversion than normal.

If the patient is young (e.g., <35 years of age), an arthroplasty may not be the optimal choice of treatment. A fascial interposition arthroplasty is another option that may help to improve function, relieve pain, and postpone or obviate the need for an arthroplasty (Fig. 1-5). This technique has been well-described for use in the elbow, with good results in selected patients (57). In the shoulder, we use an Achilles tendon allograft sutured to the glenoid labrum and augmented with transosseous sutures. Results are best when the arthrosis is primarily on the glenoid side of the joint, although the results tend to deteriorate with time. Satisfactory results using interpositional meniscal allografts have also been reported (58). In addition to providing pain relief, fascial interposition arthroplasty does not complicate a future total shoulder arthroplasty.

Subscapularis Tendon Rupture

A 19-year-old college football player presents 6 months following open Bankart repair for recurrent anterior instability. He complains of instability and pain during tackling drills with his operated arm.

An underreported complication of open anterior stabilization procedures is rupture of the subscapularis tendon following surgical tenotomy and repair. Patients generally present with pain and occasional weakness, although recurrent instability is also common. If this complication is not routinely considered, it is extremely difficult to diagnose. On physical examination, the presence of excessive passive external rotation in adduction should alert the examiner to a possible subscapularis tendon tear. Weak and/or painful internal rotation against resistance in adduction is also suggestive of injury to the subscapularis. A positive belly press test or liftoff test can help to suggest the diagnosis (Fig. 1-6). Confirmation of both the presence and degree of rupture, as well as the status of the muscle belly, can be made by MRI.

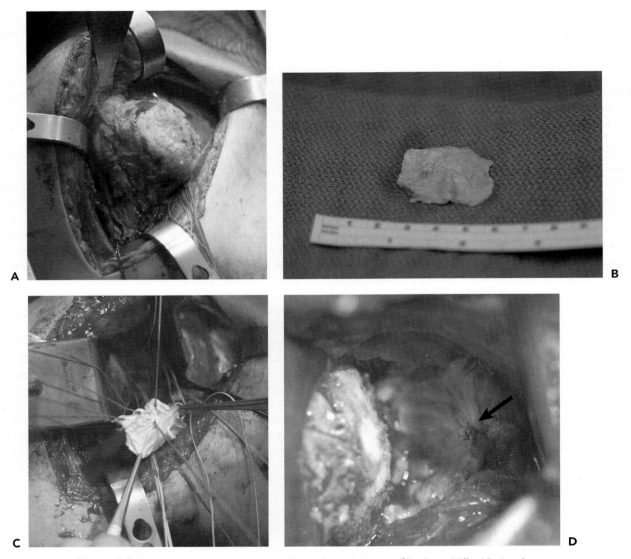

Figure 1-5 A: Osteoarthrosis in a young, active patient. (Courtesy of Dr. Peter Millet.) **B**: Autologous fascia lata graft from ipsilateral lower extremity. **C**: Suture anchors or transosseous tunnels are placed around the periphery of the glenoid rim and passed through the perimeter of the matched fascial graft. **D**: Intra-operative photo of the fascial interposition arthroplasty.

Obtaining the initial operative report is an important part of recognizing a possible subscapularis rupture. A complete tenotomy is usually performed for operative exposure during a typical Bankart repair or open inferior capsular shift. Check for an indication of how and where the tenotomy was made with respect to the lesser tuberosity, because a 10- to 15-mm stump left attached to the lesser tuberosity is typically needed to perform a strong repair. It should also be noted what type of sutures were used for the initial repair (absorbable vs. nonabsorbable, size of the sutures, simple vs. figure of eight configuration, etc.). Rupture is particularly possible when the subscapularis and capsule are released together as a single flap. In contrast, operative approaches that only split the subscapularis rather than release it, detach the subscapularis with a piece of bone,

or perform a tenotomy but leave the inferior 25% intact are much less likely to be complicated by postoperative rupture. Often, surgeons will make note of the degree of tension-free post-Bankart repair motion obtained intraoperatively. Overly tight repairs which present with full or increased external rotation should alert the examiner to a possible rupture.

Early recognition and surgical repair of a torn subscapularis tendon is essential. A delay in diagnosis can make a successful repair impossible due to either excessive medial retraction or fatty atrophy/replacement of the subscapularis muscle belly. If the tendon is not repairable or is of poor quality, a pectoralis major tendon transfer can be performed (Fig. 1-7). The procedure has been well-described by Jost et al. (59), who reported good results when there was not an

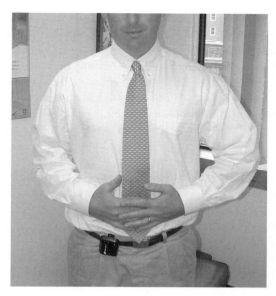

Figure 1-6 Belly press test in patient with subscapularis tear in right shoulder. Note inability to maintain elbow in forward position.

associated irreparable tear of the supraspinatus. It is important to ensure that the pectoralis major tendon is transferred under tension by placing the tendon lateral to the bicipital groove if stability and internal rotation are to be restored.

Neurologic Injury

A 23-year-old woman complains of limited motion following a Putti-Platt procedure. Physical examination reveals full passive elevation, abduction, and rotation, but marked weakness in forward elevation and abduction.

Neurologic injuries are addressed in detail in a separate chapter of this book. Such injuries are not uncommon after primary and revision anterior stabilization procedures. The most commonly injured nerves are the axillary nerve and the musculocutaneous nerve. During the operative exposure of the glenohumeral joint, retraction of the short head of the biceps and the coracobrachialis muscles can injure the musculocutaneous nerve. The injury is typically a neurapraxia and generally recovers with time. The axillary nerve is at risk due to its location at the inferior of the subscapularis tendon. It too can be damaged due to excessive surgical retraction. However, neurotomesis or axonotmesis can not be ruled out, particularly following an inferior capsular shift of Bankart procedure. An EMG obtained at baseline and at 3 months can be helpful in making the diagnosis of the injury. If there is no electrophysiologic evidence of return by 3 to 6 months (60), consideration should be given to surgical exploration of the nerve and possible nerve grafting as needed.

Brachial plexus injuries have been sustained during Putti-Platt and Bristow procedures (60). Suture material has been retrieved from around or within the musculocutaneous, ulnar, axillary, and median nerves. Lacerations to the axillary artery have also been reported. These complications are typically caused by inadequate knowledge of regional anatomy, blind clamping of vascular lacerations, and the use of axillary incisions with limited exposure.

A previous Bristow procedure presents a slightly unique situation. The musculocutaneous nerve is at-risk with the coracoid transfer. A musculocutaneous injury following a Bristow procedure may be an indication for immediate operative exploration.

In general, good recovery of motor function with variable sensory return can generally be expected following nerve surgery.

Hardware-Related

A 46-year-old woman presents 3 years following a Bristow procedure for recurrent anterior instability complaining of pain and

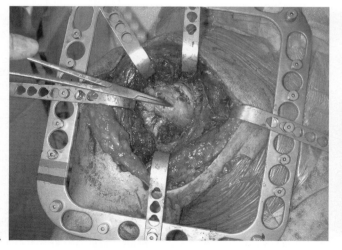
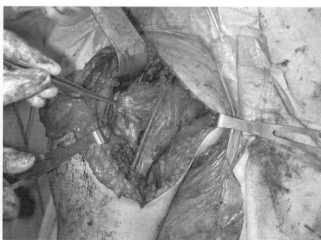

Figure 1-7 A: Subscapularis insufficiency, with torn tendon and fatty atrophy of muscle belly. B: Split pectoralis major transfer of the sternal head. Note attachment lateral to biceps groove. (Courtesy of Dr. Peter Millet.)

limited motion. She states that although she has not experienced any instability since her surgery, she has never been pain-free.

Placing hardware near the glenohumeral joint can lead to arthrosis. Metal suture anchors used for Bankart repairs can fail, loosen, migrate, or be left proud. Articular damage may be the result of direct contact of the humeral head with the transferred coracoid and screw after a Bristow procedure (15,16,42,60,61). Screws and staples can produce complications that require reoperation and are capable of causing a permanent loss of joint function. Zuckerman and Matsen (15) classified implant complications as: 1) incorrect placement of the implant, 2) migration after placement, 3) loosening, and 4) breakage of the device. Patients with implant-related complications present with anterior shoulder pain, stiffness, crepitus, or radiating paresthesias. The average time from the original operation to the onset of symptoms is 16 months. There is often a considerable delay in making the diagnosis of implant-related complications.

If complications from its use do occur, the implant should be removed and the joint should be debrided. Lastly, if significant osteoarthrosis has resulted from the use of hardware, treatment of the arthrosis can be performed as previously described.

PEARLS

The keys to treating complications of surgery for anterior instability are:

1. Make an accurate diagnosis of the patient's current problem: is there recurrent instability, loss of motion, arthrosis, or simply "pain"?
2. Understand exactly what procedure was previously performed.
3. Diagnose what anatomical pathology is present, and correlate it with the patient's symptoms.

It is important to understand how the normal anatomy was altered at the time of the previous surgery or surgeries. A good rule of thumb is to try to develop a surgical treatment plan that restores as much normal anatomy as possible.

Several generalizations can be made regarding patients and their assessments of their surgical outcomes. Patients prefer a more loose shoulder with full motion rather than a shoulder that is very tight but has restricted motion. This should be considered if an overlap capsulorraphy or a capsular shift procedure is performed in addition to a Bankart repair. There is a direct correlation between the range of motion obtained after a stabilization and the clinical outcome.

Rehabilitation is also very important. Most patients state that they wished they had worked harder on their exercises during their initial postoperative periods. The postoperative rehabilitation program that should be prescribed depends upon the type of repair that has been done, its strength, and the individual patient's requirements. In general, passive elevation to 90 degrees and external rotation to 0 degrees can be allowed in the immediate postoperative period. If the repair is strong, a sling is not needed after the first day except to protect the shoulder from unexpected motions, such as while sleeping or in a crowd. Full elevation, full internal rotation, and gradually increasing external rotation with terminal stretching are allowed at 4 to 6 weeks, at which time resistive exercises using elastic bands are initiated. Regaining external rotation requires careful attention. The goal is to achieve 50% of the external rotation of the contralateral extremity by 6 weeks and full external rotation by 12 weeks after surgery. Full range of motion and strength should be achieved by 12 weeks postoperatively. For the athlete who throws, it is desirable to regain full motion earlier than described above.

Whenever possible, the guiding principle for revision surgery to treat complications of anterior shoulder instability surgery is the restoration of normal anatomy. If a Bankart lesion is present, it should be repaired and tissues returned to their correct locations. Failure to repair a Bankart lesion is the major cause of failure if nonanatomic repairs have been employed. If the subscapularis has been ruptured, it should be anatomically repaired. If it has been excessively shortened, it needs to be lengthened. If there is arthrosis due to overtightening, the joint should be decompressed and the arthrosis treated accordingly to its severity.

REFERENCES

1. Hawkins RH, Hawkins RJ. Failed anterior reconstruction for shoulder instability. *J Bone Joint Surg Br* 1985;67:709–714.
2. Gill T, Micheli L, Gebhard F, et al. Bankart repair for anterior instability of the shoulder. Long-term outcome. *J Bone Joint Surg Am* 1997;79:850–857.
3. Zarins B, McMahon MS, Rowe CR. Diagnosis and treatment of traumatic anterior instability of the shoulder. *Clin Orthop* 1993; 291:75–84.
4. Bigliani LU, Newton PM, Steinmann SP, et al. Glenoid rim lesions associated with recurrent anterior dislocation of the shoulder. *Am J Sports Med* 1998;26:41–45.
5. Rowe CR, Patel D, Southmayd WW. The Bankart Procedure: a long-term end result study. *J Bone Joint Surg Am* 1978;60:1–16.
6. Rowe CR, Zarins B, Ciullo JV. Recurrent anterior dislocation of the shoulder after surgical repair. *J Bone Joint Surg Am* 1984;66: 159–168.
7. Sugaya H, Moriishi J, Dohi M, et al. Glenoid rim morphology in recurrent anterior glenohumeral instability. *J Bone Joint Surg Am* 2003;85:878–884.
8. Aston JW Jr, Gregory CF. Dislocation of the shoulder with significant fracture of the glenoid. *J Bone Joint Surg Am* 1973;55: 1531–1533.
9. Detrisac DA, Johnson LJ. Arthroscopic shoulder capsulorrhaphy using metal staples. *Orthop Clin North Am* 1993;24:71–88.
10. Rowe CR, Pierce DS, Clark JF. Voluntary dislocations of the shoulder: a preliminary report on a clinical, electomyographic and psychiatric study of twenty-six patients. *J Bone Joint Surg Am* 1973; 55:445–460.
11. Gill TJ, Zarins B. Open repairs for the treatment of anterior shoulder instability. *Am J Sports Med* 2003;31(1):142-53.

12. Torg JS, Balduini FC, Bonci C, et al. A modified Britow-Helfet-May procedure for recurrent dislocation and subluxation of the shoulder. Report of two hundred and twelve cases. *J Bone Joint Surg Am* 1987;69:904–914.

13. Lombardo SJ, Kerlan RK, Jobe FW, et al. The modified Bristow procedure for recurrent dislocation of the shoulder. *J Bone Joint Surg Am* 1976;58:256–261.

14. Regan WD, Webster-Bogaert S, Hawkins RJ, et al. Comparative functional analysis of the Bristow, Magnuson-Stack, and Putti-Platt procedures for recurrent dislocation of the shoulder. *Am J Sports Med* 1989;17:42–48.

15. Zuckerman JD, Matsen FA. Complications about the glenohumeral joint related to the use of screws and staples. *J Bone Joint Surg Am* 1984;66:175–180.

16. Young DC, Rockwood CA. Complications of a failed Bristow procedure and their management. *J Bone Joint Surg Am* 1991;73:969–981.

17. MacDonald PB, Hawkins RJ, Fowler PJ, et al. Release of the subscapularis for internal rotation contracture and pain after anterior repair for recurrent anterior dislocation of the shoulder. *J Bone Joint Surg Am* 1992;74:734–737.

18. Magnuson PB, Stack JK. Recurrent dislocation of the shoulder. *JAMA* 1943;123:889–892.

19. Karadimas J, Rentis G, Varouchas G. Repair of recurrent anterior dislocation of the shoulder using transfer of the subscapularis tendon. *J Bone Joint Surg Am* 1980;62:1147–1149.

20. Miller LS, Donahue JR, Good RP, et al. The Magnuson-Stack procedure for treatment of recurrent glenohumeral dislocations. *Am J Sports Med* 1984;12:133–137.

21. Lusardi DA, Wirth MA, Wurtz D, et al. Loss of external rotation following anterior capsulorraphy of the shoulder. *J Bone Joint Surg Am* 1993;75:1185–1192.

22. Nicola T. Recurrent anterior dislocation of the shoulder. *J Bone Joint Surg* 1929;11:128–132.

23. Hovelius LK, Sandström BC, Rösmark DL, et al. Long-term results with the Bankart and Bristow-Laterjet procedures: recurrent shoulder instability and arthropathy. *J Shoulder Elbow Surg* 2001;10:445–452.

24. Hovelius L, Thorling J, Fredin H. Recurrent anterior dislocation of the shoulder: results after the Bankart and Putti-Platt operations. *J Bone Joint Surg Am* 1979;61:566–569.

25. Warner JP, Gill TJ, Millet PJ, et al. Anatomical reconstruction of the glenoid for the treatment of recurrent anterior shoulder instability. *AJSM*, 2005. In press.

26. Kromberg M, Brostrom LA, Posch E. Stability in relation to humeral head retroversion after surgical treatment of recurrent anterior shoulder dislocations. *Orthopedics* 1993;16:281–285.

27. Bach BR, Warren RF, Fronek J. Disruption of the lateral capsule of the shoulder. *J Bone Joint Surg Br* 1988;70:274–276.

28. Zarins B, Kolettis G. Failed surgery for shoulder instability. In: Zarins B, Marder RA, eds. *Revision of Failed Arthroscopic and Ligament Surgery*. Oxford: Blackwell Science, 1998:98–107.

29. Gill TJ, Warren RF, Rockwood CA, et al. Complications of Shoulder Surgery. *AAOS ICL* 1999;48:359–374.

30. Itoi E, Lee SB, Berglund LJ, et al. The effect of glenoid defect on anteroinferior stability of the shoulder after Bankart repair: a cadaver study. *J Bone Joint Surg Am* 2000;82:35–46.

31. Burkhart SS, DeBeer JF, Tehrany AM, et al. Quantifying glenoid bone loss arthroscopically in shoulder instability. *Arthroscopy* 2002;18:488–491.

32. Burkhart SS, DeBeer JF. Traumatic glenohumeral bone defects and their relationship to failure of arthroscopic Bankart repairs: significance of the inverted-pear glenoid and the humeral engaging Hill-Sachs lesion. *Arthroscopy* 2000;16:677–694.

33. Gerber C, Nyffler RW. Classification of glenohumeral joint instability. *Clin Orthop* 2002;400:65–76.

34. Edelson JG. Bony changes of the glenoid as a consequence of shoulder instability. *J Shoulder Elbow Surg* 1996;5:293–298.

35. Greis PE, Scuderi MG, Mohr A, et al. Glenohumeral articular contact areas and pressures following labral and osseous injury to the anteroinferior quadrant of the glenoid. *J Shoulder Elbow Surg* 2002;11:442–451.

36. Itoi E, Lee SB, Amrami KK, et al. Quantitative assessment of classic anteroinferior Bony Bankart lesions by radiography and computed tomography. *Am J Sports Med* 2003;31:112–118.

37. Lazarus MD, Sidles JA, Harryman DT II, et al. Effect of chondral-labral defect on glenoid concavity and glenohumeral stability. A cadaveric model. *J Bone Joint Surg Am* 1996;78:94–102.

38. Lippitt SB, Vanderhooft JE, Harris SL, et al. Glenohumeral stability from concavity-compression: a quantitative analysis. *J Shoulder Elbow Surg* 1993;2:27–35.

39. Allain J, Goutallier D, Glorion C. Long-term results of the Laterjet procedure for the treatment of anterior instability of the shoulder. *J Bone Joint Surg Am* 1998;80:841–852.

40. Hovelius L, Korner L, Lundberg B, et al. The coracoid transfer for recurrent dislocation of the shoulder. Technical aspects of the Bristow-Latarjet procedure. *J Bone Joint Surg Am* 1983;65:926–934.

41. Hovelius L, Sanstrom B, Saeboe M, et al. Clinical Results of a Prospective 15 year Study on 118 Bristow-Laterjet Repairs for Recurrent Anterior Dislocation of the Shoulder. Presented at the 2003 Annual Meeting of the American Shoulder and Elbow Surgeons. New Orleans, LA.

42. Hovelius L, Körner L, Lundberg B, et al. The coracoid transfer for recurrent dislocation of the shoulder. *J Bone Joint Surg Am* 1983;65:926–934.

43. Nielsen AB, Nielsen K. The modified Bristow procedure for recurrent anterior dislocation of the shoulder. *Acta Orthop Scand* 1982;53:229–232.

44. Schauder KS, Tullos HS. Role of the coracoid bone black in the modified Bristow procedure. *Am J Sports Med* 1992;20:31–34.

45. Singer GC, Kirkland PM, Emery RJH. Coracoid transposition for recurrent anterior instability of the shoulder: a 20-year follow-up study. *J Bone Joint Surg Br* 1995;77:73–76.

46. Wredmark T, Tornkvist H, Johansson C, et al. Long-term functional results of the modified Bristow procedure for recurrent dislocation of the shoulder. *Am J Sports Med* 1992;20:157–161.

47. Miniaci A. Matched humeral head allografts for the treatment of symptomatic Hill-Sachs deformities. Presented at the American Academy of Orthopedic Surgeons. Washington, DC, 2004.

48. Connolly JF. Humeral head defects associated with shoulder dislocations—their diagnostic and surgical significance. *AAOS Instruct Course Lect* 1972;21:42–54.

49. Flatow EL, Warner JJP. Instability of the shoulder: complex problems and failed repairs. Part I. Relevant biomechanics, multidirectional instability, and severe bone of the glenoid and humeral bone. ICL. *J Bone Joint Surg Am* 1998;80:122–140.

50. Noerdlinger MA, Cole BJ, Stewart M, et al. Results of pectoralis major transfer with fascia lata autograft for scapula winging. *J Shoulder Elbow Surg* 2002;11:345–350.

51. Rosenberg BN, Richmond JC, Levine WN. Long-term followup of Bankart reconstruction: incidence of late degenerative glenohumeral arthrosis. *Am J Sports Med* 1995;23:538–544.

52. Samilson RL, Prieto V. Dislocation arthropathy of the shoulder. *J Bone Joint Surg Am* 1983;65:456–460.

53. O'Driscoll SW, Evans DC. Long-term results after staple capsulorraphy for anterior instability of the shoulder. *J Bone Joint Surg Am* 1993;75:249–258.

54. Sisk TD, Boyd HB. Management of recurrent anterior dislocation of the shoulder. DuToit-type or staple capsulorraphy. *Clin Orthop* 1974;103:150–156.

55. Hawkins RJ, Angelo RL. Glenohumeral osteoarthrosis: a late complication of the Putti-Platt repair. *J Bone Joint Surg Am* 1990;72:1193–1197.

56. Bishop JY, Flatow EL. Management of glenohumeral arthritis: a role for arthroscopy? *Orthop Clin North Am* 2003;34:559–566.

57. Cheng SL, Morrey BF. Treatment of the mobile, painful arthritic elbow by distraction interposition arthroplasty. *J Bone Joint Surg Br* 2000;82:233–238.

58. Ball CM, Galatz LM, Yamaguchi K. Meniscal allograft interposition arthroplasty for the arthritic shoulder: description of a new surgical technique. *Techniques Shoulder Elbow Surg* 2001;2(4):247–254.

59. Jost B, Puskas GJ, Lustenberger A, et al. Outcome of pectoralis major transfer for the treatment of irreparable subscapularis tears. *J Bone Joint Surg Am* 2003;85:1944–1951.

60. Richards RR, Hudson AR, Bertoia JT, et al. Injury to the brachial plexus during Putti-Platt and Bristow procedures. *Am J Sports Med* 1987;15:374–380.

61. Hill JA, Lombardo SJ, Kerlan RK, et al. The modified Bristow-Helfet procedure for recurrent anterior shoulder subluxations and dislocations. *Am J Sports Med* 1981;9:283–287.

Complications of Surgery for Posterior/Multidirectional Instability

James D. O'Holleran   **Russel F. Warren**

INTRODUCTION

Posterior instability of the shoulder has been described since the early 19th century. Historically considered a rare problem, traumatic posterior dislocation has been reported to comprise less than 4% of all shoulder dislocations (1–3). However, posterior instability is becoming increasingly recognized as an important clinical entity, alone or in combination with a multidirectional component. In 1980, Neer and Foster (4) solidified our understanding of multidirectional instability (MDI) by distinguishing it from other unidirectional instabilities, as well as by introducing the concept of the inferior capsular shift to globally tension the capsule to recreate multidirectional stability. In addition, instability manifested as subluxation, as opposed to frank dislocation, has been recognized as a separate and much more common clinical entity.

Although the treatment of multidirectional or nontraumatic posterior instability is diagnostically and therapeutically challenging, most patients can be successfully managed nonoperatively, with individually tailored strengthening and balancing of rotator cuff muscles and the scapular stabilizers. When such conservative treatment fails, anatomic restoration of the injured or insufficient structures can reliably relieve pain and restore function. A variety of treatment alternatives exists, depending on the pathologic process involved.

A thorough review of the underlying pathoanatomy of posterior instability and MDI, leading to the rationale for surgical decision-making, is beyond the scope of this chapter. However, some mention of the basis for surgical reconstruction is warranted. Posterior instability can be classified in a variety of ways, either by *degree* (subluxation, dislocation, or locked dislocation), *direction* (uni-, bi-, or multidirectional), *chronicity* (acute or chronic), *volition* (involuntary or voluntary), or *mechanism* (traumatic or atraumatic). A thoughtful assessment of the direction and the degree of instability combined with an appreciation of the anatomic abnormalities, which are reflected by a combination of the above factors, will lead the surgeon to choose the proper type of surgical reconstruction.

Open techniques have been the historical standard for stabilization. Open posterior capsular shift, with or without posterior labral repair, and with or without infraspinatus augmentation, remains the mainstay of open treatment for posterior instability (1–3,5). For true MDI, capsular shift remains the gold standard, with the direction of the capsulorrhaphy determined by the side of greatest instability (1,4,6,6a). If the instability had a primarily anterior component, then selective inferior capsular shift performed through an anterior deltopectoral approach is preferred. For MDI associated with a primarily posterior component, an inferior capsular shift is performed through a posterior approach. For posterior instability associated with excessive glenoid retroversion, an opening wedge glenoid osteotomy, performed through a posterior approach, is advocated (7). In advanced and multiple-revision cases, humeral rotational osteotomy and glenohumeral fusion are salvage options (8,9).

Currently, arthroscopic techniques are being advocated to address these forms of instability, whether a posterior labral repair in a patient with an acute, traumatic posterior labral tear (the so-called reverse Bankart), or a global arthroscopic capsular placation/shift with a rotator interval closure for the patient with MDI. These techniques and their resultant complications will be addressed in another chapter, as well as complications of the anterior approach for a capsular shift.

It has been stated that the only way to prevent surgical complications is to avoid performing surgery (10). Complications represent a diagnostic and technical challenge, as the reason for the event may be difficult to ascertain, and the revision procedure usually requires restoring normal anatomy in the face of scarred tissue planes, previously placed anchors, and possibly glenohumeral arthrosis. Surgical reconstruction may fail because of errors made during the preoperative, intraoperative, or postoperative period (11). *Preoperative errors* occur in the process of patient evaluation and surgical decision-making, and include diagnostic errors and the failure to address a patient's expectations for surgery and the resulting outcome. *Intraoperative errors* include technical pitfalls encountered during the posterior approach to the shoulder and complications involving bony procedures (hardware problems and glenoid fracture). Complications encountered in the *postoperative setting* include loss of motion with or without resulting arthrosis, recurrent instability or new-onset anterior instability, coracoid impingement syndrome, and bony fixation problems (malunion, nonunion, loss of fixation, osteonecrosis of the glenoid). For each of these complications, we evaluate their nature and incidence, assess the anatomical or technical reasons for them, provide pearls on how to avoid them, and suggest treatment options in their management.

PREOPERATIVE ERRORS

The history, physical examination, and radiographic evaluation provide the foundation for accurate surgical decision-making. Although most surgeons are comfortable and familiar with anterior instability, especially of an acute traumatic nature, many are less familiar with atraumatic multidirectional instability and isolated posterior instability. Fastidious attention to detail in the preoperative period will dramatically reduce complications encountered in the operative and postoperative periods.

Incorrect Diagnosis

When evaluating any complaint in the shoulder, a thorough history and physical examination form the foundation for an accurate diagnosis. One of the most common

sources of unrecognized referred pain to the shoulder is the cervical spine (12). In addition, other shoulder problems including rotator cuff or superior labral pathology may be responsible for painful symptoms (13). For the most part, however, improper assessment of the degree, direction, and mechanism of instability is the most common diagnostic error, leading to a failure to appreciate the true type of instability. Improper diagnosis in turn leads to vague or incorrect physical therapy orders, and ultimately to improper surgical procedures. The literature documenting the failure of posterior instability and MDI surgery is sparse compared to that assessing failed anterior surgery, but a common thread runs throughout: missed diagnosis of either unidirectional instability or MDI is responsible for failure of surgical stabilization, with rates ranging from 21% to 68% (14–17).

To avoid missing the correct diagnosis, the clinician must be thoughtful in taking the history, performing specific provocative maneuvers in the physical exam, and obtaining all necessary imaging. As noted previously, posterior instability can be classified in a variety of ways: by degree (subluxation, dislocation, or locked dislocation), mechanism (traumatic or atraumatic), chronicity (acute or chronic), direction (uni-, bi-, or multidirectional), or volition (involuntary or voluntary). A focused history will elucidate these factors and their relative contribution to the overall diagnosis.

The degree, mechanism, and chronicity of instability can often help to differentiate unidirectional from multidirectional instability. Frank dislocations that occur from a discernible acute traumatic event and require medical assistance for reduction are often associated with labral pathology and are usually unidirectional in nature. On the other hand, subtle perceptions of atraumatic subluxation that occur chronically often suggest multidirectional instability. The patient describes the shoulder as "loose" or "popping in and out," labral pathology is less common, and nonphysiologic capsular laxity is often present.

The direction of instability is usually suggested by the history. Anterior instability is perceived when the shoulder is in the abducted, externally rotated position, such as the driver of a car reaching into the backseat for an item. Posterior instability is perceived when the arm is forward flexed, as when reaching in front of the body for something. Even more sensitive is when a posteriorly directed force is applied along the arm when in this position, such as at the beginning or end of a repetition in a bench press. Inferior instability, corresponding to a sulcus sign, is perceived when an inferiorly directed force is applied to the adducted arm, such as lifting a heavy suitcase.

Lastly, voluntary subluxation is a particularly important subset of patients to recognize. Wall and Warren (11) separate volitional instability into positional and muscular types, with the former experiencing instability only in certain arm positions, and the latter being able to cause subluxation with simple muscle contraction (Fig. 2-1). Neer

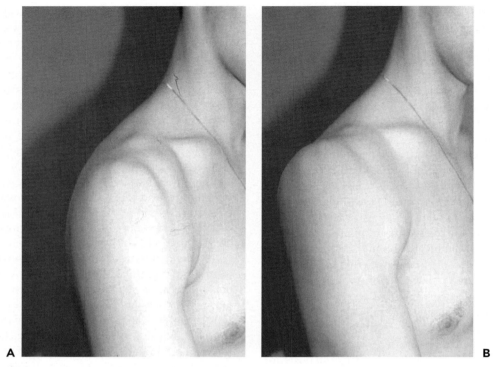

A   **B**

Figure 2-1 A patient at rest (**A**) and after muscle contraction (**B**), exhibiting voluntary muscular posterior subluxation.

(18) carefully distinguishes between the patient who can cause instability and the patient who receives secondary gain from such behavior. Although Fuchs and Gerber (19) reported satisfactory intermediate-term results with posterior-inferior capsular shift in voluntary subluxators, several reports in the literature caution the clinician to avoid surgery in the volitional instability patient who has documented psychiatric issues, exhibits muscular instability, or receives secondary gain (11,14–18,20).

The physical exam should be thorough, including the cervical spine, the neurovascular assessment of the whole extremity, and the complete shoulder exam. Specific unidirectional instability signs include evocative tests of a patient's subjective reaction to a maneuver, such as the apprehension and relocation signs, and clinician-derived objective measures of laxity, such as translation on load and shift testing. Positions similar to those mentioned in the history are recreated. Anterior instability is assessed with the arm in the abducted, externally rotated position. A subjective, uneasy feeling of instability or impending dislocation suggests a positive apprehension test. When a posteriorly directed force is applied to the humerus with the arm still in this position, the feeling of apprehension subsides, marking a positive relocation test. Anterior translation is documented by the load and shift test. The patient is placed supine to stabilize the scapula and the arm is positioned in abduction, neutral rotation, and forward flexion of approximately 30 degrees to match the plane of the scapula. An axial force is directed along the humerus and then the head is anteriorly translated.

Several variations on a grading scheme have been published; we use a 0 to 3+ grading system (21). Grade 0 indicates no increased translation over the opposite side; grade 1 indicates translation to the glenoid rim but not over; grade 2 indicates that the head can be dislocated over the glenoid rim but it spontaneously reduces; grade 3 indicates dislocation over the glenoid rim with no spontaneous reduction.

Posterior instability is assessed by placing the arm in the forward flexed position and applying a longitudinal force along the humerus, which effectively exerts a posteriorly directed force. A feeling of apprehension is again queried; however, it is far rarer to elicit the true apprehension of an impending dislocation as is seen anteriorly. Often the patient will experience pain, clicking, or vague discomfort. A posterior load and shift test is then performed to assess translation, with all factors similar to those described for anterior translation, but after axial loading, the humerus is shifted posteriorly. Grading is similar to the above.

Signs of MDI include generalized ligamentous laxity, pathologic translation anteriorly and/or posteriorly, and a positive sulcus sign (inferior translation). Although isolated anterior and posterior signs suggest unidirectional instability in that direction, the addition of a sulcus sign suggests more of a global problem. As will be discussed further, a positive sulcus sign indicates insufficiency in the rotator interval. The sulcus sign is performed with the patient standing or seated and with the arm at the side. A longitudinal force is applied to the humerus by pulling on it such that the humerus is distracted from the acromion. The magnitude of the gap observed (and palpated), the so-called sulcus, is recorded. Grade 0 is minimal, grade 1 is less than 1 cm, grade 2 is 1 to 2 cm, and grade 3 is greater than 2 cm.

A critical distinction to appreciate is that laxity does not equal instability. *Laxity* is a relative amount of humeral translation that it is asymptomatic and usually symmetrical when compared with the opposite side (Fig. 2-2). *Instability* is a symptomatic, subjective sense of unease, discomfort, or pain in the setting of excessive translation. The other shoulder should be used as a control, taking care to assess symptoms during provocative testing and to elucidate whether the day-to-day complaints are being recreated upon a specific maneuver. The patient history is very helpful at this point to aid in differentiating laxity from instability. Two seemingly identical patients may have a 2-cm sulcus sign, but if one patient perceives instability while lifting a suitcase with the adducted arm and the other patient does so without difficulty, then the former patient is more likely to suffer from instability, whereas the latter may simply have excessive laxity that is asymptomatic and therefore likely not pathologic.

Lastly, proper imaging will aid in making an accurate diagnosis. All patients should be initially evaluated with appropriate radiographs (true AP, axillary lateral) (Fig. 2-3). Cross-sectional imaging usually involves magnetic resonance imaging (MRI), in which labral pathology, cartilage wear, and glenoid version can be assessed. Depending on the quality of the MRI, computed tomography (CT) is a very useful adjunct to accurately assess glenoid version and bone stock, bony avulsions of the capsulolabral complex, and Hill Sachs/reverse Hill Sachs defects (Fig. 2-4). It has been shown that glenoid version cannot be accurately assessed on plain axillary radiographs and that more advanced imaging is necessary (22).

Failure to appreciate glenoid retroversion, hypoplasia, or avulsions, as well as large Hill Sachs lesions, is a common cause of failed instability procedures (2,7,13,23). It is crucial to evaluate the bony anatomy preoperatively, using proper imaging as above, with an appreciation of the role

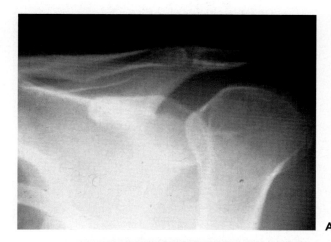

A

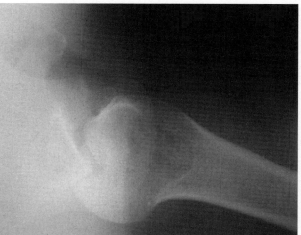

B

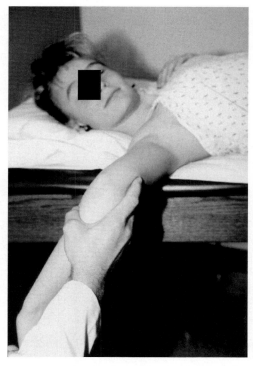

Figure 2-2 A patient exhibits excessive physiologic laxity, which is not symptomatic. Be cautious to differentiate laxity from instability.

Figure 2-3 **A:** This AP of the shoulder could be interpreted as a normal, aligned glenohumeral joint. **B:** Axillary lateral radiograph clearly demonstrates a locked posterior dislocation with a large reverse Hill-Sachs lesion of the humeral head.

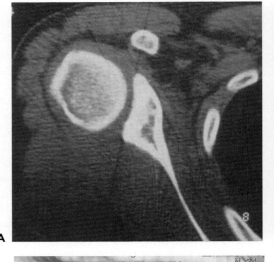

A

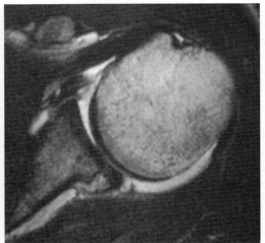

B

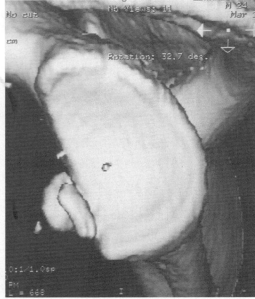

C

Figure 2-4 **A:** Axial CT image of a right shoulder demonstrating excessive glenoid retroversion. **B:** Axial MR image of a left shoulder demonstrating a posterior glenoid bony fragment in association with an injury to the capsulolabral complex. **C:** Three-dimensional CT demonstrating anterior glenoid bone loss.

of the bony articulation in overall glenohumeral stability. Traditionally, focus has centered on addressing the static and dynamic contributors to stability by attempting to rehabilitate the rotator cuff and scapular stabilizers, and to restore normal capsulolabral architecture and tension. Much work has been done on the role of the anterior inferior glenoid in recurrent anterior instability, which is covered in another chapter. Likewise, purely soft tissue procedures in the presence of excessive glenoid retroversion, hypoplasia, or other posterior bony deficiencies are doomed to fail (1,2,7,11,13,22,23).

Pearls

■ Always rule out cervical spine pathology when evaluating the shoulder.

■ Seek to classify the instability by *degree* (subluxation, dislocation, or locked dislocation), *mechanism* (traumatic or atraumatic), *chronicity* (acute or chronic), *direction* (uni-, bi-, or multidirectional), or *volition* (involuntary or voluntary).

■ Tailor your history and physical examination to specifically differentiate unidirectional instability from multidirectional instability.

■ Remember that laxity does not equal instability.

■ Use advanced imaging such as CT and MRI to carefully assess glenoid version and bone stock as well as humeral Hill-Sachs lesions.

Patient Expectations

Healthcare has gradually shifted toward a market model, with consumer satisfaction a major driving force for change. Consumers are increasingly determining how health care is delivered and administered, and traditional tools of measuring clinical outcomes are likewise evolving. Over the last decade, the outcomes assessment movement has evolved in response to these and other forces, becoming a major component of patient care. Outcomes instruments include generic measures of health quality-of-life such as the SF-36, condition-specific measures of disease such as the American Shoulder and Elbow Surgeons Score, and measures of patient satisfaction.

Commensurate with being responsive to patient outcome and satisfaction, clinicians are increasingly attuned to the need to assess a patient's preoperative expectations of a successful outcome. Mancuso and colleagues developed a 17-item Hospital for Special Surgery Shoulder Surgery Expectations Survey, which can serve as a guide to understand the patient's perspective and as a template to direct preoperative discussions and education (24). Questions assess the relative importance of such varied features as the relief of night pain, the regaining of motion, the return to employment, and the improvement of psychological well-being.

Specifically with regards to shoulder instability, patient expectations may be varied. For the professional football lineman with a history of traumatic posterior instability, the ability to return to the same level of play with stability is paramount. For the overhead athlete, regaining range of motion may even supersede stability as the primary surgical goal. Lastly, for the young female with generalized ligamentous laxity and multiple daily episodes of subtle instability, merely returning to a more normal quality of life may be the primary goal. For each patient, a careful assessment of his or her preoperative expectations will facilitate the development of shared, reasonable goals of treatment. It is important to understand and to communicate to patients that all expectations may not be attainable; the true error would be to fail to recognize and address this disparity with the patient before undertaking a surgical relationship.

Pearls

- Outcome instruments include generic measures of health quality of life, condition-specific measures of disease, and measures of patient satisfaction.
- Patient expectations regarding outcome after instability surgery, and especially after revision surgery, vary widely.
- Each patient's expectations must be addressed carefully in the initial stages to tailor a treatment strategy that is individualized and to educate him or her about reasonable expectations.

INTRAOPERATIVE ERRORS

Intraoperative complications are encountered in the surgical approach and through manipulation of the soft tissues and bony structures in the shoulder. Careful attention to patient positioning, a thorough knowledge of anatomy, familiarity with all instruments and hardware, and the use of intraoperative fluoroscopy will all serve to minimize surgical complications. Of course, a well-designed preoperative plan as discussed in the previous section will facilitate adequate preparation by assuring that all of these criteria are met.

Complications of the Posterior Approach to the Shoulder for Instability Repairs

The posterior approach to the shoulder has been well described (3,5,25,26). Several critical points warrant emphasis to avoid surgical complications.

Patient positioning is important and is often determined by the possible need for other procedures. In general, we favor the use of an arm holder, either the hydraulic arm holder (Spider Limb Positioner, Tenet Medical Engineering, Calgary, Canada) or the McConnell arm holder (McConnell Orthopaedic Manufacturing Company, Greenville, TX). These devices allow the arm to be rigidly positioned in space without the need for an additional surgical assistant for this purpose. If a combined open anterior and posterior approach is used, then either the beach chair or the lateral decubitus position on a bean bag can be used. We prefer the beach chair position, with the hemithorax clear for adequate exposure. This facilitates multiple simultaneous approaches to the shoulder, including arthroscopy. The lateral decubitus position could also be employed with an initial arthroscopic evaluation, depending on the surgeon's preferences.

The posterior skin incision should be made vertically in Langer's lines for cosmesis, centered over the glenohumeral joint. This is especially important in the female instability population, who often have generalized ligamentous laxity and surgical scars that stretch widely while healing. The deltoid should be split between its posterior and middle thirds in line with its fibers, which run obliquely in relation to the skin incision. Neurovascular injury can be avoided with a sound understanding of the anatomy of the suprascapular nerve, circumflex scapular artery, axillary nerve, and posterior circumflex humeral artery. Ball et al. (27) described the anatomy of the posterior branch of the axillary nerve as it relates to open and arthroscopic procedures of the posterior shoulder. The deltoid may be split up to 4 cm distal to the edge of the acromion, as the axillary nerve branches that supply the deltoid lie approximately 5 cm distal to the lateral edge of the acromion. These branches largely come from the anterior branch, but there is a variable (and redundant) contribution from the posterior branch. The two other contributions from the posterior branch of the axillary nerve are the branches to the teres minor and the superior-lateral brachial cutaneous nerve.

This cutaneous branch passes around the medial aspect of the deltoid, on average 8.7 cm distal to the posterolateral corner of the acromion; as it becomes a terminal branch, it is not endangered during routine surgical dissection. However, the more proximal posterior branch itself and its immediate branches lie directly adjacent to the capsule at the inferior aspect of the glenoid rim. The nerve is at particular risk during both open and arthroscopic procedures involving the posterior inferior capsule. A clinical pearl offered by Ball et al. (27) suggests that postoperative sensory changes in the distribution of the superior-lateral brachial cutaneous nerve might be a harbinger of coexistent injury to the nerve supply to the teres minor.

The internervous plane deep to the deltoid, as classically described, lies between the infraspinatus (suprascapular nerve) and the teres minor (axillary nerve), for the axillary nerve and the posterior circumflex humeral artery run in the quadrilateral space just inferior to the teres minor. Thus emphasis has been made to keep the plane of dissection superior to the teres minor. However, developing this plane between the infraspinatus and the teres minor is often difficult, as the muscle fibers coalesce medially, as do the tendonous insertions laterally on the greater tuberosity. Therefore, the surgeon may choose to split the bipennate infraspinatus between its two heads, a technique described by Jobe et al. (28). A fat stripe is usually present as a landmark for this plane (Fig. 2-5). A benefit to the infraspinatus split is that the plane of dissection, carried laterally, brings one to the equator of the glenohumeral joint as opposed to the inferior aspect of the glenoid, which is advantageous for posterior labral work. The plane between the infraspinatus and teres minor brings one inferior to the glenoid

equator, which is ideal to dissect the inferior posterior capsule for a large shift. This is our preferred approach when performing such a shift.

Once the appropriate plane is found, the dissection can be difficult as it is carried laterally towards the humeral head, as the posterior rotator cuff insertion becomes confluent with the capsule. To perform a laterally based (or humeral) shift, it is often helpful to split the infraspinatus in a T-shaped configuration, with the vertical limb approximately 1 cm medial to the rotator cuff insertion on the greater tuberosity. This will facilitate adequate exposure of the capsule and the joint, as well as provide a more robust tissue to hold sutures if the posterior capsule is attenuated (Fig. 2-6). If a medially based shift is preferred, then the infraspinatus split is usually adequate. We prefer a medially based shift, with the horizontal limb an oblique capsulotomy, from superior-lateral to inferior-medial. This facilitates a "pants-over-vest" capsular plication, by bringing the inferior medial flap superiorly (Fig. 2-7).

Whether reflecting the infraspinatus or splitting it, the position of the suprascapular nerve is critical to remember. Warner et al. (29) demonstrated in a cadaver study that the motor branches to the infraspinatus lie on average 2 cm medial to the posterior rim of the glenoid. Excessive medial dissection or retraction of the infraspinatus could endanger these motor branches.

Common sources of error in the posterior approach include the posterior labrum, the inferior capsule, and the rotator interval. Analogous to anterior instability and the Bankart lesion, the posterior labrum is critical to assess. Although it is not as robust as the anterior labrum, it should be assessed for integrity and injury. If it is detached from the glenoid, then a standard labral repair with suture anchors is indicated.

When performing a capsular shift, it is critical to dissect the posterior inferior capsule and axillary pouch as far anteriorly as the anterior band of the inferior glenohumeral

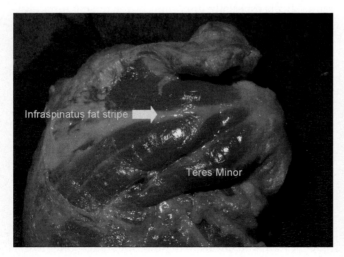

Figure 2-5 Cadaver specimen of the posterior shoulder girdle. The infraspinatus and teres minor are dissected. Note the fat stripe demarcating the two heads of the infraspinatus; this feature serves as a landmark for performing an infraspinatus split in the posterior approach to the shoulder.

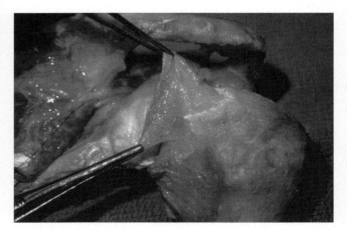

Figure 2-6 The posterior capsule of the shoulder can be quite attenuated.

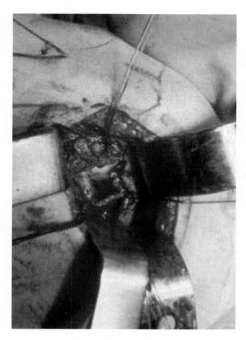

Figure 2-7 A medial-based capsulotomy is performed.

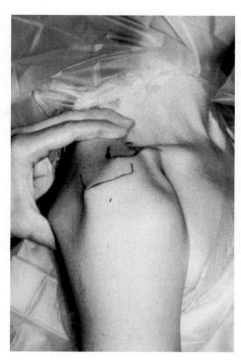

Figure 2-8 The sulcus sign is demonstrated, showing excessive inferior translation of the humeral head.

ligament. This allows adequate mobilization of the inferior flap of capsule for an effective shift. Although the axillary nerve is intimately associated with inferior capsule as noted above (27), to refrain from dissection in this area would limit the ability to perform a full shift. Blunt, gentle dissection is facilitated by pulling superiorly on the inferior flap after the capsulotomy. The axillary nerve can usually be both palpated and visualized when performing a primary surgery.

The rotator interval (RI) and its role in glenohumeral instability have been extensively studied (21,30–35). Harryman et al. (34) demonstrated that sectioning of the capsule, the superior glenohumeral ligament (SGHL), and the coracohumeral ligament (CHL) led to inferior instability in the adducted shoulder and posterior instability in the shoulder that is either forward flexed or abducted and externally rotated. Imbrication of the rotator interval caused a decrease in inferior translation of the adducted arm and a decrease of posterior translation when the arm was forward flexed. Most authors agree that true rotator interval lesions need to be addressed in instability surgery, but deciding when a pathologic lesion exists can be difficult. Clinical examination centers on the sulcus sign, when traction is applied to the adducted arm in neutral and external rotation (Fig. 2-8). Greater than 1 cm of inferior translation that does not diminish when the arm is externally rotated may be suggestive of pathologic laxity. Although we are unaware of any clinical study documenting a treatment algorithm for the rotator interval based on stability in differing rotations, it has been documented that the CHL exerts its primary restraining effect to inferior translation when

the humerus is externally rotated (36). Thus, when the sulcus sign is performed under anesthesia, it should be performed in neutral and full external rotation. A dampening of the sulcus sign in external rotation signifies a competent CHL, and careful consideration should be given to whether the RI warrants closure. Again, as mentioned previously, laxity must be differentiated from instability, and the key determinant is often subjective symptoms. A history of inferior instability, such as when picking up a piece of luggage is classic, and is analogous to posterior instability felt when reaching forward or anterior instability when in the abducted, externally rotated position. Taverna et al. (35) described six arthroscopic findings that were consistent with a lesion of the rotator interval. These included capsular redundancy or tearing in the interval, fraying of the biceps tendon as it exits the joint, tearing of the SGHL, fraying of the superior border of the subscapularis, and flattening and medial dislocation of the biceps tendon.

In summary, there currently exists no agreement among surgeons and no clear data in the literature to determine the exact role of RI closure. The senior author performs a closure in the patient with MDI when there is less than 1 cm sulcus sign that does not diminish in external rotation. In addition, if a patient is symmetrically unstable anteriorly, inferiorly, and posteriorly, all to a grade of 1+, then an isolated rotator interval closure will be performed arthroscopically, with superior shifting of the anterior capsule and ligaments as was described by Fitzpatrick et al. (37). If a rotator interval closure is to be performed in conjunction with a posterior capsular shift, an arthroscopic interval closure is preferred, followed by the posterior shift as described. The closure may also be performed as a mini-open procedure through a superior deltopectoral split.

As mentioned previously, the preferred surgical approach to address multidirectional instability is dependent upon the direction of greatest instability. If this is posterior, then a posterior inferior capsular shift is preferred. If anterior instability is primary, then a selective anterior inferior capsular shift through an anterior deltopectoral approach is warranted. This technique will be addressed in another chapter.

Pearls

- Careful consideration must be given to patient positioning in planning for the possible need for multiple exposures or a combination of open and arthroscopic procedures.
- Neurovascular injury can be avoided with a sound understanding of the anatomy of the suprascapular nerve, circumflex scapular artery, axillary nerve, and posterior circumflex humeral artery.
- The deep interval of the posterior approach may be modified to accommodate different surgical goals and exposures; that is, to dissect between the infraspinatus and teres minor or to split the two heads of the teres minor.
- We prefer a medially based shift posterior capsular shift, with the horizontal limb an oblique capsulotomy, from superior-lateral to inferior-medial.
- Common sources of error in the posterior approach include the posterior labrum, the inferior capsule, and the rotator interval.
- When performing a capsular shift, it is critical to dissect the posterior inferior capsule and axillary pouch as far anteriorly as the anterior band of the inferior glenohumeral ligament.
- Rotator interval lesions certainly contribute to glenohumeral instability, and failure to address them can lead to recurrent instability. However, no consensus exists to guide the surgeon on when to perform a rotator interval closure. The sulcus sign in neutral rotation and external rotation is the most reliable test, combined with an associated history.
- The preferred surgical approach to address multidirectional instability is dependent upon the direction of greatest instability.

Intraoperative Complications of Bony Procedures

Any hardware placed in or around the shoulder can potentially loosen, migrate, break, or impinge on adjacent structures, thus placing the articular surfaces in jeopardy. Most hardware complications have been reported for anterior procedures (11,13–17,25). Hardware problems may manifest in the immediate postoperative period or at any point thereafter. Zuckerman and Matsen (38) reported on the

myriad complications encountered with hardware: incorrect placement, migration, loosening, and breakage. Screws and staples used for coracoid transfer or anterior capsular plication were most commonly responsible (Fig. 2-9). Patients present with pain, crepitus, mechanical symptoms, or radiating paresthesias. Most patients required some form of reoperation and 41% had significant injury to the articular cartilage (38). In addition, migration of hardware used in the Bristow procedure had lead to injury to the brachial plexus and the axillary artery (39,40). These issues will be pursued in detail in another chapter.

Procedures for posterior instability requiring fixation include posterior capsular shift plus possible bone block augmentation, posterior opening wedge glenoid osteotomy, rotational humeral osteotomy, and glenohumeral arthrodesis. As mentioned for surgical complications in general, the only assured way to avoid hardware complications is to avoid the use of hardware. Posterior soft tissue procedures should avoid the use of staples, and the type of suture anchors used around the glenoid should be carefully considered. Bioabsorbable anchors have the advantage of avoiding metal in and around the articular surfaces; in the event of anchor pullout, there would be no metal to abrade the joint. As a practical measure, the true source of recurrent or persistent postoperative symptoms can be difficult to elucidate in the patient with a prominent or slightly mispositioned metal suture anchor visible on x-rays, even if the anchor is outside of the true glenohumeral joint. On the other hand, biodegradable implants have been associated with synovitic reactions and are not without potential complication (41). Whatever anchor material is chosen, the same principles must apply. The geometry of the glenoid is one of a truncated cone, with bone stock rapidly tapering deep to the inferior glenoid. The angle of anchor placement must be carefully considered to assure that it rests in bone, deep to the chondral surface.

Posterior bone block augmentation is rarely performed (Fig. 2-10). It may be necessary in the setting of posterior glenoid insufficiency where soft tissue procedures alone would not restore stability. The graft is taken from the scapular spine or the iliac crest. This technique carries the risks of hardware failure or migration, bone block nonunion or breakage, and impingement of the construct at the end range of motion. For all of these reasons, it is rarely performed by most surgeons.

Posterior opening wedge osteotomy of the glenoid has been advocated by some authors to address posterior instability secondary to glenoid hypoplasia or extreme glenoid retroversion. These reports describe a recurrence rate from 14% to 100%, a complication rate of 30%, and a glenohumeral arthrosis rate of 30% (42–46). Walch et al. (46) discusses this procedure in the clinically stable population but with static posterior subluxation of the humeral head, a potential precursor to primary glenohumeral arthritis. The other reports focus on the clinically unstable patient whose posterior instability is thought to result from excessive glenoid retroversion. In all reports, the numbers of patients

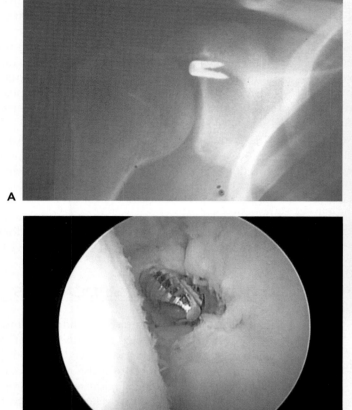

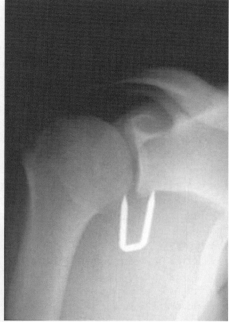

Figure 2-9 A,B: Staples used around the joint have the potential to loosen and migrate, thereby jeopardizing the articular cartilage and other local and possibly remote structures. C: A screw used in an anterior stabilization has penetrated the joint and caused severe erosive changes on the glenoid and humeral articular cartilage.

were small and the variability of procedures performed is large. Hawkins (47) analyzed the technique using CT, where he noted several potential complications, including under correction of version, intra-articular fracture, graft extrusion, and osteoarthritis. Although no conclusive evidence exists in the literature regarding the role of this proce-

dure, it is clearly technically demanding and associated with a high rate of complications, recurrence, and glenohumeral arthrosis.

The procedure of posterior glenoid opening wedge osteotomy has been described in detail (42–46). The most devastating intraoperative complications are completion of the osteotomy through the anterior cortex, thus producing a floating glenoid, and prematurely wedging the glenoid open, resulting in an intra-articular fracture into the glenoid face (48). The exposure is through the same approach as for a posterior capsular shift. The glenoid is exposed subperiosteally 1 to 1.5 cm medially, keeping in mind the position of the suprascapular nerve 2 cm medial to the glenoid rim as described above. A Fukuda humeral head retractor is used to displace the head anteriorly to visualize the articular surface, a critical step to aid in determining the proper depth of penetration of the saw and osteotomes. Intraoperative fluoroscopy can be used as well to determine depth. A 2-mm drill is used to score the osteotomy site, approximately 1 cm medial to the articular surface. The drill may be advanced through the anterior cortex to provide a perforated line for hinging the glenoid open. A depth gauge is used to measure the anterior–posterior dimensions of the glenoid for planning the depth of cutting. An oscillating

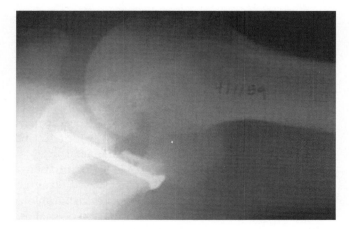

Figure 2-10 Posterior glenoid bone block placed to restore posterior glenoid anatomy.

saw is used to cut the posterior cortex, stopping approximately halfway towards the anterior cortex. Broad, flat, low-profile osteotomes are used to make the remaining portion of the osteotomy, with progressive wedging of them one after another to gradually open the osteotomy posteriorly and to elevate the articular surface to the desired level, as determined by preoperative imaging and careful planning. Although to our knowledge no studies exist that have assessed the optimal depth of penetration, an approximate guideline of 5 mm short of the anterior cortex allows for hinging on the cortex while preventing premature propagation of a fracture line into the glenoid face. Tricortical iliac crest bone or a wedge of bone from the scapular spine is placed into the osteotomy without hardware fixation, provided the anterior cortical hinge is intact. A capsular shift and closure are then performed.

Rotational humeral osteotomy and glenohumeral arthrodesis are salvage procedures in the patient for whom more traditional methods of stabilization have failed (Fig. 2-11) (49,50). The use of these procedures and their technical aspects are beyond the scope of this text. As with any case involving bony fixation, complications can be minimized by careful preoperative planning, the use of intraoperative fluoroscopy, the application of the principles of internal fixation, and appropriate postoperative rehabilitation.

Pearls

■ Any hardware placed in or around the shoulder can potentially loosen, migrate, break, or impinge on adjacent structures, thus placing the articular surfaces in jeopardy.

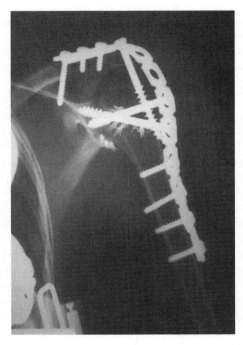

Figure 2-11 Glenohumeral arthrodesis can be a viable salvage option to stabilize the glenohumeral joint in certain situations.

■ Posterior soft tissue procedures should avoid the use of staples, and the type of suture anchors used around the glenoid should be carefully considered.

■ Whatever anchor material is chosen, the same principles must apply. The geometry of the glenoid is one of a truncated cone, with bone stock rapidly tapering deep to the inferior glenoid. The angle of anchor placement must be carefully considered to assure that it rests in bone, deep to the chondral surface.

■ The techniques of posterior glenoid bone block augmentation and opening wedge osteotomy have specific indications, but they are clearly technically demanding procedures that associated with a high rate of complications.

■ Rotational humeral osteotomy and glenohumeral arthrodesis are salvage procedures in the patient for whom more traditional methods of stabilization have failed.

POSTOPERATIVE COMPLICATIONS

The majority of complications encountered in instability surgery occur in the postoperative setting. Loss of motion, recurrence, coracoid impingement syndrome, bony complications, and glenohumeral arthrosis all may occur in the months or years following surgical reconstruction. Some complications like infection are general risks of any surgery and are unavoidable in a small percentage of patients, even in the setting of meticulous technique. Relative factors such as skill in handling tissues, length of operation, and intrinsic patient factors such as general nutritional status or immunocompromise all may play a role, but infection is never 100% preventable. Appropriate informed consent in the preoperative period will help patients prepare for this rare but devastating complication. As in all cases of postoperative infection, the *sine qua non* to a successful outcome is close follow-up, immediate recognition, and appropriate expeditious treatment. Further discussion of the management of postoperative infection will be deferred to other sources.

Loss of Motion and Arthrosis

Postoperative assessment of motion is important, as some degree of limitation is often a goal of surgery for instability. Excessive nonphysiologic restriction of motion, however, can lead to both early and late morbidity. The literature is abundant with reports on the consequences of overtightening the anterior capsule and subscapularis, with resultant loss of motion, pain, and eventual glenohumeral arthritis. This will be addressed in the chapter on anterior instability.

Although little is published in peer-reviewed literature on the sequelae of overtightening a posterior stabilization, many of the concepts we have learned from anterior stabilizations would certainly apply. Harryman et al. (30,31) described obligate humeral translation, where capsular tight-

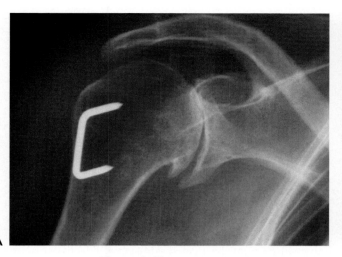
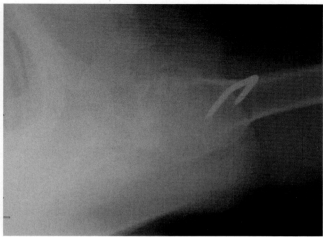

A   B

Figure 2-12 AP (A) and axillary (B) views demonstrating arthrosis secondary to an overly-tight anterior stabilization.

ening on one side of the joint led to humeral translation in the other direction at certain arm positions. Any procedure that leads to a nonphysiologic posterior tightening (such as the so-called reverse Putti-Platt procedure, where the posterior rotator cuff muscles are sectioned, overlapped, and tightened to limit internal rotation) would likely lead to obligate anterior translation and disproportionate contact stresses across the anterior articular surfaces. This relationship and the glenohumeral arthrosis that results have been well-documented in the Putti-Platt procedure for anterior instability (Fig. 2-12)(51,52); a similar outcome would be expected in overly tight posterior repairs.

Even in procedures designed to recreate normal anatomy rather than overtighten the tissues, postoperative stiffness is a frequent concern. Careful attention to detail intraoperatively will minimize the potential to overly tighten the tissues and thus overly constrain motion. When performing a posterior capsular shift, the tendency is toward limiting internal rotation, and the posterior capsule is tethered. To avoid this tendency, we recommend placing the arm in neutral rotation and in 30 to 40 degrees of abduction when securing the capsular shift. Open anterior capsular shift for MDI can present with motion loss that is similar to open procedures for direct anterior instability, covered in another chapter. External rotation is lost as the anterior capsule is tethered. Similar to the technique for a posterior shift, the fundamental technique to avoid overconstraint of the joint is to place the arm in a functional position before shifting the capsule. This is usually about 30 to 40 degrees of external rotation and a similar amount of abduction for an anterior inferior capsular shift.

The primary goals of postoperative rehabilitation are dichotomous in balancing stiffness and motion. It is important to allow enough immobilization to facilitate healing and to regain physiologic constraint of the joint, while at the same time slowly regaining normal preoperative mo-

tion. In trying to find this balance, some patients will lose motion.

The evaluation of the patient with postoperative stiffness is important. Passive versus active motion loss must be differentiated. Muscle weakness or rupture will cause a disparity, with passive motion greater than active motion. Contracture and stiffness will lead to equal losses of both passive and active motion. A goniometer should be used for documentation with comparison made to the opposite side. Scapulothoracic substitution should be recognized, as a patient with loss of motion through the glenohumeral joint can accommodate through scapular motion. Examination with the patient lying supine can aid to minimize the role of the scapula, as it becomes trapped between the thorax and the examination table (Fig. 2-13). External and internal rotation should be evaluated with the arm ad-

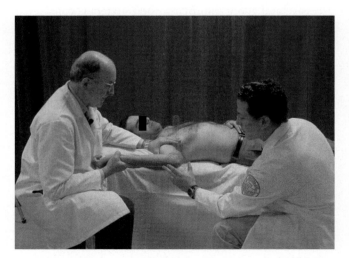

Figure 2-13 The supine position limits scapulothoracic substitution and allows for a more precise examination of the glenohumeral joint.

ducted and in 90 degrees of abduction. A relative loss of motion of less than 80% compared to the opposite side has been defined as significant.

The mainstay of treatment of postoperative stiffness is conservative, as physical therapy will restore motion in the vast majority of patients. Indeed, the most assured way to manage loss of motion is to prevent it. Although a thorough discussion of physical therapy programs for the postoperative period is beyond the scope of this text, some principles should be considered. The therapy should be phasic and progressive, with each phase building on the previous one. The initial phase should focus on gentle passive motion while still protecting the repair. The progression to active and active-assisted motion should occur once reasonable gains in passive motion have been achieved; this is usually at the 4- to 6-week mark. Strengthening can commence at approximately 10 to 12 weeks postoperatively. A close working relationship with the therapist, with clear instructions as to the exact surgery performed and the rehabilitation plan, will assure an appropriate and safe progression.

In some instances, however, motion will be lost. Initial treatment should be through physical therapy. Once this fails, operative treatment should be considered. It is important to distinguish the treatment of postoperative adhesions from that of idiopathic adhesive capsulitis, which is usually a self-limiting process that responds well to conservative treatment that often lasts 1 year or more. In the postoperative setting, motion gains plateau after a few months, and the freezing-frozen-thawing progression that many are familiar with in idiopathic frozen shoulder does not apply. Although no rigid guidelines exist, we usually consider surgical release at approximately 4 to 6 months postoperatively in the patient who has lost external rotation with the arm at the side. If internal rotation is lost with the arm at the side (most commonly after a posterior procedure), surgical release should be considered at approximately 6 to 9 months postoperatively. If motion loss is excessive and is not improving, then surgery is considered earlier. If gains are being made through therapy, albeit slowly, then further therapy can be considered. Keep in mind that physical therapy in and of itself does not necessarily imply less trauma to the tissues; a carefully planned and executed surgical release can be far safer than aggressive efforts at manipulation. For this reason, we do not advocate the routine use of closed manipulation under anesthesia for the postoperative loss of motion.

Once the decision is made for operative release, then the choice must be made between arthroscopic and open techniques. As a general principle, large open procedures involving intracapsular and extracapsular scarring respond less well to arthroscopic release, which predominantly addresses the capsule. The addition of tissue releases in the subacromial and subdeltoid spaces to the arthroscopic capsulectomy, however, can often provide enough tissue release that a gentle closed manipulation can then be sufficient to restore the last few degrees of motion. If gains are

inadequate after this arthroscopic technique, then a formal open release may be performed in the same surgical setting. Preoperative planning for anesthesia, patient positioning, and instrumentation will facilitate this transition if necessary. The results of arthroscopic capsular release in this patient population have been favorable and comparable to the well-documented successful outcomes in the treatment of idiopathic frozen shoulder (53,54). Holloway et al. (53) demonstrated that arthroscopic capsular release was as effective for improving range of motion in patients with postoperative contracture of the shoulder as it was in patients with idiopathic and postfracture contracture. However, there was less improvement in the subjective scores for pain, function, and patient satisfaction in the postoperative group. Gerber et al. (54) showed similarly that postoperative stiffness can be treated with equal effectiveness, and that the ultimate outcome is related directly to the severity of stiffness, regardless of the etiology.

Pearls

- Any procedure that leads to a nonphysiologic posterior tightening to limit internal rotation would likely lead to obligate anterior translation and disproportionate contact stresses across the anterior articular surface, placing the joint at risk for arthrosis.
- Even in procedures designed to recreate normal anatomy, as opposed to overtightening the tissues, postoperative stiffness is a frequent concern.
- To avoid excessive limitation of internal rotation, we recommend placing the arm in neutral rotation and in 30 to 40 degrees of abduction when securing the posterior capsular shift.
- Scapulothoracic substitution should be recognized in the evaluation of the patient with a postoperative loss of motion.
- The mainstay of treatment of postoperative stiffness is conservative, as physical therapy will restore motion in the vast majority of patients.
- In the event of failure of conservative treatment, we usually consider surgical release at approximately 4 to 6 months postoperatively in the patient who has lost external rotation, and at approximately 6 to 9 months in the patient who has lost internal rotation.
- Surgical release can be accomplished either open or arthroscopically. In general, the more extracapsular contracture that exists, the less effective arthroscopic release will be.

Recurrent Instability or New Anterior Instability after Posterior Surgery

The incidence of recurrence after open posterior instability repair is variably reported in the literature (25). Recurrence after soft tissue procedures has seen the widest range. Boyd et al. (55) reported no recurrences at the 2-year follow-up of patients treated with posterior capsular plication. Bowen and Warren (3) reported an overall 9% recurrence rate (1 of 11 patients) of open posterior capsular plication. Hurley noted a recurrence rate of 72% for soft tissue reconstructions (56). Bony procedures have also been reported with variable success. In a follow-up to the mentioned group, Bowen and Warren (3) reported an overall recurrence rate of 12% in 26 patients treated with a capsular shift. Seventeen of these patients were augmented by the infraspinatus tendon and seven by a posterior bone block. The results of posterior glenoid osteotomy were described above; recurrence rates have been reported from 14% to 41% (42,57,58).

Recurrence after stabilization for MDI has historically been low. Neer and Foster (4) reported 1 out of 40 failures after inferior capsular shift for MDI. Altchek and Warren (59) also reported that only 1 of 40 patients suffered a recurrence, which was actually posterior. Cooper and Brems (60) noted four recurrences out of 49 patients with an inferior capsular shift.

To our knowledge there are no formal clinical reports on postoperative anterior instability after posterior capsular shift. However, as noted above, data exist that demonstrate obligate humeral translation in the opposite direction of the side overconstrained (30,31). Again, accurate diagnosis is paramount. The fundamental concept to understand is that multidirectional instability caused by underlying global laxity cannot be successfully treated with unidirectional stabilization. An anatomic reconstruction for isolated unidirectional instability is highly unlikely to lead to *de novo* instability in the opposite direction. However, in the face of global laxity, a patulous capsule, and some degree of heightened tissue elasticity, tightening the capsule in only one direction will allow the humeral head to take the path of least resistance at certain points in the arc of motion. Numerous clinical reports have documented this scenario in failed anterior stabilizations, with the common thread being a failure to recognize MDI (14–17,61).

When confronted with the patient with recurrent instability or new instability in the opposite direction, a systematic approach is warranted. The final section of this chapter addresses the key components of the history, physical exam, and diagnostic studies. Once the diagnosis is reached and the decision is made for revision stabilization, careful consideration must be given to the etiology of the new instability. Tendon failure of the infraspinatus after surgical repair, analogous to subscapularis failure after an anterior procedure, is possible. Abnormal glenoid version (usually beyond 20 degrees) might have been missed, as well as a glenoid fracture or insufficiency. Capsular failure is possible and must be considered. Even in a person with normal collagen, the capsular tissues might be insufficient after several revision stabilizations, and some sort of augmentation might be necessary. Achilles tendon allograft has been successfully used in instability of native shoulders and in arthroplasty (62). There

are also a variety of new synthetics or xenografts that are designed to augment a deficient capsule.

Pearls

- Recurrence after stabilization for MDI has historically been low.
- Multidirectional instability caused by underlying global laxity cannot be successfully treated with unidirectional stabilization.
- When confronted with the patient with recurrent instability or new instability in the opposite direction, a systematic approach is warranted.

Coracoid Impingement Syndrome

The entity of coracoid impingement syndrome, whether idiopathic or secondary to lesions of the rotator cuff or instability, has been described by many authors (25, 63–65) and refers to abnormal contact between the anterior humeral head and the coracoid process. Gerber et al. (64) described iatrogenic subcoracoid impingement resulting from posterior glenoid osteotomy. If the version of the glenoid is overcorrected, then theoretically the humeral head will drift anteriorly and medially at certain points in the arc of motion, resulting in painful impingement between the anterior humeral head and the coracoid process. In a corresponding cadaver study, this anatomic impingement was recreated with glenoid osteotomy, and similar to reports of treatment of other forms of coracoid impingement, resection of the coracoacromial ligament and bone from the inferolateral coracoid process eliminated the abnormal contact (25,64).

On physical exam, pain will be elicited exactly at the coracoid process upon horizontal adduction of the forward flexed arm. A diagnostic injection may be preformed for confirmation.

Postoperative Complications of Bony Procedures

Hardware complications have been addressed previously in this chapter. As mentioned, complications can be minimized by careful preoperative planning, the use of intraoperative fluoroscopy, the application of the principles of internal fixation, and appropriate postoperative rehabilitation. Nevertheless, the utilization of bony procedures with hardware can lead to malunion, nonunion, loss of fixation, or osteonecrosis of the glenoid in glenoid osteotomy. All of these complications are rare, and to our knowledge no data exist in the literature on the true incidence in posterior shoulder stabilization procedures. Rather, sound clinical evaluation and routine follow-up are the tools of the prepared surgeon. Mechanical symptoms of catching or grinding, new symptoms of pain, new trauma to the shoulder, or failure of expected postoperative progression should all alert the physician that further evaluation is necessary. For any patient who had undergone bony work or who had metal hardware in place, plain radiographs at a minimum are required. Further evaluation with CT or MRI may be necessary to evaluate nonunion or osteonecrosis.

The use of bioabsorbable implants eliminates many of the problems of metal around the shoulder, but introduces the risk of reactive synovitis in response to the biomaterials (41). Arthroscopic procedures will be addressed further in Section II of this book.

THE EVALUATION OF THE PATIENT WITH A FAILED INSTABILITY REPAIR

The preceding discussion highlights some of the most common errors made in the preoperative, intraoperative, and postoperative periods when treating posterior shoulder instability and multidirectional instability. Clearly, the evaluation of the patient with a complication or a new symptom or complaint can be difficult, as the breadth of possible diagnoses is expansive. Lazarus and Guttmann described principles for the office evaluation of such a patient (25).

History

The most important factor in the history is the nature of the initial instability event. Improper diagnosis leading to improper treatment is the most likely source of error. The position of the arm during instability events and the nature and severity of antecedent trauma (or the lack of trauma) are critical factors to assess. Likewise, current symptoms, including arm position during new instability episodes, the existence of a new postoperative traumatic event, and the presence (or absence) of a period of time postoperatively that was free from these symptoms will aid the examiner in reaching a new diagnosis.

In the patient with a loss of motion, the extent of impairment on activities of daily living and sports or hobbies is important to ascertain. The degree of compliance and the progression of restoration of motion during rehabilitation are both important factors.

Operative notes should be carefully reviewed to determine what was done, what was not done, and what potential complications are likely. A patient with a glenoid osteotomy will likely have different reasons for stiffness, recurrence, or pain than a patient who was treated with a posterior capsular shift.

Physical Examination

A thorough physical exam as described previously in this chapter is vital. Specifically in the postoperative patient, previous scars should be assessed to aid in determining what procedures were performed. Careful assessment of range of motion with a goniometer, compared to the opposite side, is important. Instability tests may be clouded by pain, an important distinction as these two findings might have a common source or two different sources (e.g., painful hardware and a failed labral repair). Laxity must be assessed with the arm at the side and in 90 degrees of abduction, to assess the relative role of the rotator interval. Mechanical locking and catching from a displaced labrum or from loose hardware should be evaluated. Rotator cuff function is important to assess, especially the status of the subscapularis for an anterior deltopectoral approach for MDI and the infraspinatus/teres minor for a posterior approach. For a patient with instability and pain or stiffness, full internal rotation required for a proper liftoff test is often difficult for a patient to achieve. Gerber described the belly-press sign for this scenario (66), and its validity and reliability were confirmed by Tokish et al. (67). Nerve injury should be ruled out, including the axillary, suprascapular, and musculocutaneous nerves.

Diagnostic Tests

Imaging performed prior to the index operation is invaluable in the workup of these patients. Plain radiographs are important to evaluate glenohumeral arthrosis and the presence of hardware complications. Advanced imaging such as CT or MRI can be very helpful in evaluating the bony anatomy, the soft tissues, and the articular cartilage. Special MRI pulse sequences to evaluate the cartilage and to minimize metal artifact may be necessary, and communication with the radiology department before the scans will optimize the amount of information obtained from these studies.

Pearls

- The most important factor in the history is the nature of the initial instability event.
- Improper diagnosis leading to improper treatment is the most likely source of error.
- The position of the arm during instability events and the nature and severity of antecedent trauma (or the lack of trauma) are critical factors to assess.
- Operative notes should be carefully reviewed to determine what was done, what was not done, and what potential complications are likely.
- Instability tests may be clouded by pain, an important distinction, as these two findings might have a common source or two different sources.
- Use proper imaging, including CT and MRI, to evaluate hardware, bony anatomy, and soft tissue structures.
- Always consider indolent infection as a possible source of postoperative pain, loss of motion, or other symptoms, even in the setting of a clinically benign appearing shoulder.

CONCLUSION

Posterior and multidirectional instability are difficult problems for the patient and physician alike. Obtaining the correct diagnosis is the most assured way to provide successful treatment and to avoid complications. In addition, meticulous preoperative preparation and a sound knowledge of anatomy, instrumentation, and proper surgical techniques will serve to minimize errors made during the preoperative and intraoperative periods. Nevertheless, unanticipated results occur in surgery and the only way to reduce the impact of these events on the lives of our patients is to anticipate them, identify them, and aggressively treat them upon recognition. The goals of instability surgery are to obtain glenohumeral stability while maintaining physiologic motion through the recreation of normal anatomy. It is the aim of this chapter to assist the surgeon to accomplish these goals.

REFERENCES

1. Warner JJP, Schulte KR, Imhoff AB. Current concepts in shoulder instability. *Adv Oper Orthop* 1995;3:217–248.
2. Pollock RG, Bigliani LU. Recurrent posterior shoulder instability: diagnosis and treatment. *Clin Orthop* 1993;291:85–96.
3. Bowen MK, Warren RF. Surgical approaches to posterior instability of the shoulder. *Oper Tech Sports Med* 1993;1:301–310.
4. Neer CS II, Foster CR. Inferior capsular shift for involuntary inferior and multidirectional instability of the shoulder. *J Bone Joint Surg Am* 1980;62:897–907.
5. Bowen MK, Warren RF. Recurrent posterior subluxation: open surgical treatment. In: Warren RF, Craig EV, Altchek DW, eds. *The Unstable Shoulder*. Philadelphia: Lippincott-Raven Press 1999: 237–247.
6. Yamaguchi K, Flatow EL. Management of multidirectional instability. *Clin Sports Med* 1995;14:885–902.
6a. Cohen SB, Altchek DW, Warren RF. Selective capsular shift approach for treatment of anterior and multidirectional shoulder instability. *Tech Shoulder Elbow Surg* 2001;2:225–233.
7. Graichen H, Koydl P, Zichner L. Effectiveness of glenoid osteotomy in atraumatic posterior instability of the shoulder associated with excessive retroversion and flatness of the glenoid. *Int Orthop* 1999;23:95–99.
8. Diaz JA, Cohen SB, Warren RF, et al. Arthrodesis as a salvage procedure for recurrent instability of the shoulder. *J Shoulder Elbow Surg* 2003;12:237–241.
9. Surin V, Blader S, Markhede G, et al. Rotational osteotomy of the humerus for posterior instability of the shoulder. *J Bone Joint Surg Am* 1990;72:181–186.
10. Sherman OH, Fox JM, Snyder SJ, et al. Arthroscopy—no problem surgery. *J Bone Joint Surg Am* 1986;68:256–265.
11. Wall MS, Warren RF. Complications of shoulder instability surgery. *Clin Sports Med* 1995;14:973–1000.
12. Heller JG. The syndromes of degenerative cervical disease. *Orthop Clin North Am* 1992;23:381–394.
13. Flatow EL, Miniaci A, Evans PJ, et al. Instability of the shoulder: complex problems and failed repairs: Part II. Failed repairs. *Instr Course Lect* 1998;47:113–125.
14. Hawkins RH, Hawkins RJ. Failed anterior reconstruction for shoulder instability. *J Bone Joint SurgBr* 1985;67:709–714.
15. McAuliffe TB, Pangayatselvan T, Bayley I. Failed surgery for recurrent anterior dislocation of the shoulder. *J Bone Joint Surg Br* 1988; 70:798–801.
16. Norris TR, Bigliani LU. Analysis of failed repair for shoulder instability—a preliminary report. In: Bateman JE, Welsh RP, eds. *Surgery of the Shoulder*. Philadelphia: BC Decker, 1984:111–116.
17. Rockwood CA Jr, Gerber C. Analysis of failed surgical procedures for anterior shoulder instability. *Orthop Trans* 1985;9:48.
18. Neer CS II. *Shoulder Reconstruction*. Philadelphia: WB Saunders, 1990.
19. Fuchs B, Jost B, Gerber C. Posterior-inferior capsular shift for the treatment of recurrent, voluntary posterior subluxation of the shoulder. *J Bone Joint Surg Am* 2000;82:16–25.
20. Kuroda S, Sumiyoshi T, Moriishi J, et al. The natural course of a traumatic shoulder instability. *J Shoulder Elbow Surg* 2001;10: 100–104.
21. Cole BJ, Rodeo SA, O'Brien SJ, et al. The anatomy and histology of the rotator interval capsule of the shoulder. *Clin Orthop* 2001; 390:129–137.
22. Nyffeler RW, Jost B, Pfirrmann CW, et al. Measurement of glenoid version: conventional radiographs versus computed tomography scans. *J Shoulder Elbow Surg* 2003;12:493–496.
23. Walch G, Ascani C, Boulahia A, et al. Static posterior subluxation of the humeral head: an unrecognized entity responsible for glenohumeral osteoarthritis in the young adult. *J Shoulder Elbow Surg* 2002;11:309–314.
24. Mancuso CA, Altchek DW, Craig EV, et al. Patients' expectations of shoulder surgery. *J Shoulder Elbow Surg* 2002;11:541–549.
25. Lazarus MD, Guttmann D. Complications of instability surgery. In: Iannotti JP, Williams GR, eds. *Disorders of the Shoulder*. Philadelphia: Lippincott Williams & Wilkins, 1999:361–393.
26. Schwartz E, Warren RF, O'Brien SJ, et al. Posterior shoulder instability. *Orthop Clin North Am* 1997;18:409–419.
27. Ball CM, Steger T, Galatz LM, et al. The posterior branch of the axillary nerve: an anatomic study. *J Bone Joint Surg Am* 2003;85: 1497–1501.
28. Shaffer BS, Conway J, Jobe FW, et al. Infraspinatus muscle-splitting incision in posterior shoulder surgery: an anatomic and electromyographic study. *Am J Sports Med* 1994;22:113–120.
29. Warner JP, Krushell RJ, Masquelet A, et al. Anatomy and relationships of the suprascapular nerve: anatomical constraints to mobilization of the supraspinatus and infraspinatus muscles in the management of massive rotator-cuff tears. *J Bone Joint Surg Am* 1992;74:36–45.
30. Harryman DT II, Sidles JA, Clark JM, et al. Translation of the humeral head on the glenoid with passive glenohumeral motion. *J Bone Joint Surg Am* 1990;72:1334–1343.
31. Harryman DT II, Sidles JA, Matsen FA III. The role of the coracohumeral ligament in range of motion and obligate translation in the shoulder. *Orthop Trans* 1990;14:727.
32. Wolf RS, Zheng N, Iero J, et al. The effects of thermal capsulorrhaphy and rotator interval closure on multidirectional laxity in the glenohumeral joint: a cadaveric biomechanical study. *Arthroscopy* 2004;20:1044–1049.
33. Fitzpatrick MJ, Powell SE, Tibone JE, et al. The anatomy, pathology, and definitive treatment of rotator interval lesions: current concepts. *Arthroscopy* 2003;19(Suppl 1):70–79.
34. Harryman DT II, Sidles JA, Harris SL, et al. The role of the rotator interval capsule in passive motion and stability of the shoulder. *J Bone Joint Surg Am* 1992;74:53–66.
35. Taverna E, Sansone V, Battistella F. Arthroscopic rotator interval repair: the three-step all-inside technique. *Arthroscopy* 2004; 20(Suppl 2):105–109.
36. Itoi E, Berglund LJ, Grabowski JJ, et al. Superior-inferior stability of the shoulder: role of the coracohumeral ligament and the rotator interval capsule. *Mayo Clin Proc* 1998;73:508–515.
37. Fitzpatrick MJ, Powell SE, Tibone JE, et al. The anatomy, pathology, and definitive treatment of rotator interval lesions: current concepts. *Arthroscopy* 2003;19(Suppl 1):70–79.
38. Zuckerman JD, Matsen FA II. Complications about the glenohumeral joint related to the use of screws and staples. *J Bone Joint Surg Am* 1984;66:175–180.
39. Iftikhar TB, Kaminski RS, Silva I. Neurovascular complications of the modified Bristow procedure. *J Bone Joint Surg Am* 1984;66: 951.
40. Artz T, Huffer JM. A major complication of the modified Bristow procedure for recurrent dislocation of the shoulder. *J Bone Joint Surg Am* 1972;54:1293–296.
41. Freehill MQ, Harms DJ, Huber SM, et al. Poly-L-lactic acid tack synovitis after arthroscopic stabilization of the shoulder. *Am J Sports Med* 2003;31:643–647.

42. Hawkins RJ, Koppert G, Johnson G. Recurrent posterior instability (subluxation) of the shoulder. *J Bone Joint Surg Am* 1984;66:169.

43. Norwood LA, Terry GC. Shoulder posterior subluxation. *Am J Sports Med* 1984;12:25.

44. Wilkinson JS, Thomas WG. Glenoid osteotomy for recurrent posterior dislocation of the shoulder. *J Bone Joint Surg Br* 1985;67:496.

45. Graichen H, Koydl P, Zichner L. Effectiveness of glenoid osteotomy in atraumatic posterior instability of the shoulder associated with excessive retroversion and flatness of the glenoid. *Int Orthop* 1999;23:95–99.

46. Walch G, Ascani C, Boulahia A, et al. Static posterior subluxation of the humeral head: an unrecognized entity responsible for glenohumeral osteoarthritis in the young adult. *J Shoulder Elbow Surg* 2002;11:309–314.

47. Hawkins RH. Glenoid osteotomy for recurrent posterior subluxation of the shoulder: assessment by computed axial tomography. *J Shoulder Elbow Surg* 1996;5:393–400.

48. Johnston GH, Hawkins RJ, Haddad R, et al. A complication of posterior glenoid osteotomy for recurrent posterior shoulder instability. *Clin Orthop* 1984;187:147–149.

49. Diaz JA, Cohen SB, Warren RF, et al. Arthrodesis as a salvage procedure for recurrent instability of the shoulder. *J Shoulder Elbow Surg* 2003;12:237–241.

50. Kronberg M, Brostrom LA. Rotation osteotomy of the proximal humerus to stabilize the shoulder. Five years' experience. *J Bone Joint Surg Br* 1995;77:924–927.

51. Kiss J, Mersich I, Perlaky GY, et al. The results of the Putti-Platt operation with particular reference to arthritis, pain, and limitation of external rotation. *J Shoulder Elbow Surg* 1998;7:495–500.

52. Hawkins RJ, Angelo RL. Glenohumeral arthrosis. A late complication of the Putti-Platt repair. *J Bone Joint Surg Am* 1990;72:1193–1197.

53. Holloway GB, Schenk T, Williams GR, et al. Arthroscopic capsular release for the treatment of refractory postoperative or post-fracture shoulder stiffness. *J Bone Joint Surg Am* 2001;83:1682–1687.

54. Gerber C, Espinosa N, Perren TG. Arthroscopic treatment of shoulder stiffness. *Clin Orthop* 2001;390:119–128.

55. Boyd HD, Sisk TD. Recurrent posterior dislocation of the shoulder. *J Bone Joint Surg Am* 1972;54:779–786.

56. Hurley JA, Anderson TE, Dear W, et al. Posterior shoulder instability: surgical vs. nonsurgical results. *Orthop Trans* 1987;11:458.

57. Scott DJ. Treatment of recurrent posterior dislocations of the shoulder by glenoplasty. *J Bone Joint Surg Am* 1967;49:471–476.

58. Kretzler HH. Scapular osteotomy for posterior shoulder dislocation. *J Bone Joint Surg Am* 1974;56:197–200.

59. Altchek DW, Warren RF, Skyhar MJ, et al. T-plasty modification of the Bankart procedure for multidirectional instability of the anterior and inferior types. *J Bone Joint Surg Am* 1991;73:105–112.

60. Cooper RA, Brems JJ. The inferior capsular shift procedure for multidirectional instability of the shoulder. *J Bone Joint Surg Am* 1992;74:1516–1521.

61. Burkhead WZ Jr, Richie MF. Revision of failed shoulder reconstruction. *Contemp Ortho* 1992;24:126–133.

62. Moeckel BH, Altchek DW, Warren RF, et al. Instability of the shoulder after arthroplasty. *J Bone Joint Surg Am* 1993;75:492–497.

63. Gerber C, Terrier F, Ganz R. The role of the coracoid process in the chronic impingement syndrome. *J Bone Joint Surg Br* 1985;67:703–708.

64. Gerber C, Ganz R, Vinh TS. Glenoplasty for recurrent posterior shoulder instability. An anatomic reappraisal. *Clin Orthop* 1987;216:70–79.

65. Dines DM, Warren RF, Inglis AE, et al. The coracoid impingement syndrome. *J Bone Joint Surg Br* 1990;72:314–316.

66. Gerber C, Hersche O, Farron A. Isolated rupture of the subscapularis tendon. *J Bone Joint Surg Am* 1996;78:1015–1023.

67. Tokish JM, Decker MJ, Ellis HB, et al. The belly-press test for the physical examination of the subscapularis muscle: electromyographic validation and comparison to the lift-off test. *J Shoulder Elbow Surg* 2003;12:427–430.

Complications of Rotator Cuff Repair

3

Joseph Iannotti   Michael Codsi

Pain or disability following a rotator cuff repair is not always due to a recurrent tear. In fact, subjective outcomes after recurrent tears can be quite good. Common complications of rotator cuff repair include failed repairs, stiffness, deltoid injury, persistent subacromial impingement, and infection. Other issues include heterotopic ossification, acromial fractures, and anterosuperior humeral head subluxation. A precise diagnosis of the etiology of the patient's complaints is the key to the treatment of complications of rotator cuff repair.

FAILED REPAIR

Successful open repair of the rotator cuff depends on many patient factors including cuff tear size, patient age, tendon quality, tendon retraction, and degree of muscle atrophy. The clinical success rate varies between 85% and 90% when measured in terms of patient satisfaction or patient outcome scores. These high success rates, however, do not directly correlate well with the rate at which tendon repairs heal when measured by postoperative imaging. Harryman et al. (1) described their findings in a series of 105 rotator cuff repairs, which were followed by an ultrasound exam to document the integrity of the repair. In all, 80% of the supraspinatus repairs were intact, 57% of the supraspinatus/infraspinatus repairs were intact, and 32% of three tendon tears were intact at an average of 5-years follow-up. Older patients with larger tears were more likely to have a recurrent defect. Nineteen patients in this series had revision cuff repair and they were more likely to have a recurrent defect than the primary repairs. Patients who had an intact repair had better function, motion, and pain relief, and the patients with recurrent defects had worsening

function, motion and strength with increasing cuff defects. Overall, 94% of patients were satisfied with the repairs; this did not correlate with cuff integrity.

The lack of correlation between rotator cuff integrity and clinical outcome is commonly seen. Jost et al. (2) prospectively evaluated a series of 65 rotator cuff repairs and found 20 reruptures by magnetic resonance imaging (MRI) scan. Sixteen were smaller than the initial repair. Atrophy, fatty degeneration, and glenohumeral osteoarthritis progressed in all 20 patients, yet only three patients were not satisfied with the procedure and one patient underwent revision surgery. In the 20 reruptures, the average Constant score, adjusted for age- and sex-related normal values, increased from 49% preoperatively to 83% postoperatively; the scores did correlate with the number of tendons retorn.

An even larger disparity between patient satisfaction and cuff integrity was reported in the series by Galatz et al. (3). Eighteen patients underwent arthroscopic repair of large and massive tears and ultrasound evaluation of the cuff 12 months after surgery. Recurrent tears were seen in 17 patients. Despite the high rate of failed repair, 16 patients had an Adult Self-Expression Scale (ASES) score lower than 90, 12 patients had no pain, and all patients regained above shoulder motion to an average of 152 degrees. All patients were satisfied with the procedure. At the 2-year follow-up exam, the ASES scores decreased by 5 points and their forward elevation decreased 10 degrees. Outcome scores were not correlated with number of tendons retorn.

Etiology of Failed Repairs

The causes of a failed repair have been correlated to cuff tear size (number of tendons and amount retraction), degree of muscle atrophy (which in turn is related to size of the tear), and chronicity of the tear. All of these factors influence the quality of the tendon tissue. In addition, other factors associated with failure of the tendon repair to heal can be attributed to inadequate subacromial decompression, poor tendon mobilization, excessive tendon tension, inappropriate suture technique, patient age, improper physical therapy, and patient compliance.

There are several main risk factors for rerupture following rotator cuff repair. Jost et al. (2) reported that in their series of 80 revision repairs, the initial tear was massive in 28% and large in 35% of the revisions. In all, 49 patients had an inadequate subacromial decompression and four patients underwent complete lateral acromionectomy. Twenty-four patients had inadequate tissue for a secure repair of the cuff at the initial repair, resulting in 17 repairs requiring arm abduction in order to bring the tendon to its insertion site. Also, nine patients had inappropriate rehabilitation because they either initiated strengthening too early or neglected passive motion exercises too late. The active motion before revision was 105 degrees of forward flexion, 39 degrees of external rotation, and internal rotation to the 11th thoracic vertebrae.

Similarly, Bigliani et al. (4) reviewed 31 patients who underwent revision surgery for their failed rotator cuff repairs. In all, 97% of the patients had large or massive tears at the initial procedure and 90% of the patients had persistent subacromial impingement before their revision procedure. Fifteen patients did not have adequate mobilization of the cuff tendon for attachment to the bone at the initial repair.

DeOrio et al. (5) attributed the failure of rotator cuff repairs to the size of the tears, inadequate subacromial decompression, and possibly inadequate postoperative external support. The average patient age was 52 years and 66% of the patients had a large or massive tear. Seven patients had tenderness over the supraspinatus tendon, a painful arc of motion, and a positive impingement sign, suggesting that the subacromial pathology was still present after the initial repair.

These three studies all had a retrospective study design and it is not known the frequency in which these presumed negative factors were present in successful surgery (2,4,5). The data and conclusion presented are suggestive but not definitive for a correlation between initial tear size, subacromial pathology, and clinical outcome.

In addition to these factors, Davidson et al. (6) studied the effects of rotator cuff tension on the subjective and objective outcomes after 67 rotator cuff repairs. A tissue tensiometer was used to measure the tension on the tendon after it was stretched to its insertion site on the humerus. ASES scores, isokinetic strength measurements, and visual analog pain scores were all worse if the tension of the repair was greater than 8 pounds.

Effect of Fixation Technique

Many studies have evaluated the effects of suture techniques on the strength of rotator cuff repairs. Gerber et al.

(7) used the modified Mason-Allen stitch and a simple stitch to repair the cuff tendons in sheep. He found that the simple stitch pulled out of the tendon in all cases, whereas the Mason-Allen stitch failed in only 2 of 17 repairs. The fixation through the bone was also varied between augmentation with cortical-bone polylactide plate and no augmentation. The augmented group never failed, whereas the nonaugmented group failed in 8 of 16 cases.

The mode of failure for rotator cuff repairs was prospectively evaluated by Cummins et al. (8) in a series of 342 patients who underwent repair with suture anchors. Repairs were done with either one or two rows of anchors, depending on the size of the tears. Horizontal mattress sutures were used in all repairs. In all, 21 repairs failed and underwent revision surgery, and 19 of those failed at the suture-tendon junction. One suture anchor pulled out of the bone and two retears occurred at a different location.

The results of tendon repair found in the animal model were tested in a clinical trial by Gerber et al. (9). Repair of 29 massive rotator cuff tears involving complete detachment of at least two tendons was performed using no. 3 braided polyester sutures placed in a modified Mason-Allen technique. Both ends of the sutures were brought through the greater tuberosity and tied over a titanium plate used for cortical bone augmentation. After a minimum 2-year follow-up, the Constant score improved from 49% to 85%. The overall rate of retears according to MRI was 34%. The Constant score was 91% in group with an intact repair compared to 61% in the group with a retear ($p = 0.016$).

Workup

Clinical Evaluation

Patients with recurrent rotator cuff tears may complain of pain and weakness in the shoulder. It is imperative that the clinical assessment of a patient with persistent pain after rotator cuff surgery include an evaluation of all possible causes of shoulder pain beyond that of an anatomic finding of a persistent cuff defect. This includes symptomatic biceps tendon, acromioclavicular arthritis, cervical spine disease, or frozen shoulder. The importance of this fact is underscored by the extensive literature that clearly demonstrates that many patients with persistent cuff defects after rotator cuff repair have subjective outcome (using patient directed outcome assessment tools) equal to that of patients without persistent defects.

Many patients require narcotics before their revision surgery (4). The pattern of pain may help differentiate between a recurrent tear and persistent subacromial pathology, but this is often unreliable. Weakness, especially when it is not caused by pain, can predict which cuff tendon remains functional. The external rotation lag sign tests the integrity of the external rotators (10). If the arm cannot be actively held at maximum passive external rotation, then the infraspinatus tendon is substantially involved in the tear.

Testing the subscapularis can be done with the lift-off test or the belly-press test (Napoleon test). The lift-off test is the most reliable, but if the patient has pain or lacks sufficient internal rotation to get the hand to the lumbar spine, then the test is not reliable. The belly-press test is positive if the patient is unable to push their hand against their belly while keeping their elbow at or anterior to the coronal plane of the body. If the wrist flexes or the elbow extends behind the patient, then the test is positive. This test is sometimes difficult to perform for the patient and it can give a false-positive result if there is loss of passive internal rotation. A study of 25 patients with subscapularis tendon tears by Burkhart et al. (11) described the abdominal compression or Napoleon test and its relationship to the operative findings. Eight of nine patients with a positive Napoleon test had complete tears of the subscapularis, whereas seven patients with a negative Napoleon test had a tear of the upper half only. The authors warn that the reliability of the Napoleon test is altered if the patient lacks passive internal rotation.

Imaging

Radiographic evaluation of a patient with a suspected rotator cuff retear should start with plain films, including an outlet view to look for subacromial spurs, a Greise view or true anteroposterior view of the shoulder joint to evaluate the joint space, and an axillary lateral view to inspect the acromion for possible fracture or os acromiale. Findings particular to rotator cuff pathology include displaced suture anchors. Pearsall et al. (12) showed that greater tuberosity sclerosis, osteophytes, subchondral cysts and osteolysis are associated with rotator cuff tears, but these changes are not reliable in the postoperative setting. Significant superior migration of the humeral head is associated with large and massive chronic rotator cuff tears. When the acromial humeral space is less than 7 mm, the tear is often irreparable or, if reparable, has a low chance to heal.

Ultrasound can effectively evaluate the rotator cuff in patients who have sufficient pain-free motion to expose the cuff tendons from underneath the acromion. Pricket et al. (13) reported the results of 44 rotator cuff repairs that underwent both ultrasound and MRI exams. The ultrasound sensitivity was 91% and the specificity was 86%. The accuracy was 89%. Another study by Teefey et al. (14) compared the ultrasound findings and arthroscopic findings of 100 patients with shoulder pain who did not undergo surgery. All full thickness tears were correctly diagnosed with ultrasound, resulting in a specificity of 100%. There were 17 true-negative and 3 false-negative ultrasounds, resulting in a specificity of 85%.

Gaenslen et al. (15) compared the findings of MRI exams to the operative findings of 30 shoulders that had failed rotator cuff repairs. The sensitivity for full-thickness tears was 84% and the specificity was 91%. The sensitivity for partial-thickness tears was 83% and the specificity was 83%. The positive-predictive value for full-thickness tears was 94% and the negative predicted value was 77%. The MRI scans in this study also diagnosed articular cartilage damage and a ganglion cyst in the supraspinatus muscle, both of which could not be diagnosed with ultrasound.

Results of Revision

The results of revision rotator cuff repairs in patients without concomitant pathology, such as deltoid injury or acromioclavicular arthritis, are not easily found in the literature. The first published report of revision cuff repairs by DeOrio et al. (5) included 27 patients with a minimum 2-year follow-up. In all, 37 percent of patients had no, slight, or moderate pain, and 76% of patients had a reduction in pain. Seven patients had a third attempt to repair the rotator cuff and three of those patients went on to have a shoulder fusion. Overall, only four patients were considered to have a good result.

Bigliani et al. (4) reported slightly better results in their series of revision cuff repairs. Thirteen patients had attempts at mobilization and repair of the detached deltoid origin in addition to revision repair of the rotator cuff. At the time of revision, a massive tear was found in 12 patients, a large tear in 10 patients, a medium tear in seven patients, and a small tear in two patients. The results were excellent in 19%, good in 32%, fair in 23%, and poor in 26% of patients. An inferior result was associated with previous lateral acromionectomy, detached deltoid origin, and poor tendon quality at the time of revision.

Neviaser et al. (16) reported their results after reoperation for failed rotator cuff repairs in 50 patients. The patients included 39 men and 11 women with an average age of 54.5 years. The average number of previous operations was 1.6. Six patients had deltoid dysfunction. In all, 28 of 50 patients started resistance exercises within the first 3 months of their first rotator cuff repair. There were 6 small tears, 23 large tears, and 21 massive tears in the group. After operative fixation of the tear through bone troughs, the patients were allowed to do passive shoulder motion for 6 weeks, followed by active motion until 3 months after the repair. Resistive exercises were then started. After a mean follow-up of 30 months, 19 patients had no pain and 27 patients had only slight shoulder pain. Four patients had no change in pain. Improved motion was found in 26 patients, whereas 22 patients had the same shoulder motion.

Revision rotator cuff repair in 80 patients was more recently reported by Djurasovic et al. (17). The average initial tear size was massive in 22, large in 28, medium in 10, and small in 13 patients. In all, 45% of repairs required an anterior interval slide to aid in cuff mobilization and 24 patients had additional procedures to repair the deltoid to the acromion. The overall results were excellent in 33%, good in 25%, fair in 9%, and poor in 31% of patients. The average pain rating improved from 3 to 7.4 points out of a maximum pain score of 10. A satisfactory outcome was reported in 78% of patients with an intact deltoid origin, compared to 57% of patients who did not have a deltoid injury. Other factors related to outcome were cuff tendon tissue quality, preoperative active motion, and number of prior procedures.

The most recent report of revision rotator cuff repairs was done by Lo and Burkhart (18). They arthroscopically repaired 14 failed repairs that consisted of 11 massive, one large, and two medium tears. Seven patients were involved in worker's compensation claims and five patients had superior migration of the humeral head. Concomitant pathology found at the revision surgery included five patients with persistent acromial spurs, two superior labrum anterior posterior (SLAP) lesions requiring repair, and three biceps tendonopathies. Four patients were found to have a U-shaped tear repaired directly to bone instead of using a margin convergence technique. The University of California Los Angeles (UCLA) scores improved from 13.1 to 28.6, which translated into four excellent, five good, four fair, and one poor result. Five patients returned to previous level of work activity, two patients returned to less strenuous work activity, and one patient did not return to work.

Pearls

Postoperative pain needs a systematic evaluation that includes a combination of clinical examination and imaging studies. The first step is to determine if the pain is from the shoulder or from some other source outside of the shoulder such as the brachial plexus, cervical spine, or a nonorganic cause. If the pain is thought to come from the shoulder, then selective injections can on occasion help localize the pain to the glenohumeral joint, subacromial space, or acromioclavicular joint. It also helps in some cases validate that the pain is organic and localized to the shoulder. Addressing all of the causes of shoulder pain both within the shoulder, outside of the shoulder, organic, and nonorganic is critical to both determining operative versus nonoperative treatment and, if surgery is indicated, the nature of the surgery to be performed.

When a persistent rotator cuff tear is present, the questions that need to be addressed for treatment include:

1. Is it the source of pain?
2. What are the patient's primary objectives: pain relief or return of strength?
3. What are the patient's functional goals?
4. Can these goals be achieved with a reasonable degree of success (75%)?
5. Is the cuff repairable?
6. What is the likelihood that the cuff will heal if reparable?
7. What are the consequences if a second repair is attempted and it does not heal (i.e., will the results of surgery be a failure to achieve some of the goals of surgery)?

If the MRI arthrogram demonstrates a persistent tear that is large or massive with retraction medial to the midhumeral head and there is associated moderate to severe atrophy, then it is likely that the tear is irreparable or, if reparable, the repair will not heal. If strength is a primary objective of surgery, then a muscle transfer (latissimus and or teres major for a posterior superior defect or a sternocostal portion of the pectoralis major for an anterior superior cuff tear) should be planned as part of the revision surgery. The best results of muscle transfer surgery is for a patient with tolerable pain, good passive range of motion, good deltoid function, an intact cuff on the side opposite to the transfer, a nonarthritic joint, active elevation to shoulder height, ability to control the arm in decent when placed in a full elevated position, an intact coracoacromial arch, and physiologic youthfulness both in mind and activity level. Multiple negative attributes in these categories are, in the senior author's experience, associated with poor clinical results.

Candidates for arthroscopic debridement are patients with a large or irreparable tear, pain as a primary indication for surgery, the ability to actively elevate the arm to shoulder height, the ability to control the decent of the arm from a passively fully elevated arm, and an intact coracoacromial arch. Arthroscopic debridement includes smoothing of the arch (do not decrease the anterior-posterior dimension of the acromion or remove the coracoacromial ligament) and removal of all greater tuberosity osteophyte (tuberoplasty) and foreign material (sutures, loose anchors, etc.). The response (pain and function) to a preoperative injection of lidocaine into the glenohumeral joint is often a good indicator of the response to a limited-goal arthroscopic debridement.

When a persistent tear is repairable and the patient is symptomatic, then the tear should be repaired. All causes of persistent pain should be addressed at the time of surgery and/or with the pre- and postoperative rehabilitation program.

For a massive cuff tear with coracoacromial arch deficiency in a patient of advanced age (greater than 70 years), with anticipated postoperative activity level to include only activities of daily living, the only surgery that the senior author has found to be reliable in providing pain relief and improvement in functions is a reverse total shoulder replacement. This surgery should be reserved for this older and lower-activity level patient.

For revision rotator cuff repair or muscle transfer, the authors always use a postoperative abduction brace for 4 to 6 weeks after surgery. During this time, the brace is removed for dressing and washing and eating activities, as well for the exercise program, which includes pendulum, passive range-of-motion in supine forward flexion. Other than for these activities, the brace is worn during the day and through the night. No. 2 fiberwire suture or its equivalent is used through bone tunnels as in a primary open rotator cuff repair; bone augmentation with a plastic button is used if the bone quality is poor. The principles of scar excision and cuff mobilization are achieved to the maximum extent possible.

DELTOID INJURY

The deltoid can be injured during open rotator cuff repair by an overaggressive subacromial decompression, inadequate deltoid origin repair, injury to the axillary nerve, or compression from retractors. Early reports of complete acromionectomy or lateral acromionectomy for the treatment of impingement syndrome detailed the disadvantages of trading a treatable pathology for an untreatable condition. Patients no longer complained of anterior shoulder pain, but some patients lost the ability to elevate the arm. Neer and Marberry (19) treated 30 patients who previously underwent a radical acromionectomy and all the patients had poor results. The authors concluded that the acromion allowed for a mechanical advantage necessary for forward elevation of the arm, and that loss of the deltoid muscle integrity resulted in significant disability.

Bosley (20) reported his results after treating 38 shoulders with total acromionectomy between 1969 and 1989. Six patients were laborers and 19 shoulders also had a concomitant rotator cuff repair. The age range was from 31 to 70 years, 10 patients were women, and 21 patients were men. Postoperatively, the shoulders were immobilized in abduction for 5 to 9 weeks, which depended on status of the rotator cuff repair. After a minimum 2-year follow-up, 25 shoulders had excellent results, four shoulders had good results, three shoulders had fair results, and one had a poor result. Poor results of complete acromionectomy are often associated with persistent cuff tears and deltoid problems. That being said, a complete or even subtotal acromionectomy is not advocated by the authors, but this article is cited to give a balanced review of the literature.

Reports of revision rotator cuff repair all included patients who had concomitant deltoid injuries, and these patients had significantly worse outcomes compared to patients with similar-sized tears without deltoid injury.

Groh et al. (21) reported the results of 36 patients who lost deltoid function after open acromioplasty and rotator cuff repair (n = 20), shoulder arthroplasty (n = 9), revision shoulder arthroplasty (n = 3), open reduction with internal fixation (n = 1), and Bristow and Magnuson-Stack procedures (n = 3). In all, 33 patients suffered detachment of the deltoid from the origin, 3 patients had an axillary nerve injury, 20 patients had a deltoid-splitting approach, and 13 patients had a long deltopectoral approach. All patients were referred to the authors from other surgeons and no further surgery was performed. Function assessment of the patients revealed no excellent results, five good results, six fair results, and 25 poor results. All patients were dissatisfied with the previous surgery.

Sher et al. (22) evaluated 24 patients who underwent surgical treatment for postoperative deltoid origin disrup-

tion. The injury occurred during rotator cuff surgery in 12 patients, acromioplasty in four patients, and lateral acromionectomy in eight patients. Fifteen patients had isolated injury to the anterior deltoid, whereas nine patients had deficiencies of the middle and anterior deltoid. Four patients had direct repair of the deltoid defects and the remaining patients underwent a rotationplasty of the middle deltoid to the origin of the anterior deltoid (Fig. 3-1). After an average follow-up of 39 months, one patient had excellent results, seven had good results, and 16 had unsatisfactory results. Twelve patients had minimal pain, which correlated with the integrity of the deltoid repair. Eleven patients had a healed repair. A poor outcome was associated with prior lateral acromionectomy, middle deltoid injury, massive rotator cuff tear, and a deltoid defect larger than 2 cm after an attempted repair.

Splitting the deltoid beyond the level of the axillary nerve can cause anterior deltoid paralysis. The safe distance for a deltoid split is approximately 4 to 7 cm distal to the acromion (23). The surgeon may also use the distal extent of the subacromial bursa as a marker for the location of the axillary nerve.

Workup

Deltoid origin disruptions are easily seen as a defect at the acromion with a retracted mass distal to the acromion. This

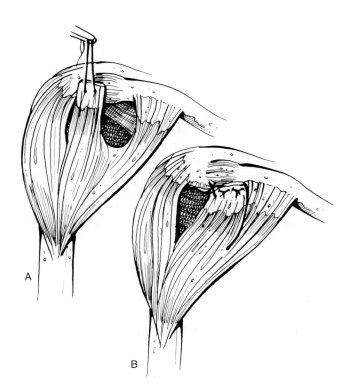

Figure 3-1 Line drawing representing a defect in the anterior deltoid. **A:** Portion of the middle deltoid is detached from the acromion and split in line with the muscle fibers without injuring the axillary nerve. **B:** The middle deltoid is then reattached medially with nonabsorbable sutures through the clavicle.

is best seen with active elevation of the arm-to-shoulder height. In patients with an abundance of subcutaneous fat, the defect is harder to see but can often be palpated. Some deltoid defects are isolated to the area surrounding the incision, which can occur secondary to excessive retraction against the deltoid. The most notable finding on the physical examination is the patient's weakness with forward elevation. When a deltoid injury is suspected, an MRI can confirm the diagnosis and even determine the cause. Assessment of the degree of fat atrophy in the teres minor would suggest an injury to the axillary nerve proximal to its trifurcation. The MRI can also show the degree of detachment from its origin. An electromyelogram (EMG) is the study of choice if an axillary nerve injury is suspected, which should be done at least 3 weeks after the injury. If complete transaction of the nerve is suspected by EMG, immediate repair is indicated. If the nerve remains intact, repeat EMG should be performed 2 months later to assess the amount of nerve regeneration. Reports of axillary nerve repairs after trauma indicate that delayed repair more than 5 months can decrease the success rate from 81% to 53% (24). There are no reports of surgical repair of axillary nerve injuries after rotator cuff repair.

Pearls

Chronic deltoid detachment larger than 4 cm, middle deltoid involvement, and association with a persistent rotator cuff tear of more than one tendon has not been amenable to soft tissue repair and, in the senior author's practice, is an unsolved problem. Smaller defects when found early should be repaired as soon as possible and if a persistent tear is noted than it should be rerepaired. Patients should be protected in an abduction brace for 4 to 6 weeks after surgery with limited passive range of motion exercise (pendulums only during the first 4 weeks).

Deltoid denervation involving a portion of the deltoid (injury of the intramuscular portion of the axillary nerve) is not a surgically correctable problem in most cases. Salvage surgery for a complete or near complete deltoid denervation in a young and active patient with an intact and functional rotator cuff can be treated with a bipolar latissimus dorsi transfer. The ideal indications for the complex surgery are very limited compared to the number of patients with deltoid denervation that occurs after open rotator cuff repair.

PERSISTENT SUBACROMIAL IMPINGEMENT

One cause of shoulder pain after rotator cuff repair is persistent subacromial spurs, which impinge on the rotator cuff during shoulder elevation and may lead to a retear in future. Many articles have documented the efficacy of subacromial decompression for the treatment of impingement syndrome and for the treatment of rotator cuff tears (25-27). Reports of rotator cuff repair failures have been attributed to incomplete subacromial decompression. Bigliani et al. (4) reported that 5 of 31 patients did not undergo appropriate acromioplasty during their initial rotator cuff repair, and the 27 other patients in the series underwent revision acromioplasty. In the review by Djurasovic et al. (17), 66% of the revisions underwent repeat acromioplasty either because of inadequate removal of bone or because of failure to address acromial morphology at all during the initial procedure.

Patients with persistent impingement will complain of pain with shoulder forward elevation and a Neer or Hawkins sign will be positive on physical exam. Subacromial injection of lidocaine (impingement test) will relieve the pain with active forward elevation, but a recurrent rotator cuff tear cannot be ruled out. Outlet views should be obtained to assess the acromial morphology. A positive impingement test can be positive with other causes of persistent shoulder pain other than boney impingement. Other causes include excessive scar tissue (captured cuff), biceps, or other intra-articular pathology when a full thickness cuff tear is present.

Some authors have questioned the benefit of subacromial decompression for the treatment of rotator cuff tears, given the risk of deltoid detachment and coracoacromial ligament resection. In a study of 27 rotator cuff repairs done without acromioplasty, Goldberg et al. (28) report an average improvement in the ability to perform 8 of 12 Simple Shoulder Test functions to the ability to perform 10 of 12 functions.

A recent study by Gartsman et al. (29) randomized subacromial decompression for the treatment of rotator cuff repairs in 93 patients. The age and preoperative ASES scores were similar in each group of patients. The tear size was 2.4 mm larger in the group that did not undergo subacromial decompression. Only patients with type II acromial morphology and with a full-thickness supraspinatus tear were included in the study. At an average follow-up of 2 years, the mean ASES score in the decompression group was 91.5 and in the group without decompression was 89.2, which were not statistically significant.

INFECTION

Infection complicating open rotator cuff repair is rare, but often leads to poor results because of irreversible damage to soft tissue, tendons, bone, and cartilage. The incidence of infection ranges from 0.27% to 1.9%. Prevention is the best treatment of this complication, which consists of optimizing preoperative risk factors for infection such as malnutrition, smoking cessation, avoiding elective procedures during active infection in other areas, shaving the skin the night before surgery, and high glucose levels in diabetics. Other factors that increase the risk of infection are immunodeficiency, hypothyroidism, prior exposure to radiation (such as in breast cancer survivors), and lymphedema, which can result from radical lymph node resection of the axilla. Chen et al. (30) reported a series of 30 type I diabetic patients with a matched control group who all underwent rotator cuff repair. The infection rate was 10% in the diabetic group and 0% in the control group.

Patients present with persistent shoulder pain, poorly controlled by narcotics, erythema, and wound drainage. Laboratory studies often reveal a normal white blood cell count and normal neutrophil percentage. The most reliably elevated studies are the erythrocyte sedimentation rate, which rises 2 days after the infection begins, and C-reactive protein, which rises hours after the start of the infection. Radiographs may show lesions in the bone if the infection is long-standing, but the most important finding on plain radiographs may be subcutaneous air resulting from anaerobic bacteria.

A review of 16 patients with infection complicating open rotator cuff repair was done by Settecerri et al. (31). Eight of the repairs were performed at their institution, which calculates to a complication rate of 0.27%. Only one patient had a preoperative risk factor for immunocompromise, which was seronegative rheumatoid arthritis. Ten patients did not receive preoperative antibiotics. The average time from the index procedure to presentation was 21.5 days. *Propionibacter* was isolated in seven patients, coagulase-negative *Staphylococcus* was isolated in five patients, *Staphylococcus aureus* in four patients, and *Peptostreptococcus magnus* in one patient. The number of debridements ranged from two to eight, and five rotator cuffs could not be repaired at the time of closure. Satisfactory results according to the patient or final UCLA scores were found in 5 of the 16 shoulders.

A study by Mirzayan et al. (32) reviewed the cases of 13 infected open rotator cuff repairs. Risk factors for infection included one patient with diabetes, one with immunoglobulin A deficiency, two with hypothyroidism, six smokers, two alcoholics, and two with prior mastectomies. Nine patients presented with a draining sinus, and the humeral head was exposed in three patients. The average sedimentation rate was 57 (range 6 to 135) and only one patient had a normal value. Culture results showed five *Staphylococcus aureus*, four *Staphylococcus epidermidis*, three *Propionibacterium*, one *Diptheroids*, and one coagulase-negative *Staphylococcus* infections. At the final 3-year follow-up, two patients had reflex-sympathetic dystrophy and two patients had persistent deltoid defects. Eight patients could sleep comfortably and perform activities below shoulder level.

Herrera et al. (33) reported the results of seven patients who developed postoperative infections after arthroscopy and mini-open rotator cuff repairs. *Propionibacter acnes* was isolated in six of seven cases. After irrigation and debridement of all cases, and revision repair in four cases, all patients had an ASES score of 95. Since the authors review of their infections, they routinely performed a second prep and drape between the arthroscopy and the mini-open procedures and have not encountered another infection. Although these authors advocate this procedure, the risk of infection for mini-open rotator cuff repair has not been reported to be any higher than that of standard open surgery and the need of a second prep and draping can not be substantiated. Given the many variables that could be associated with infection, the lack of a control group, and the small sample size in the Herrera study, the need for a second prep cannot be supported.

Pearls

Postoperative infections should be treated early with open debridement. When a persistent rotator cuff tear is present, the tear is not repaired until a second or subsequent debridement shows no evidence of infection after at least 1 week on intravenous (IV) antibiotic. When the persistent tear is repaired or a transfer is performed for an irreparable tear, the patient is kept on IV antibiotic for at least an additional 4 weeks with oral antibiotic for an additional 4 weeks. If a persistent rotator cuff tear is not seen at the time of the first debridement, then a second-look debridement is not required unless clinically indicated. For patients with an intact rotator cuff with an acute infection (less than 6 weeks), cuff debridement may be done with an arthroscopic technique, as long as mechanical debridement of the synovial tissue and subacromial space is accomplished. It is important in all cases to open the biceps tendon sheath distal to the groove to be sure that the purulent material is removed from this space. In chronic infections, arthroscopy can still be performed but dense adhesions may require a portion of the surgery in the subacromial space to be performed by open technique. Debridement of the subacromial space by either technique should remove all suture material, any visible or loose anchors, or any anchor that is surrounded by soft infected bone. Anchors not visible in dense bone are left in place as removal would likely create a very large defect in the humeral head or greater tuberosity.

HETEROTOPIC OSSIFICATION

Postoperative ossification of the shoulder was first reported by Smith in 1835. Since that time, many theories have been written to explain how heterotopic bone forms after shoulder surgery. Some believe trauma to the muscle causes calcification of the tissues, whereas others believe bone dust from acromioplasty and rotator cuff repairs incites the formation of heterotopic ossification (HO).

Berg et al. (34) reported a series of 40 patients who developed postoperative HO after acromioplasty and distal clavicle excision. Other concomitant surgeries included rotator cuff repair, Weaver-Dunn, Bankhart, and labral repair. The incidence of HO for the operating surgeon was 3.2% of all patients who underwent shoulder surgery. The authors did not find any correlation between the incidence of HO and the use of an osteotome, which generates little bone debris, or the use of a burr, which creates a lot of bone debris. Sixteen patients with acromial HO underwent surgical excision, one of which required a second excision procedure, and three others required a third surgical exision. In all, 60% of the patients in this series had chronic pulmonary disease, and the authors recommended prophylaxis for HO in these patients.

Erggelet et al. (35) reviewed a series of 131 patients with preoperative and postoperative radiographs who underwent open rotator cuff repairs and open acromioplasty. HO was found in 26.7% of cases, 28 after rotator cuff repair and seven after acromioplasty. A good to excellent result was found in 89% of the patients without HO and in 80% of those with HO. The duration and complexity of the procedure correlated with the existence of HO.

Treatment

Heterotopic ossification is excised when mature. Heterotopic bone is not removed for 1 year after the index surgery. This is followed by postoperative single dose of irradiation of 400 Gy within the first 24 hours after surgery.

POSTOPERATIVE STIFFNESS

Postoperative shoulder stiffness after rotator cuff repair causes significant pain in addition to the loss of shoulder motion (36). The spectrum of stiffness can range from an inability to internally rotate a few vertebral levels to the inability to move the arm away from the patient's belly. The first step of the physical exam starts with a comparison to the opposite arm for both active and passive motion. Generally, a difference between the active and passive motion on the same shoulder indicates a loss of muscle function secondary to a rotator cuff tear or deltoid dysfunction. If the patient's active motion is limited to the same extent as the passive motion, either soft tissue or bony lesions are inhibiting motion. Because an apparent loss of postoperative motion can be caused by pain that inhibits the patient from moving their shoulder completely, other causes of pain must be evaluated. This includes subacromial impingement, acromioclavicular (AC) joint pathology, biceps tendonopathy, and a persistent rotator cuff tear.

Postoperative stiffness secondary to capsular contracture follows a recognizable pattern. If the rotator interval is contracted, the patient will lose external rotation with the arm adducted at the side. Loss of internal rotation is caused by posterior capsule contracture. When the inferior capsule is contracted, the patient loses both abduction, forward elevation, and external rotation. Combinations of capsular contractions occur depending on the etiology of the stiffness. In most cases after rotator cuff repair, the loss of motion

is in all planes of motion and the scar that forms is within the capsule and in the subacromial subdeltoid space.

Workup

Postoperative stiffness should be worked up according to the findings on the physical exam. Plain radiographs should include an anteroposterior (AP) image of the shoulder to evaluate the joint surface, a supraspinatus outlet view to look for residual acromial spurs, and an axillary lateral view to look for an unrecognized os acromiale or iatrogenic acromial fracture. If a rotator cuff tear is suspected because of a difference between the patient's active and passive motion, an MRI with contrast should be obtained. In addition, EMG studies should be obtained if a nerve injury is suspected because of muscle atrophy or postoperative deltoid dysfunction.

Etiology

Loss of shoulder motion after rotator cuff surgery can be caused by a variety of lesions. A review of the literature reveals a prevalence rate of 21 out of 500 patients (4%) who develop stiffness postoperatively (37). Most commonly, the capsule stiffens and adheres to the surrounding tissues secondary to postoperative immobilization. Repairs should be secure enough to withstand passive elevation of the shoulder, even if they are immobilized in an abduction position using a brace or pillow. Assistance may be required depending on patient factors, but patients should perform passive or active-assisted range-of-motion exercises immediately postoperatively to avoid this complication. Risk factors such as diabetes and keloid scar formation, which are associated with idiopathic adhesive capsulitis, also increase a patient's risk of developing postoperative stiffness (30,38,39).

Adhesions between the rotator cuff and the deltoid can also cause postoperative stiffness. Mormino et al. (40) reported the results of 13 patients who developed restrictive subdeltoid adhesions after arthroscopic acromioplasty and open rotator cuff repair. The incidence of this complication was 4.8% of all rotator cuff repairs. Manipulation under anesthesia yielded little motion. Arthroscopic treatment included resection of the scarred subacromial bursa and glenohumeral joint inspection, which revealed a humeral articular lesion in every case. All rotator cuff repairs were intact at the second surgery. UCLA scores at 6-months follow-up increased from 14.8 to 30.1, and the forward flexion increased 17 degrees, the internal rotation increased 22 degrees, and the external rotation increased 21 degrees.

Inferior capsule contracture may also cause postoperative pain without a perceptible loss of motion by physical exam. Hata et al. (41) compared 22 patients who had no postoperative pain after rotator cuff surgery to a group of 28 patients who had residual pain and who did not have a retear, impingement, or acromioclavicular arthritis. Fluoroscopy exam revealed a 10-degree loss of forward elevation in the group with persistent pain, and intra-articular contrast exam revealed less inferior joint volume in the group with persistent pain.

Another common cause of shoulder stiffness is uncontrolled postoperative pain. Some patients experience significant pain after their surgery and any shoulder motion exacerbates that pain. This leads to capsular stiffness and scar formation in the normally mobile tissue planes. Once the stiffness sets in, the patient experiences more pain once they are instructed to work harder to break through the adhesions. A viscous cycle begins and pain management intervention may be necessary to break the cycle. Prevention is difficult because many surgeons are reluctant to increase their narcotic doses. A more common problem than shoulder stiffness caused by pain inhibition is prolonged narcotic use, which can sometimes lead to narcotic addiction. This reluctance to enable unnecessary narcotic use must be balanced with reasonable pain control in a small subgroup of patients who are predisposed to a low pain tolerance. Another confounding problem is reflex sympathetic dystrophy, which may also inhibit full participation in the postoperative rehabilitation program. In this case, the use of an indwelling cervical epidural catheter for 4 to 6 weeks can provide extraordinary pain relief while maintaining full motor function of the upper extremities, thereby allowing more aggressive and effective rehabilitation. The use of an epidural cervical catheter requires an experienced chronic pain management team for insertion, dosing, and monitoring of the catheter and medications to provide safe and effect pain relief.

Specific operative procedures can lead to loss of motion in specific planes. Repairs that include the subscapularis tendon can limit external rotation for two reasons. First, if the tendon is a chronic tear, the muscle-tendon unit will be contracted and shortened. Once it is repaired to its insertion site, the shoulder motion will be limited from the time of surgery. A second cause occurs postoperatively. During the healing process, scar formation can inhibit the normal gliding motion between the capsule, rotator cuff, and the subacromial bursa. The postoperative immobilization can also play a role if the surgeon limits external rotation to protect the repair. In some cases where the repaired tissue is not strong, a balance must be made between ensuring strong tendon fixation through immobilization and maximizing shoulder motion through early mobilization.

Results of Stiffness Treatment

Gerber et al. (38) treated 45 stiff shoulders with arthroscopic capsulotomy, 21 of which were secondary to operative procedures. After a minimum of 12 months, the Constant-Murley score improved from 41% to 75%. Patients with idiopathic stiffness had better scores than patients with postoperative stiffness, and the worst scores were found in patients with posttraumatic stiffness. In the post-

operative group, three patients lost an average 18 degrees of forward elevation and four patients substantially decreased their participation in sports activities. The only common finding is this group was the loss of internal rotation. Flexion improved by 30 degrees and external rotation improved by 25 degrees.

Holloway et al. (42) studied the results of arthroscopic capsular release for treatment of postoperative stiffness that was refractory to postoperative rehabilitation. In a group of 50 cases, 33 were treated for stiffness after rotator cuff repair. In these cases, both a capsular release and debridement of scar in the subacromial space was equally effective in restoring passive and active range of motion (average change of 26 degrees of forward flexion), but was less effective than treatment of idiopathic frozen shoulder in relief of preoperative shoulder pain.

Pearls

Surgical management for postoperative stiffness after rotator cuff surgery should not be considered before 6 months after the procedure. Between 6 and 12 months after surgery, further surgical intervention can be considered when there has been at least 3 months of home-based daily and weekly supervised physical therapy for aggressive stretches without any significant improvement in passive arcs of motion in any plane. So long as there is objective evidence of progress, surgical intervention for treatment of postoperative stiffness should be delayed for 1 year after the index procedure. When an arthroscopic release is performed, it requires complete 360-degree release of the capsule; it is this author's preference to resect about 5 to 7 mm of the capsule at the site of the capsular release. Removal of all subacromial and subcoracoid scar with complete release and resection of the scarred and shortened coracohumeral ligament is as important as the capsular release. If a persistent rotator cuff tear larger than 2 cm is seen at the time of the capsular release, it is not repaired at that time as it will not likely heal given the nature of the postoperative rehabilitation that is required to maintain passive arcs of motion. Postoperative pain management is critical to clinical success, along with a daily home-based passive range-of-motion exercise program. The authors preferred postoperative pain management includes the use of an indwelling cervical epidural catheter for 4 weeks. This catheter is placed and maintained by the anesthesia pain management group.

PERSISTENT OS ACROMIALE AND ACROMIAL FRACTURE

Acromial fracture after arthroscopic or open acromioplasty is an infrequent complication. In a small case series of six patients reported by Matthews et al. (42a), most patients had sudden onset of pain during physical therapy. The diagnosis was delayed until an axillary radiograph revealed the pathology and the patient's disability varied from mild pain to severe functional impairment. Treatment ranged from conservative measures to total acromionectomy. Risk factors cited by the authors included osteopenia and overzealous bone resection.

An asymptomatic os acromiale may become a symptomatic lesion after an acromioplasty because the stable fibrous tissue is destabilized. Axillary radiographs should be obtained before acromioplasty to insure that a postoperative acromial fracture is not simply a destabilized os acromiale. In a study by Lee et al. (43), the double-density sign found on anteroposterior radiographs was seen in 82.4% of shoulders that had an os acromiale, compared to the axillary lateral radiograph, which revealed an os acromiale on 95.6% of the radiographs. The double-density sign is produced by the overlap of two transversely elongated radiographic cortical densities. One density represents the os acromiale fragment, and the second density represents the anterior cortical margin of the remaining acromial process. MRI scans will also show the lesion, and it is best seen on the transverse images through the acromion.

Warner et al. (44) reported their results of 11 patients treated with tension band fixation and screw fixation with autogenous iliac-crest bone graft. In all, 58% of patients achieved union at an average 9 weeks. Five of seven successful unions required hardware removal for persistent pain. Four patients with tension band fixation alone failed and required screw fixation to achieve union.

Hertel et al. (45) treated 15 symptomatic os acromiale with tension-band techniques through both an anterior deltoid-off approach and a transacromial approach, which protected the anterior blood supply to the acromion. Three of seven treated with the deltoid-off approach healed, whereas seven of eight through the deltoid preserving approach achieved union.

Peckett et al. (46) reported the results of internal fixation of 26 symptomatic os acromiales. One patient in the series had a previous acromioplasty without relief of symptoms, whereas the others failed conservative treatment alone. Open reduction, bone grafting, and fixation with screws, wires, or combination of the two was performed on all patients. The anterior blood supply was protected during the surgery. At 1-year follow-up, 96% of patients had clinical and radiographic union, and 92% of patients were satisfied with the procedure. Eight patients underwent removal of the hardware for persistent discomfort.

Wright et al. (47) reported the results of arthroscopic resection of 13 symptomatic os acromiales that did not respond to conservative management. Four shoulders had partial thickness rotator cuff tears treated with concomitant debridement, and one shoulder had a partial thickness tear treated with mini-open rotator cuff repair. The UCLA scores improved from 17 to 31 after 12 months follow-up. Five patients had excellent results, six patients had good results, and two patients had unsatisfactory results. There were no deltoid detachments in any patients. The authors recommended arthroscopic excision because of the poor results

reported in the literature after open resection or open fixation of the os acromiale. If excision is performed, it is important that the cuff is functionally intact with a centered humeral head and that the delto-trapezius in kept intact to avoid compromise in the deltoid attachment.

ANTERIOR SUPERIOR HUMERAL HEAD SUBLUXATION

Anterior superior humeral head subluxation, or superior escape of the humeral head, is a consequence of a massive rotator cuff tear and insufficiency of the coracoacromial arch. In the postoperative setting, the coracoacromial arch may have been disrupted secondary to overaggressive acromionectomy or complete excision of the coracoacromial ligament during the open procedure. Patients often complain of pain along with the inability to elevate their arm because they have lost the functional fulcrum necessary for the deltoid to elevate the arm. The humeral head subluxes anteriorly when the deltoid fires, revealing an obvious arch defect, and often the anterior deltoid is thinned secondary to the chronic pathology (Fig. 3-2).

Treatment options for this difficult problem are based on the anatomical defects associated with the superior escape. The extent of the rotator cuff defect must be assessed by MRI or prior operative visual examination. If the primary defect in the rotator cuff is the subscapularis, then a pectoralis major transfer may keep the head centered during active shoulder elevation. This soft tissue procedure is predicated on the force couple mechanism of the rotator cuff that keeps the head centered in the glenoid. Restoring the anterior couple with the pectoralis major will keep the head centered during active elevation only if the posterior couple, namely the

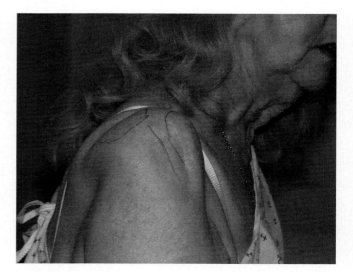

Figure 3-2 This patient has superior escape of the humeral head out of the coracoacromial arch. This abnormality can be seen more easily while the patient attempts to actively elevate the arm from 0 to 45 degrees.

infraspinatus and teres minor, is also intact. If the external rotators are not functional, then a pectoralis major transfer alone is not indicated. For patients who have a rupture of both the external and internal rotators, then a combined muscle transfer is indicated. Both the latissimus dorsi transfer in combination with the pectoralis major transfer will act to center the humeral head during active shoulder elevation, thus eliminating superior escape (48–50).

Galatz et al. (51) described their results of pectoralis major transfer alone in a heterogeneous population with superior escape. The patients had undergone a mean of 2.3 prior surgical procedures, including three total shoulders, one revision total shoulder, six rotator cuff repairs, two debridements for infection, and three hemiarthroplasties. After 17 months of follow-up, the ASES score improved from 27 to 48 and the mean active elevation improved from 28 degrees to 60 degrees. Seven patients had a contained head at final follow-up, whereas six patients had intermediate instability and one patient had complete instability.

Reconstruction of the coracoacromial ligament has been reported by Flatow et al. (52) in six patients who had multiple prior surgeries, including hemiarthroplasty in three patients and coracoacromial ligament excision in all six cases. The ligament was reconstructed with an autologous fascia lata graft, and three patients underwent concomitant latissimus dorsi muscle transfer. Only two patients were satisfied with their reconstruction and the average active and passive ranges of motion were unchanged. Wiley (53) reported four cases of superior humeral dislocation. Two occurred after hemiarthroplasty and two occurred following debridement of the subacromial bursa to treat an irreparable rotator cuff tear. The two hemiarthroplasty cases were treated with reconstruction of the coracacromial arch with bone graft, which prevented further superior dislocation; however, forward elevation was severely limited. Based on these anecdotal reports and our clinical experience, we do not recommend reconstruction of the coracoacromial arch.

In patients who are not candidates for muscle transfers because of their age, reverse total shoulder prostheses may be used to restore active shoulder elevation (54,55). This prosthesis restores the fulcrum between the humerus and glenoid, thus allowing the deltoid to elevate the arm. The long-term failure rate is unknown and the complication rate remains higher than traditional total shoulder arthroplasty. The most common complications include instability, acromion fracture, and glenoid notching.

For patients who cannot undergo muscle transfer and are too young to have a reverse total shoulder prosthesis, arthrodesis of the shoulder may be the only other option. This procedure sacrifices motion for pain relief and improved strength.

REFERENCES

1. Harryman DT II, Mack LA, Wang KY, et al. Repairs of the rotator cuff. Correlation of functional results with integrity of the cuff. *J Bone Joint Surg Am* 1991;73:982–989.
2. Jost B, Pfirrmann CW, Gerber C, et al. Clinical outcome after structural failure of rotator cuff repairs. *J Bone Joint Surg Am* 2000;82:304–314.
3. Galatz LM, Ball CM, Teefey SA, et al. The outcome and repair integrity of completely arthroscopically repaired large and massive rotator cuff tears. *J Bone Joint Surg Am* 2004;86:219–224.
4. Bigliani LU, Cordasco FA, McIlveen SJ, et al. Operative treatment of failed repairs of the rotator cuff. *J Bone Joint Surg Am* 1992;74:1505–1515.
5. DeOrio JK, Cofield RH. Results of a second attempt at surgical repair of a failed initial rotator-cuff repair. *J Bone Joint Surg Am* 1984;66:563–567.
6. Davidson PA, Rivenburgh DW. Rotator cuff repair tension as a determinant of functional outcome. *J Shoulder Elb Surg* 2000;9:502–506.
7. Gerber C, Schneeberger AG, Perren SM, et al. Experimental rotator cuff repair. A preliminary study. *J Bone Joint Surg Am* 1999;81:1281–1290.
8. Gerber C, Fuchs B, Hodler J. The results of repair of massive tears of the rotator cuff. *J Bone Joint Surg Am* 2000;82:505–515.
9. Cummins CA, Murrell GA. Mode of failure for rotator cuff repair with suture anchors identified at revision surgery. *J Shoulder Elb Surg* 2003;12:128–133.
10. Hertel R, Ballmer FT, Lombert SM, et al. Lag signs in the diagnosis of rotator cuff rupture. *J Shoulder Elb Surg* 1996;5:307–313.
11. Burkhart SS, Tehrany AM. Arthroscopic subscapularis tendon repair: Technique and preliminary results. *Arthroscopy* 2002;18:454–463.
12. Pearsall AW IV, Bonsell S, Heitman RJ, et al. Radiographic findings associated with symptomatic rotator cuff tears. *J Shoulder Elb Surg* 2003;12:122–127.
13. Prickett WD, Teefey SA, Galatz LM, et al. Accuracy of ultrasound imaging of the rotator cuff in shoulders that are painful postoperatively. *J Bone Joint Surg Am* 2003;85:1084–1089.
14. Teefey SA, Hasan SA, Middleton WD, et al. Ultrasonography of the rotator cuff. A comparison of ultrasonographic and arthroscopic findings in one hundred consecutive cases. *J Bone Joint Surg Am* 2000;82:498–504.
15. Gaenslen ES, Satterlee CC, Hinson GW. Magnetic resonance imaging for evaluation of failed repairs of the rotator cuff. *J Bone Joint Surg Am* 1996;78:1391–1396.
16. Neviaser RJ, Neviaser TJ. Reoperation for failed rotator cuff repair: analysis of fifty cases. *J Shoulder Elb Surg* 1992;2:283–286.
17. Djurasovic M, Marra G, Arroyo JS, et al. Revision rotator cuff repair: factors influencing results. *J Bone Joint Surg Am* 2001;83:1849–1855.
18. Lo IK, Burkhart SS. Arthroscopic revision of failed rotator cuff repairs: technique and results. *Arthroscopy* 2004;20:250–267.
19. Neer CS II, Marberry TA. On the disadvantages of radical acromionectomy. *J Bone Joint Surg Am* 1981;63:416–419.
20. Bosley RC. Total acromionectomy. A twenty-year review. *J Bone Joint Surg Am* 1991;73:961–968.
21. Groh G, Simoni M, Rolla P, et al. Loss of the deltoid after shoulder operations: an operative disaster. *J Shoulder Elbow Surg* 1994;3:243–253.
22. Sher JS, Iannotti JP, Warner JJ, et al. Surgical treatment of postoperative deltoid origin disruption. *Clin Orthop* 1997;343:93–98.
23. Burkhead WZ, Scheinberg, RR, Box G. Surgical anatomy of the axillary nerve. *JSES* 1992;1:31–36.
24. Bonnard C, Anastakis DJ, van Melle G, et al. Isolated and combined lesions of the axillary nerve. A review of 146 cases. *J Bone Joint Surg Br* 1999;81:212–217.
25. Neer CS II. Anterior acromioplasty for the chronic impingement syndrome in the shoulder: a preliminary report. *J Bone Joint Surg Am* 1972;54:41–50.
26. Galatz LM, Griggs S, Cameron BD, et al. Prospective longitudinal analysis of postoperative shoulder function: a ten-year follow-up study of full-thickness rotator cuff tears. *J Bone Joint Surg Am* 2001;83:1052–1056.
27. McKee MD, Yoo DJ. The effect of surgery for rotator cuff disease on general health status. Results of a prospective trial. *J Bone Joint Surg Am* 2000;82:970–979.

28. Goldberg BA, Lippitt SB, Matsen FA III. Improvement in comfort and function after cuff repair without acromioplasty. *Clin Orthop Relat Res* 2001;390:142–150.

29. Gartsman GM, O'Connor DP. Arthroscopic rotator cuff repair with and without arthroscopic subacromial decompression: a prospective, randomized study of one-year outcomes. *J Shoulder Elb Surg* 2004;13:424–426.

30. Chen AL, Shapiro JA, Ahn AK, et al. Rotator cuff repair in patients with type I diabetes mellitus. *J Shoulder Elb Surg* 2003;12:416–421.

31. Settecerri JJ, Pitner MA, Rock MG, et al. Infection after rotator cuff repair. *J Shoulder Elb Surg* 1999;8:1–5.

32. Mirzayan R, Itamura JM, Vangsness CT Jr, et al. Management of chronic deep infection following rotator cuff repair. *J Bone Joint Surg Am* 2000;82:1115–1121.

33. Herrera MF, Bauer G, Reynolds F, et al. Infection after mini-open rotator cuff repair. *J Shoulder Elb Surg* 2002;11:605–608.

34. Berg EE, Ciullo JV. Heterotopic ossification after acromioplasty and distal clavicle resection. *J Shoulder Elb Surg* 1995;4:188–193.

35. Erggelet C, Eggensperger G, Steinwachs M, et al. Postoperative ossifications of the shoulder. Incidence and clinical impact. *Arch Orthop Trauma Surg* 1999;119:168–170.

36. Warner JJ, Greis PE. The treatment of stiffness of the shoulder after repair of the rotator cuff. *Instr Course Lect* 1998;47:67–75.

37. Nagels J, Valstar ER, Stokdijk M, et al. Patterns of loosening of the glenoid component. *J Bone Joint Surg Br* 2002;84:83–87.

38. Gerber C, Espinosa N, Perren TG. Arthroscopic treatment of shoulder stiffness. *Clin Orthop Relat Res* 2001;390:119–128.

39. Ide J, Takagi K. Early and long-term results of arthroscopic treatment for shoulder stiffness. *J Shoulder Elb Surg* 2004;13:174–179.

40. Mormino MA, Gross RM, McCarthy JA. Captured shoulder: a complication of rotator cuff surgery. *Arthroscopy* 1996;12:457–461.

41. Hata Y, Saitoh S, Murakami N, et al. Shrinkage in the inferior pouch of the scapulohumeral joint is related to postoperative pain after rotator cuff repair: radiographic and arthrographic comparison between patients with postoperative pain and those without it. *J Shoulder Elbow Surg* 2001;10:333–339.

42. Holloway GB, Schenk T, Williams GR, et al. Arthroscopic capsular release for the treatment of refractory postoperative or post-fracture shoulder stiffness. *J Bone Joint Surg Am* 2001;83:1682–1687.

42a. Matthews LS, Burkhead WZ, Gordon S, et al. Acromial fracture: a complication of arthroscopic subacrimal decompression. *J Shoulder and Elbow* 1994;3:256–261.

43. Lee DH, Lee KH, Lopez-Ben R, et al. The double-density sign: a radiographic finding suggestive of an os acromiale. *J Bone Joint Surg Am* 2004;86:2666–2670.

44. Warner JJ, Beim GM, Higgins L. The treatment of symptomatic os acromiale. *J Bone Joint Surg Am* 1998;80:1320–1326.

45. Hertel R, Windisch W, Schuster A, et al. Transacromial approach to obtain fusion of unstable os acromiale. *J Shoulder Elbow Surg* 1998;7:606–609.

46. Peckett WR, Gunther SB, Harper GD, Hughes JS, Sonnabend DH. Internal fixation of symptomatic os acromiale: a series of twenty-six cases. *J Shoulder Elbow Surg* 2004;13:381–385.

47. Wright RW, Heller MA, Quick DC, et al. Arthroscopic decompression for impingement syndrome secondary to an unstable os acromiale. *Arthroscopy* 2000;16:595–599.

48. Warner JJ, Parsons IM IV. Latissimus dorsi tendon transfer: a comparative analysis of primary and salvage reconstruction of massive, irreparable rotator cuff tears. *J Shoulder Elbow Surg* 2001;10:514–521.

49. Aoki M, Okamura K, Fukushima S, et al. Transfer of latissimus dorsi for irreparable rotator-cuff tears. *J Bone Joint Surg Br* 1996;78:761–766.

50. Warner JJ, Parsons IM IV. Latissimus dorsi tendon transfer: a comparative analysis of primary and salvage reconstruction of massive, irreparable rotator cuff tears. *J Shoulder Elbow Surg* 2001;10:514–521.

51. Galatz LM, Connor PM, Calfee RP, et al. Pectoralis major transfer for anterior-superior subluxation in massive rotator cuff insufficiency. *J Shoulder Elbow Surg* 2003;12:1–5.

52. Flatow EL, Connor PM, Levine WN, et al. Coracoacromial arch reconstruction for anterosuperior subluxation after failed rotator cuff surgery: A preliminary report. *J Shoulder Elbow Surg* 1997;6:228.

53. Wiley A. Superior humeral dislocation. A complication following decompression and debridement for rotator cuff tears. *Clin Orthop* 1991;263:135–141.

54. Sirveaux F, Favard L, Oudet D, et al. Grammont inverted total shoulder arthroplasty in the treatment of glenohumeral osteoarthritis with massive rupture of the cuff. Results of a multicentre study of 80 shoulders. *J Bone Joint Surg Br* 2004;86:388–395.

55. Rittmeister M, Kerschbaumer F. Grammont reverse total shoulder arthroplasty in patients with rheumatoid arthritis and nonreconstructible rotator cuff lesions. *J Shoulder Elbow Surg* 2001;10:17–22.

Complications of Total Shoulder Arthroplasty

George F. Hatch, III   *John G. Costouros*
Peter J. Millett   *Jon J.P. Warner*

INTRODUCTION

Shoulder arthroplasty is a widely accepted procedure for the treatment of arthritis, fracture, nonunion, malunion, tumor, and rotator cuff arthropathy. More than 20,000 shoulder arthroplasty surgeries were performed annually in the United States in 2000 and 2001 (1). Since 1998, the total number of shoulder arthroplasties has increased by 43%. In 2003, the total number increased to approximately 25,000 shoulder arthroplasties (16,840 hemiarthroplasties and 8,150 total arthroplasties) in the United States (2). Despite these numbers, surgeons doing only one to two shoulder replacements a year perform approximately 85% of the procedures (1,2). A recent study by Jain et al. (3) reported that complications and poor outcomes of both total and hemishoulder arthroplasty were inversely proportional to the shoulder arthroplasty volume of the surgeon and the institution. As expected, surgeons and centers that had higher volumes had lower complication rates. Therefore, it is conceivable that the number of complications and the need for possible revision surgery may increase as the number of shoulder arthroplasties increases.

Accurately defining the complication rate for either total or hemishoulder arthroplasty is very difficult due to the heterogeneous populations of patients and the differences in implants used, methods of fixation, and reporting. Several authors have pooled together multiple series and have estimated complication rates for total shoulder arthroplasty (TSA) ranging from 0% to 62%. The overall mean complication rate appears to be somewhere between 8% to 16% for total shoulder arthroplasty (4–6). Godeneche et al. (4) recently reported on a homogenous series of 268 anatomically designed shoulder arthroplasties implanted for primary arthritis only, with a mean follow-up of 30 months. The authors reported an overall complication rate of 8.6%, with a 4.9% of all shoulders needing revision surgery (4).

Although the exact incidence of complications can vary depending on the initial diagnosis, several types of complications can occur with any shoulder arthroplasty. This chapter will review the most commonly seen complications with shoulder arthroplasty such as prosthetic loosening, glenohumeral instability, rotator cuff tears, periprosthetic fracture, infection, implant failure or dissociation, deltoid dysfunction, and neurovascular injury. The chapter will also provide the authors' opinions regarding decision-making in the face of complications and approach to revision surgery.

PROSTHETIC LOOSENING

Component loosening is caused by multiple factors, often in combination. Although the shoulder joint is a typically nonweight-bearing joint, high loads can still be placed across it. For example, with the arm abducted to 90 degrees during active elevation, the load transmitted across the glenohumeral joint is approximately 90% of body weight (1). An ideal prosthetic reconstruction should minimize the risks of component wear and loosening by anatomically reconstructing the native glenohumeral geometry (Fig. 4-1). If the shoulder joint's original center of rotation is restored, then normal kinematics and joint reactive forces are permitted, forces across the implants are minimized, and the soft tissues can perform optimally. Factors that adversely affect joint mechanics, such as component malpositioning, will alter joint function and contact stresses across the articular surface and predispose the implant to loosening.

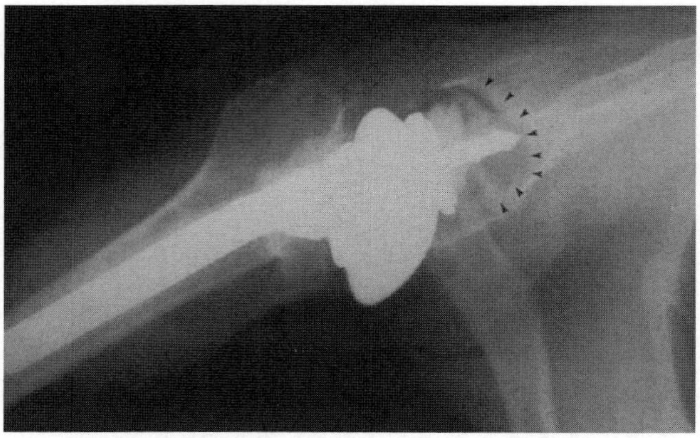

Figure 4-2 Radiograph of glenoid loosening.

GLENOID COMPONENT LOOSENING

Glenoid component loosening, which is a common indication for revision surgery, occurs in approximately 2% of patients with total shoulder arthroplasty (7–16). Glenoid loosening is a multifactor process that can be associated with component malposition, rotator cuff tears, stiffness, infection, and instability (7,17–19).

One of the main concerns with regard to glenoid loosening is the frequency of radiolucent lines around the glenoid component at follow-up (Fig. 4-2). Analysis of the literature shows a radiolucency rate ranging from 30% to greater than 90% (4,20–23). In a review of 20 reported series of total shoulder arthroplasty, 38.6% of all shoulder arthroplasties had glenoid lucent lines at an average follow-up of 5 years (24). Among those shoulders with periprosthetic lucency, revision surgery was performed in only 7.7%.

Although radiolucent lines around the glenoid are com-

mon (30% to 96%), there is currently no direct evidence linking immediate radiolucent lines and clinical loosening (25,26). Reports from the Mayo Clinic have found the probability of implant survival to be 93% at 10 years and 87% at 15 years (27). At final follow-up, 79% of glenoid components developed bone-cement radiolucencies and 44% were considered to have radiographic evidence of definite glenoid loosening. The authors found a statistically significant association between loosening and increase in pain ($p = 0.0001$) (27). However, although the radiographic frequency of glenoid loosening was high, clinical need for revision remained low.

Glenoid loosening that is symptomatic enough to require revision surgery is uncommon, but technically challenging. Therefore, all attempts to reduce the incidence of component loosening should be made. The surgeon has little control over the bone quality of the individual. Due to the limited amount of bone in the glenoid, every attempt

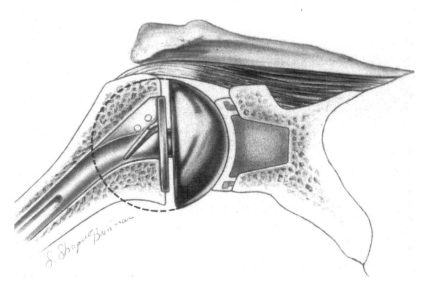

Figure 4-1 Restoration of native glenohumeral geometry.

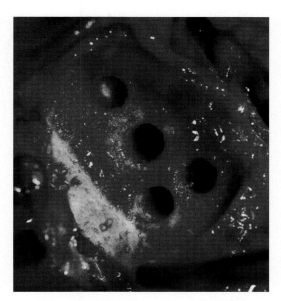

Figure 4-3 Intraoperative photograph of a concentrically reamed glenoid.

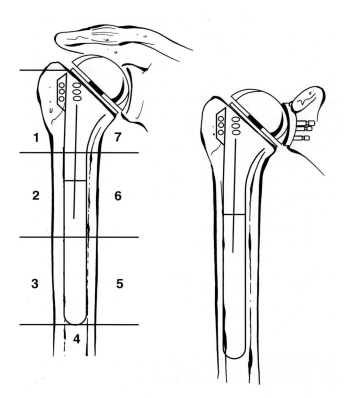

Figure 4-4 Radiograph of humeral prosthesis loosening.

should be made to preserve as much bone as possible for implant insertion. Preparation of the glenoid requires precision and meticulous attention to detail to preserve the subchondral bone while removing only enough bone to allow proper implant insertion and seating. Concentric glenoid reaming is also necessary to reduce displacement and deformation of the glenoid component (Fig. 4-3) (28). Further preparation includes pulsatile water lavage, thorough drying of glenoid bone, with or without the use of thrombin soaked gelfoam, using a vacuum system or centrifugation while mixing the bone cement to diminish porosity, pressurization of bone cement, impaction of the component into position, and maintaining stability of the component against the bone until the cement completely hardens.

HUMERAL COMPONENT LOOSENING

Although the majority of complications related to aseptic loosening in total shoulder arthroplasty appear to be attributed to difficulties with glenoid fixation, in short- and mid-term follow-up studies radiographic evaluations reveal a 5% incidence of implant subsidence or complete radiolucent lines measuring ≥2 mm about the humeral prosthesis (Fig. 4-4) (6,26,29–32). Uncemented humeral components, as opposed to cemented humeral components, are more frequently associated with complete radiolucent lines, but clinical loosening accounted for symptoms in fewer than 2% of patients (21,22,26,29–31,33).

Cofield and colleagues (5,27) reported a 17% incidence of radiolucent line lines (≥1.5 mm) surrounding press-fit humeral head components placed for osteoarthritis. In patients with rheumatoid arthritis, 9% of the press-fit humeral components demonstrated lucent lines of ≥1.5 mm surrounding the humeral stem, with 28% of components demonstrating subsidence down the humeral canal.

Interestingly, the Mayo study (27) demonstrated no clear association between the development of symptoms and the radiographic appearance of the humeral component. The authors point out that the frequency of radiographic changes surrounding the press-fit, smooth Neer components was quite high and recommended that fixation with bone-cement be used with this type of implant.

It is apparent that press-fitting the typical designs of humeral components that do not have surface texturing or surface in-growth capabilities is not advisable. These components are generally designed for use with bone cement and therefore this is the preferred method of fixation. Although loosening of a cemented humeral component is exceedingly rare, cemented humeral components can be difficult to remove should revision surgery be necessary. Therefore, in an attempt to address this issue, new generation press-fit designs have texturing or in-growth capabilities.

IMPLANT WEAR

The correlation between osteolysis and polyethylene debris, with macrophage-induced destruction of periprosthetic bone, has been well documented in arthoplasty literature (34). Wirth et al. (35) have described both the size and shapes of polyethylene wear debris, associated with osteolysis and recovered from failed total shoulder arthroplasty. When compared with particulate wear debris specimens from total hip revisions, polyethylene debris from total shoulder arthroplasty specimens are less round and more fibrillar (35).

Recently, Gunther and colleagues (36) described a new classification system for wear analysis of glenoid components. The authors describe evidence of both surface wear and fatigue failure in retrieved glenoid components. Surface wear was noted on low-power magnification as scratching, burnishing, and abrasion, whereas fatigue failure produced component pitting, delamination, and fracture. This study demonstrates how shoulder implants can develop both surface wear and fatigue failure. These findings differ from hip and knee implants, where the modes of failure are typically wear and fatigue failure, respectively (1).

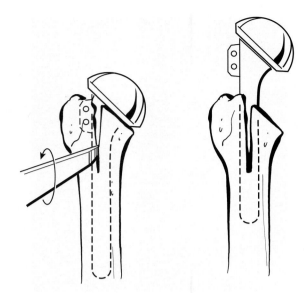

Figure 4-5 Osteotomy of humeral shaft.

AUTHORS' SURGICAL TECHNIQUE FOR COMPONENT LOOSENING

Removal of well-fixed components can be challenging and technically difficult. The need for careful preoperative planning in revision TSA surgery cannot be overstressed. Prior to entering the operating room, all attempts should be made to have complete knowledge of the previous procedure including component type/brand, fixation used, in addition to all previous incisions and complications. Bone and cement removal for humeral component revision surgery requires the immediate availability of high-speed, low-torque motorized drills, multiple osteotomes of different sizes and shape, ultrasonic removal equipment, and intraoperative fluoroscopy.

Although removal of a loose humeral stem can be quite easy with minimal damage to the humerus, extracting a well-fixed cemented or biologically in-grown prosthesis can be extremely difficult without great damage to the humeral shaft. Porous-coated stems, specifically ones where the coating extends distally, can be the most challenging of all cases. Specifically designed stem extraction devices can be of great help when removing humeral prostheses. Slap hammers and extraction devices allow the force to be applied parallel the humeral shaft, thereby decreasing the risk of humeral fracture. If the humeral stem cannot be easily removed, then a controlled osteotomy is preferred to avoid an uncontrolled iatrogenic fracture of the humerus. This is accomplished by a longitudinal anterior osteotomy just lateral to the bicipital groove of the humeral shaft, which extends approximately three-quarters of the length of the stem (Fig. 4-5) (37). Care is taken to preserve a laterally based soft-tissue hinge, which will facilitate proper closure

of the osteotomy site and healing. This technique can be used for both well-fixed cemented or porous in-growth humeral stems. By slotting only the proximal aspect of the humerus, the risk of radial nerve injury can be minimized. This is due to the fact that the majority of standard-length stems lie above the spiral groove of the humerus. After the cemented stem has been removed, we either recement within the existing mantle (nonseptic failure) or remove all remnants of the cement mantle, including the cement restrictor if possible. An ultrasonic cement removal device operated under fluoroscopic guidance can be helpful. All attempts are then made to remove loose particles by pulsatile lavage and suction, followed by meticulous hemostasis. After complete preparation of the humerus, the osteotomy is secured by using multiple cerclage sutures or wires.

Prior to injecting cement, hand reaming is used to prepare the humeral canal to avoid the risk of shaft fracture. We have had two cases of radial nerve palsies during revision surgeries involving a well-fixed humeral prosthesis. One case occurred secondary to cement extrusion, and the other resulted from humeral shaft fracture during placement of the new humeral implant. For these reasons we feel intraoperative fluoroscopy is critical for evaluation of the integrity of the humeral shaft during cement removal and new prosthesis placement. If we still have doubt regarding the integrity of the shaft after fluoroscopic evaluation, we will inject saline mixed with radio-opaque dye down the shaft and look for extrusion under fluoroscopy.

Based on the quality of the remaining bone in the proximal humerus, a long-stem prosthesis is often used in revision cases. In the case of bone deficiencies, cancellous bone-grafting is used in the proximal metaphysis, and allograft fibular struts secured with cerclage wires are used to

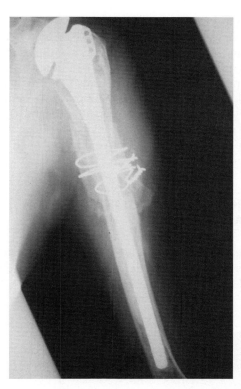

Figure 4-6 Radiograph of humeral prosthesis revision procedures with long-stem component, allograft struts, and cerclage wires.

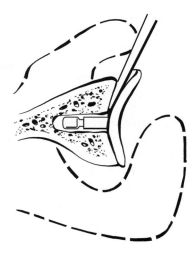

Figure 4-7 Illustration of cutting the glenoid component with an osteotome.

location and severity (Fig. 4-8) (7). The classification system and recommendations by Antuna et al. (7) give useful guidelines for surgical decision making when dealing with glenoid bone deficiencies. In cases where there are mild to moderate central or peripheral glenoid bone deficiencies,

re-enforce the fixation distally (Fig. 4-6). During placement of the new humeral prosthesis, low-viscosity cement is inserted to avoid excessive canal pressurization.

Access to the glenoid, in the presence of a well-fixed humeral component, can be a difficult situation. In cases where the well-fixed humeral stem is not modular, the techniques described earlier must often be used to gain adequate access to the glenoid component. However, in cases where a modular humeral prosthesis does not need to be revised, removal of the head alone allows for inspection of the glenoid. Here adequate soft-tissue release is the key to allowing optimal glenoid visualization while minimizing the risk of fracturing the humeral proximal metaphysis and/ or humeral shaft.

Often, a loose glenoid implant can easily be extracted from the glenoid vault without much difficulty. When a well-fixed glenoid component needs to be revised, a sharp-curved osteomes can be used to cut the articulating component away from the underlying pegs or keel (Fig. 4-7) (38). Once the articulating surface of the glenoid implant has been detached and removed, small-curved curettes, thin-curved osteomes, and/or a high-speed drill are used to address the remaining pieces. Glenoid bone loss after removal of the glenoid component is not uncommon, but every effort should be made to preserve the underlying bone-stock during component and cement removal.

Glenoid bone loss has been categorized on the basis of

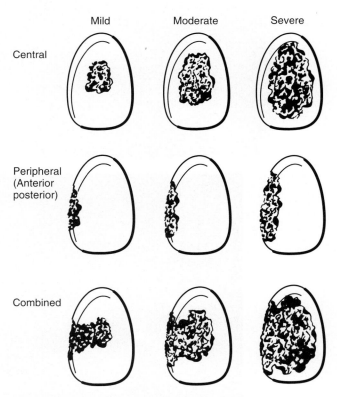

Figure 4-8 Classification of glenoid bone deficiencies after glenoid component removal. Mild and moderate deficiencies are often suitable for component reimplantation with or without bone grafting of glenoid. Severe central or combined deficiencies often preclude implantation of new component.

primary replacement of a new glenoid component, with or without bone-grafting, is often done. However, when severe central or combined deficiencies exist, implantation of a new component may not be possible. In these cases, staged grafting procedures are used by placing cancellous autograft and/or allograft into glenoid bone defects (Fig. 4-9). Therefore, a hemiarthoplasty is performed without placing a glenoid component. After graft consolidation is evident by radiographs, typically in 6 to 12 weeks, a new glenoid component can be placed. In some cases, immediate solid fixation possible primary glenoid reconstruction can be accomplished, without the need for a staged procedure (Fig. 4-10).

Extreme care is needed when preparing the glenoid vault, and every effort should be made to protect the glenoid cavity wall from penetration. Palpation with the index finger of the opposite hand on the anterior aspect of the scapular neck can give the surgeon a better idea with regard to glenoid orientation and cavity thickness (Fig. 4-11). The glenoid cancellous bed is then cleaned of debris with pulse lavage and careful drying prior to cement insertion. A syringe is used to insert the cement in a liquid state and to obtain pressurization. Cement is also directly applied to the back of the glenoid component prior to insertion. The glenoid component is then inserted and lightly impacted into the glenoid canal. Manual thumb pressure is then used to compress the implant in place until polymerization of the cement is complete.

GLENOHUMERAL COMPONENT INSTABILITY

Instability following shoulder arthroplasty is a relatively common and potentially devastating complication with reports of frequency varying from 0% to 35% (1,5,6,39–42).

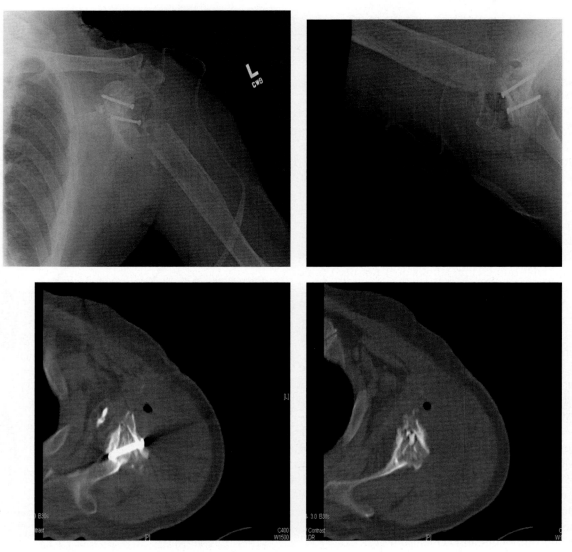

Figure 4-9 Intraoperative and postoperative radiograph of stage glenoid reconstruction.

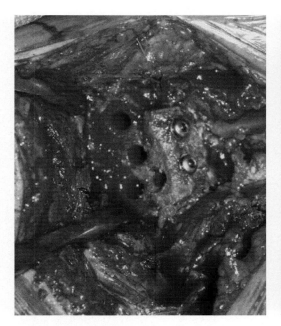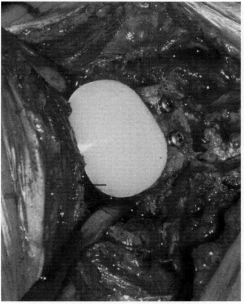

Figure 4-10 Intraoperative picture of bone grafting and fixation of glenoid defect prior to glenoid component placement.

In a literature review of 23 shoulder arthroplasty series, instability was the most commonly reported complication with a combined rate of 5.2% (43). Instability can occur acutely in the postoperative period or present slowly after several months to years. Instability following shoulder arthroplasty can range from mild subluxation to complete and fixed dislocation (Fig. 4-12). Chronic fixed dislocations occur, as do recurrent dislocations. Like nonprosthetic instability, several authors have classified the direction of instability based on the primary direction: anterior, superior, posterior, or inferior (5,6,44,45). As in nonprosthetic instability, there is debate between authors regarding classification and etiology. For example, superior instability resulting from dynamic muscle dysfunction, isolated tears and attenuation of the supraspinatus, failed rotator cuff repair, and complete rupture of the insertion of the rotator cuff

are also included into the category of glenohumeral instability by some authors (15). However, other authors feel that although superior instability can be conceptually included in the instability category, superior instability along with inferior instability should be more appropriately analyzed in the setting of massive cuff deficiency and insufficient bone-stock, respectively (46). For organizational sake, this chapter will group both superior and inferior instability in the glenohumeral instability section, realizing there can be inherent differences in the mechanisms that lead to different types of instabilities.

An extensive review of the existing literature on instability following shoulder unconstrained total shoulder arthroplasty and hemiarthroplasty have been reported by different authors (5,6,15,43,47). When broken down by direction of instability, reported rates of anterior instability

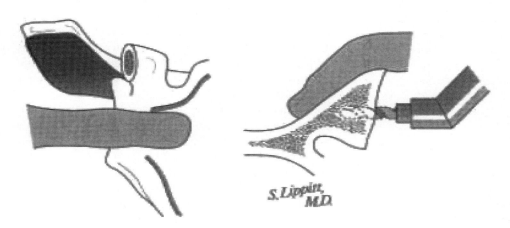

Figure 4-11 Illustration of obtaining proper glenoid orientation.

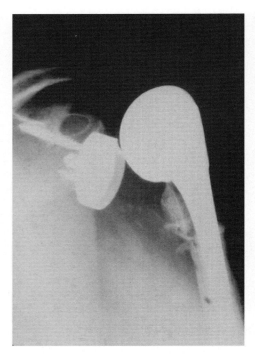

Figure 4-12 Photograph and radiograph of superiorly dislocated prosthesis.

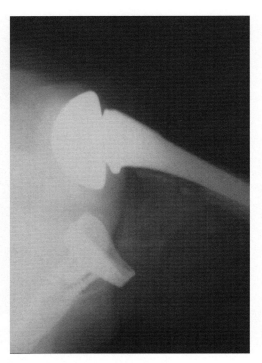

Figure 4-13 Radiograph of anterior dislocation of arthroplasty secondary to subscapularis tear.

range from 18% to 43% of cases (5,6,23,33,45,48–52); superior instability ranges from 22% to 29% of cases (5,29,53); posterior instability ranges from 20% to 27% (5,17,26,30,33,45,54–57); inferior instability ranged from 4% to 5% of cases (5,58,59); and multidirectional instability ranged from 3% to 4% (5,27,60).

It is important to note that due to the relatively small number of cases of shoulder arthroplasty, the complication rates often quoted are typically from pooled series with heterogeneous populations with regard to initial patient diagnosis, indications for surgery, and implants used. It is also important to note that complication rates for constrained total shoulder prostheses should not be included when discussing results regarding complications of total shoulder arthroplasty and hemishoulder arthoplasty. Constrained total shoulder prostheses have had only limited clinical success and have been associated with more complications than unconstrained prostheses (15). Due to the overwhelming number of complications reported in the literature, many authors question the efficacy of constrained total shoulder arthroplasty, even as a salvage procedure (15).

ANTERIOR INSTABILITY

Anterior instability after shoulder arthroplasty should be considered a subscapularis tear until proven otherwise (Fig. 4-13). Subscapularis disruption after shoulder arthroplasty has been attributed to poor tissue quality, poor technique

of subscapularis release and reattachment, oversized components that increase lateral humeral offset and create increased tension on the cuff, and inappropriate or overly aggressive physical therapy in the early postoperative period (5,6,15). Other causes of anterior instability include relative anteversion of the humeral component, anteversion of the glenoid component, an oversized humeral head, and anterior deltoid dehiscence (5,15).

Patients undergoing shoulder arthroplasty who develop osteoarthritis secondary to multiple procedures for anterior instability are at increased risk for complications postoperatively, when compared to patients undergoing arthroplasty without a history of instability. Matsoukis et al. (61) recently reported a complication rate of 18% for shoulder arthroplasty performed for osteoarthritis after anterior instability procedures; over half the complications were related to prosthetic instability. The type of prior instability surgery and preoperative active external rotation was not predictive of outcome. Factors correlated significantly with poor outcome were fatty degeneration of the rotator cuff muscles, particularly the subscapularis.

Matsoukis et al. (62) recently expanded on their previous study to include patients with a history of anterior instability, but without prior stabilization surgery, who underwent shoulder arthroplasty for osteoarthritis. No significant differences in demographic factors, prearthroplasty function, postarthroplasty function, prearthroplasty radiographic findings, postarthroplasty radiographic findings, complication rate, or reoperation rate were noted between the patients treated with a prior operation for the anterior instability and those treated nonoperatively. Negative prognosticators included an older age at the time of the initial dislocation and rotator cuff tear. This investigation demonstrated that good results are obtainable with shoulder arthroplasty for the treatment of arthritis following anterior shoulder instability.

Recently, Sanchez-Sotelo and colleagues at Mayo (46) reported on 33 shoulder arthroplasties revised for anterior instability (19 shoulders) and posterior instability (14 shoulders) following shoulder arthroplasty between 1985 and 1999. The subscapularis was ruptured in 79% (15 of 19) of shoulders with anterior shoulder instability. All cases with anterior instability also had abnormal capsular compliance of some form (either too tight or too loose), two cases showed excessive glenoid component anteversion, and one case demonstrated anterior and superior instability associated with a neck cut angled too posterior and inferiorly.

To the best of our knowledge, the recent study by Sanchez-Sotelo et al. (46) has the largest number of reported anterior instability cases (19) and posterior instability cases (14) postarthoplasty from a single series to date. Of concern is the fact that more than 50% of the shoulders (23 out of 33) remained unstable despite revision surgery. Of these, 19 of 23 shoulders (83%) were considered failures. Of the 19 shoulders that were considered to be failures, 14 (74%) were cases of anterior instability. The preoperative direction of instability (anterior instability) was the only factor that was significantly associated with the final outcome of revision surgery ($p = 0.04$) (46). Based on these findings, the authors concluded that surgical treatment for instability, primarily in the anterior or posterior direction, following shoulder arthroplasty is associated with only limited success.

AUTHORS' SURGICAL TECHNIQUE FOR ANTERIOR INSTABILITY

In our view, anterior instability represents a subscapularis tear until proven otherwise. In addition to addressing the subscapularis tear, the cause of the tear must also be sought and corrected if possible. The best method is primary prevention. We perform a lesser tuberosity ostetomy, which we have shown to be biomechanically superior to other methods of fixation (Fig. 4-14) (unpublished data, manuscript in preparation). Osteotomy of the lesser tuberosity permits bone-to-bone healing and decreases our risk of subscapularis disruption and dysfunction postoperatively. In addition, an anatomical head is preferred to avoid overstuffing and placing undue stress upon the rotator cuff.

When subscapularis ruptures do occur, tears are commonly found in association with oversized humeral heads, where the increased strain on the tendon can lead to attenuation and frank tearing. In addition, overly aggressive physical therapy in the early postoperative period is also has a high association with subscapularis tears (38). Therefore, both of these possible causes must be investigated. Traumatic cause such as after a fall or during heavy lifting can usually be elicited from the history.

If a tear is identified, particularly if it occurs in the early postoperative period, we advocate primary surgical repair without undue delay. Repair of a subscapularis rupture entails aggressive circumferential mobilization of the subscapularis and repair with nonabsorbable sutures (Fig. 4-15). We do not lengthen the subscapularis through Z-lengthening techniques or other methods, as this thins out and weakens the tendon. Instead we attempt to fully mobilize the remaining tendon and muscle belly by a 360-degree circumferential release of all adhesions, after isolating and protecting the axillary nerve (Fig. 4-16). Although described by Moeckel et al.

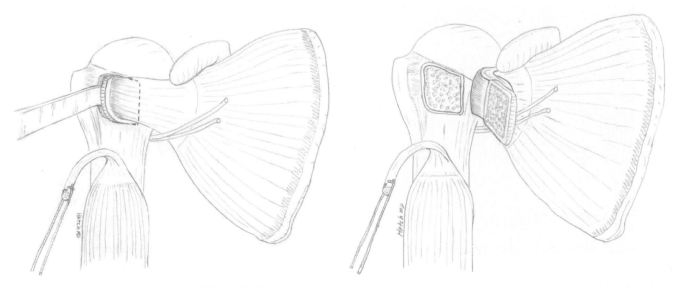

Figure 4-14 Illustration of lesser tuberosity osteotomy.

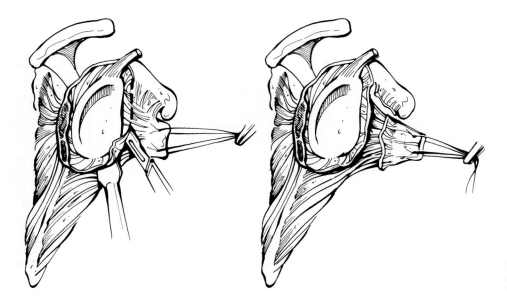

Figure 4-15 Illustration of release and 360-degree mobilization of subscapularis muscle.

(52), we have not had success with the use of bone-tendon allograft for subscapularis reconstruction. Instead, if the subscapularis remains insufficient after complete mobilization, we opt to transfer the pectoralis major muscle to the lesser tuberosity (Fig. 4-17) (63).

As stated earlier, instability following arthroplasty is typically a multifactor process. Therefore, success at revision surgery will only be achieved with a careful evaluation of the existing arthroplasty, including the soft tissue, bone stock, and components version and fixation, so that the cause of the instability can be determined.

Evaluation of component positioning and stability is performed with standard shoulder radiographs, which should always include an axillary view. A malpositioned

humeral component in anteversion increases anterior humeral head translation and the possibility of anterior instability (Fig. 4-18) (64). Computed tomography (CT) scan aids in the evaluation of the unstable arthroplasty, and in our opinion is a mandatory study prior to undertaking a revision arthroplasty procedure. Because ultimately the component version is best assessed by intraoperative evaluation, final decision regarding the need to change component version is made on the operating table. Therefore all instrumentation for component revision must be available, even if only soft-tissue issues are believed to be the primary cause of instability.

SUPERIOR INSTABILITY

Superior humeral head migration is a common complication after shoulder arthroplasty. Progressive superior humeral head migration is suggestive of superior instability. Superior instability can be associated and/or caused by dynamic muscle dysfunction, attenuation of the supraspinatus muscle-tendon unit, frank rupture of the rotator cuff, failed rotator cuff repair, and coracoacromial arch insufficiency (1,5,6,15,21,26,29,53).

Boyd and associates (39) noted proximal humeral migration in 29 (22%) of 131 total shoulder arthroplasties. Rotator cuff tears were present in only 7 (24%) of the 29 cases of proximal humeral migration. Proximal humeral migration in shoulders without rotator cuff tears was attributed to an imbalance in the force couple between the strong deltoid and a weak, poorly rehabilitated rotator cuff. Boyd and associates (39) also noted that in patients with proximal humeral migration and rotator cuff tears, the amount of proximal component migration was independent of tear size. However, there was a direct correlation between proxi-

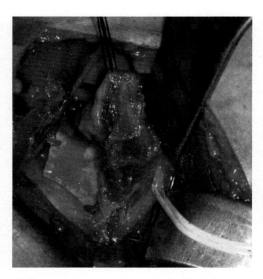

Figure 4-16 Intraoperative photograph of 360-degree mobilization of subscapularis. Notice identification and protection of axillary nerve with vessel loop.

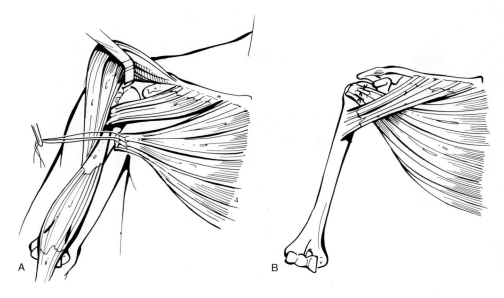

Figure 4-17 Illustration of split pectoralis major transfer. **A:** Harvest of sternal head. **B:** Transfer of sternal head to greater tuberosity.

mal humeral component migration and poor preoperative function in the setting of rotator cuff deficiency.

Cofield and associates (5) analyzed 50 shoulders which required revision surgery for instability; superior instability accounted for 17 (34%) of the cases. The causes for superior instability were supraspinatus tearing or stretching, greater tuberosity nonunion, excessive humeral component anteversion, and polyethylene dissociation (5). Unfortunately, following surgical treatment for instability in the superior direction, four patients continued to have moderate subluxation and 13 patients had severe subluxation. The results were rated as satisfactory in two patients and unsatisfactory in 15 patients.

Some authors have found that with hemiarthroplasty,

progressive proximal humeral head migration was not directly related to the development of pain or prosthesis failure (39). When comparing total shoulder versus hemiarthroplasty, several authors (6,39) have noted no increased pain with proximal migration of the humeral head in patients with humeral arthoplasty alone. However, with total shoulder arthroplasty, progressive proximal migration of the humeral component causes glenoid component loosening due to eccentric loading of the component (65). Based on their observations, Barrett and associates(26) hypothesized that a superiorly migrating humeral component results in an eccentrically applied glenoid compressive force, which causes increased stress at the glenoid bone-cement interface, and therefore eventual loosening of the glenoid implant within the glenoid fossa. An association between completely irreparable rotator cuff tears, superior humeral head migration, and glenoid component loosening was also reported in seven cases of failed total shoulder arthroplasty by Franklin and colleagues (18). The authors found that the amount of proximal humeral migration positively correlated with the degree of superior glenoid component tilting and loosening. The authors coined the term the "rocking horse" (18) of the glenoid component to describe this phenomenon. Several authors have noted the association between symptomatic loosening of the glenoid component, irreparable rotator cuff tears, and glenohumeral instability (26, 56,65–67). For the reasons mentioned above, it is therefore generally agreed that, in the setting of a massive irreparable rotator cuff tear, a traditional glenoid component should not be implanted (5,6,68).

AUTHORS' SURGICAL TECHNIQUE FOR SUPERIOR INSTABILITY

Superior instability is directly correlated with dynamic shoulder muscle dysfunction, especially the rotator cuff. In

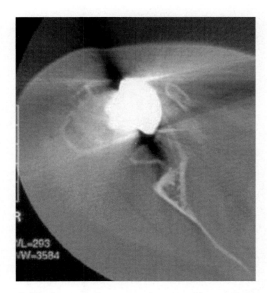

Figure 4-18 Computed tomography scan of humeral component in excessive anteversion.

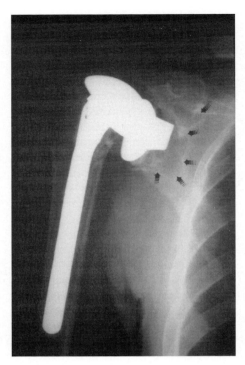

Figure 4-19 Radiograph of superior instability with glenoid lucency evident.

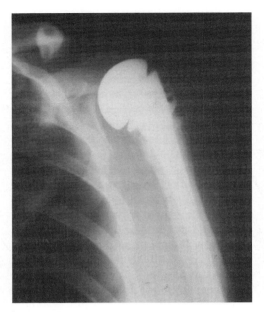

Figure 4-21 Radiograph of patient with significant superior migration of humeral head but without pain and being treated with observation.

our experience, less common causes of superior instability are malposition of humeral head height and/or inferior placement of the glenoid component. Often, mild to moderate superior instability is not associated with discomfort or pain in patients with total shoulder arthroplasty (39). However, the eccentric loading of the glenoid that results from humeral head migration, of any direction, can lead to component loosening secondary to edge-loading and the so-called rocking horse phenomenon (Fig. 4-19) (18). Cases of severe superior instability (typically with an anterior component) represent failure of the coracoacromial arch and rotator cuff (Fig. 4-20). In cases of mild to moderate superior instability without discomfort or dysfunction, we tend to follow the patients conservatively with yearly radiographic evaluation of component fixation and migration (Fig. 4-21).

We have not found reconstruction of the coracoacromial

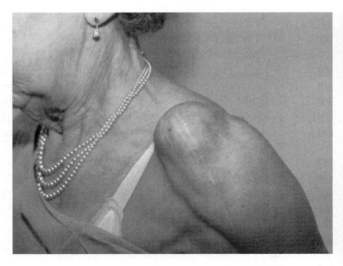

Figure 4-20 Photograph of patient with massive rotator cuff tear, failure of coracoacromial arch, and severe superior migration of humeral component.

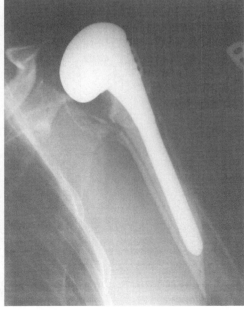

arch to be of much benefit, especially because failure of the arch virtually always is associated with a massive irreparable rotator cuff tear. Because the rotator function is also needed to prevent superior migration, addressing the arch alone does not solve the problem. Therefore, in cases of severe superior migration or moderate migration with pain and dysfunction, we recommend conversion to an inverted, reverse ball-and-socket total shoulder prosthesis (Fig. 4-22). The reverse prosthesis solves the problem of superior migration and restores function to the shoulder. Its unique design allows for a lowered, medialized center of rotation of the glenohumeral joint, which in turn results in an increased moment arm for the deltoid. Although approved by the U.S. Food and Drug Administration (FDA) in the spring of 2004, the Grammont inverted total shoulder prosthesis has been used for over 15 years in Europe. We have performed approximately more than 50 cases at the Harvard Shoulder Service with very encouraging early results.

Recently, Sirveaux et al. (69) reported their findings of a multicenter trial involving 80 shoulders with a mean follow-up of 44 months (range, 24 to 97 months). The authors reported an improvement in mean constant scores from 22.6 points preoperatively to 65.8 points postoperatively. The mean active elevation improved from 73 degrees to 138 degrees. In 96% of the shoulders, there was no or only minimal pain. Three implants (4%) failed and had to be revised. The study by Sirveaux et al. (69) demonstrated that the inverted prosthesis is a viable option in older patients with cuff-tear arthropathy and pseudoparalysis.

POSTERIOR INSTABILITY

Posterior instability accounts for 34% to 61% of all cases of instability following shoulder arthroplasty (5,15,46). Posterior instability is associated with excessive posterior capsule and posterior rotator cuff laxity, detachment of the rotator cuff by the humeral osteotomy, a malpositioned humeral head, rotator cuff tearing, posterior glenoid erosion, a malpositioned glenoid component, polyethylene dissociation from the glenoid metal tray, rotator cuff tearing, and excessive retroversion of either or both the humeral or glenoid component (1,5,6,15,46).

Several reports (2,5,15,46,70) have concluded that shoulder instability after arthroplasty is multifactoral. Subsequently, to allow the best chance at restoring shoulder stability, all implicated factors must be addressed at the time of reoperation. If any contributing factors are not corrected, the instability is likely to recur after treatment and/or another direction of instability may be manifested (46,70). However, even when seemingly all underlying factors have been addressed, stability following the revision procedure is still often not achieved. Because instability often results from more than one cause, authors stress that the treatment must include addressing all soft-tissue imbalances (including possible posterior capsulorrhaphy), restoring normal humeral component version, and reestablishing proper glenoid component version (5,15,46).

Unfortunately, the results of surgical revision for posterior instability are often disappointing. Overall, several large series (5,46) have found the results of revision surgery

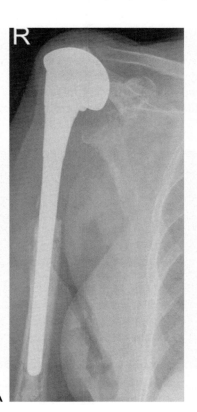
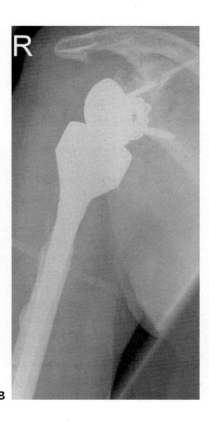

Figure 4-22 Radiograph showing conversion of superiorly displaced humeral arthroplasty converted to reverse prosthesis. **A:** Preoperative. **B:** Postoperative.

for instability (both posterior and anterior) following shoulder arthroplasty to be disappointing. In one recent series (46), 42% (14 shoulders) had one reoperation after the initial revision procedure; at final follow-up, more than 50% of the shoulders remained unstable despite attempts at revision surgery.

AUTHORS' SURGICAL TECHNIQUE FOR POSTERIOR INSTABILITY

In our experience, the majority of cases of posterior instability can be attributed to technical errors during the initial procedure. Prior to the initial procedure, marked restriction of external rotation on physical exam and radiographic evidence of posterior glenohumeral subluxation should alert the shoulder surgeon of the possibility of uneven posterior glenoid wear. Failure to recognize posterior glenoid erosion can result in the placement of a glenoid component in excessive retroversion, and therefore result in a propensity for posterior instability. In our preoperative evaluation of candidates for shoulder arthroplasty, we routinely obtain CT scans in addition to axillary radiographs to evaluate the axial plane version of the glenoid (Fig. 4-23). CT scans, optimally with three-dimensional reconstructions when available, allow the surgeon to precisely quantify the degree of glenoid deficiency and version. In addition, the CT scan gives the most accurate assessment of available glenoid bone stock. By carefully reaming the anterior glenoid and/or decreasing the amount of glenoid component retroversion, minor deficiencies of the posterior glenoid can be corrected without the need for glenoid augmentation (Fig. 4-24) (6,71–73). However, bone grafting of the glenoid is sometimes required in cases with severe posterior glenoid deficiency (74,75).

In our experience, in the majority of cases of posterior

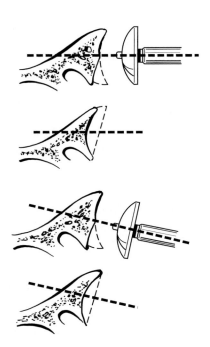

Figure 4-24 Illustration of high-side or anterior reaming of glenoid with excessive retroversion.

instability, excessive retroversion of the humeral component, the glenoid component, or both is usually present. Malposition typically occurs on the glenoid side of glenohumeral joint, with the component being placed in excessive retroversion (Fig. 4-25). This can result from failure to recognize and compensate for excessive posterior glenoid wear at the index procedure. Therefore, failure to ream down the high anterior side of the glenoid results in placement of a retroverted component and increases the chances of posterior instability.

When glenoid component retroversion is less than 15 to 20 degrees, correction may be accomplished by remov-

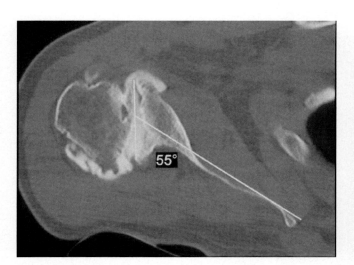

Figure 4-23 Computed tomography scan showing severe glenoid retroversion.

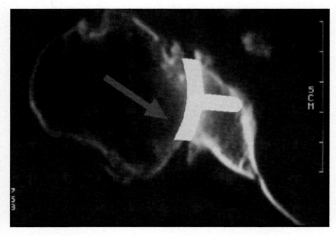

Figure 4-25 Radiograph of malpositioned glenoid component in excessive retroversion resulting in posterior instability.

ing the original component and cutting down and lowering the higher anterior side. Unfortunately, there is often little bone available anteriorly before the base of the coracoid is reached, and often this is not enough to correct the version to neutral. Therefore, glenoids retroverted greater than 15 degrees may require posterior augmentation with a bone graft (76). Glenoid bone grafting can be accomplished by securing a tricortical iliac crest autograft of appropriate height and shape to the scapula with 4.0 mm AO/ASIF cannulated screws (Fig. 4-26). If the shape or location of the glenoid defect precludes the use of bone screws, the bone graft may be wedged into the defect like a keystone, and nonabsorbable sutures are then used to secure the graft to the remaining glenoid as described by Neer and Morrison (74). In some cases with severe posterior bone deficiency and retroversion, staged bone grafting procedures are needed, with placement of the glenoid component at a future date (Fig. 4-9).

In addition to addressing the posterior bone defects, the surgeon must recognize that the prolonged posterior subluxation, often seen in patients with osteoarthritis who develop posterior glenoid deficiency, can result in excessively posterior capsule and soft-tissue laxity. Here again, this problem is best addressed at the primary procedure, where excessive posterior capsular laxity can be reduced by plication of the posterior capsule. When posterior capsular laxity is encountered during a primary total shoulder arthroplasty, the surgeon must resist the urge to oversize the humeral head to place tension on the posterior capsular tissues. Although an oversized humeral head can often reduce a patulous posterior capsule, overstuffing the glenohumeral joint can lead to several complications such as loss of motion, pain, and rotator cuff tears; therefore, this temptation must be avoided.

If a lax posterior capsule is found at the time of revision surgery, we will plicate the posterior tissue from inside the capsule with simple mattress stitches, which reduce the capsular volume by taking multiple tiny tucks of tissue. Postoperatively, the patient must be protected in a brace that holds the arm in neutral to slight external rotation. Forward flexion and cross-arm adduction are also avoided for approximately 4 to 6 weeks.

Due to the association of posterior instability with rotator cuff tearing, the rotator cuff is also thoroughly evaluated at the revision procedure and all attempts are made at repairing any tears found as best as possible. An excessively retroverted or distal humeral head cut can lead to a disruption of the posterior rotator cuff insertion and this can lead to posterior instability. If this is encountered acutely, primary repair should be attempted. In the chronic case, soft tissue reconstruction or tendon transfers may be performed although in older or lower demand individuals, conversion to a reverse type shoulder arthroplasty may be preferable (Fig. 4-22).

In the clinical workup of an arthroplasty complicated by posterior instability, all possible explanations for instability must be investigated. In turn, at the time of revision procedure, all possible factors must then be addressed. Intraoperatively, the surgeon must evaluate for factors that could be contributing to the instability but were not foreseen in the preoperative evaluation (e.g., excessive humeral component retroversion, posterior capsular, and rotator cuff tears).

INFERIOR INSTABILITY

Inferior instability most commonly results from the failure to restore humeral length, especially when the arthroplasty

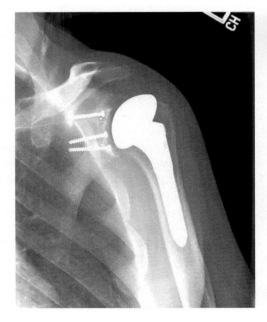
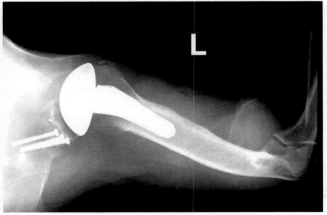

Figure 4-26 Radiograph of bone grafting with femoral head allograft for severe posterior glenoid wear.

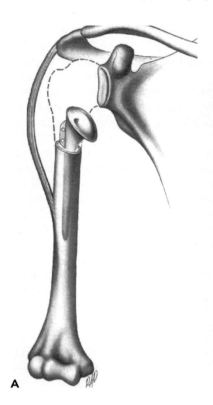

A

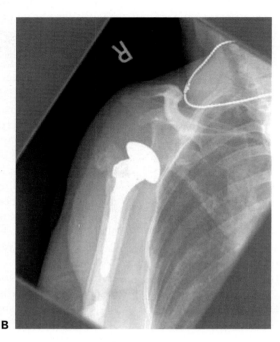

B

Figure 4-27 Inferior instability resulting for insufficient prosthesis length. **A:** Illustration. **B:** Radiograph.

is performed for the treatment of acute fracture or reconstruction following tumor excision. However, inferior instability has also been noted after total shoulder arthroplasty for prosthetic revision, previous osteosynthesis, chronic fracture, and uncomplicated osteoarthritis or rheumatoid arthritis (32,58,67,77,78). Often with inferior instability, deltoid muscle function is hindered due to shortening of the humerus with a loss of the normal length tension relationship (Fig. 4-27). Clinically, patients with this complication are unable to raise their arm above the horizontal plane, and therefore lack adequate range of motion. The importance of re-establishing correct humeral length, which restores the resting tension in the rotator cuff and deltoid, has been well documented (5,32,59,78). Correct humeral length optimizes deltoid function while minimizing inferior stability and subsequent weakness during elevation. Inferior instability can also occur after axillary nerve injury either iatrogenic or traumatic. This can be evaluated with an electromyelogram (EMG) and is usually managed nonoperatively.

AUTHORS' SURGICAL TECHNIQUE FOR INFERIOR INSTABILITY

Patients with inferior instability typically complain of persistent pain, weakness, and inability to raise their arm above the horizontal. Proper treatment involves the restoration of humeral height, which in turn restores tension in the myofascial sleeve. To accomplish this, the humeral component must be removed (as described in the section

on component loosening) and the bony deficiency evaluated. Often, bone graft is used to fill the space between the head of the prosthesis and the humeral shaft. In addition, the component must be cemented high in order to obtain proper tension in the myofascial sleeve.

The tuberosities and rotator cuff must always be evaluated in the setting of inadequate humeral length, either with or without prior proximal humerus fracture. If the tuberosities have disappeared and a massive contracted cuff tear is present, restoration of humeral height alone will not solve suffice; in these cases, the best chance at restoring stability and arm motion is conversion to a reverse ball and socket total arthroplasty prosthesis (Fig. 4-28). Patients with inferior instability typically complain of persistent pain, weakness, and inability to raise their arm above the horizontal. Proper treatment involves the restoration of humeral height, which in turn restores tension in the myofascial sleeve. To accomplish this, the humeral component must be removed (as described above) and the bony deficiency evaluated. Often, bone graft is used to fill the space between the head of the prosthesis and the humeral shaft. In addition, the component must be cemented high to obtain proper tension in the myofascial sleeve.

Evaluation of the proper humeral component length in fracture cases is extremely difficult due to alteration of the humeral head anatomy and bony landmarks secondary to fracture. We address this problem by obtaining an x-ray of the contralateral extremity and measuring the insertion of the pectoralis major muscle insertion to the top of the humeral head (Figs. 4-29 and 4-30). We have demonstrated

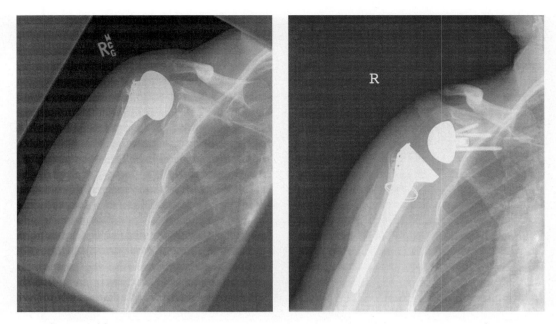

Figure 4-28 Radiograph of patient with failed hemiarthroplasty for proximal humerus fracture treated with conversion to reverse prosthesis.

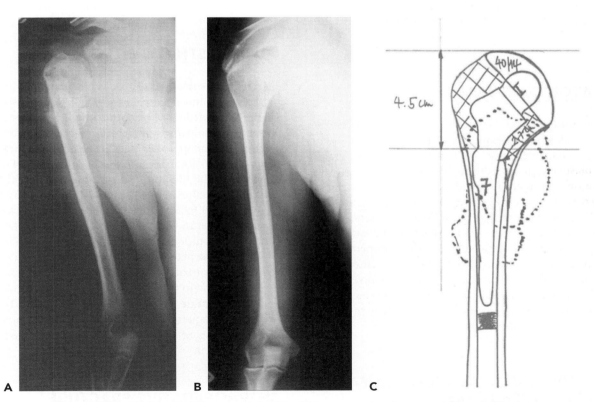

Figure 4-29 The length of the normal shoulder (x) is measured and corrected for magnification to compare to the contralateral (fractured) side. The length of the humerus on the fractured side, from the elbow to the diaphyseal edge of the fracture, is (y). The height of the prosthesis to restore the correct length is then (z), where (x) − (y) = (z).

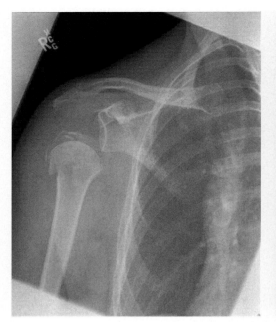
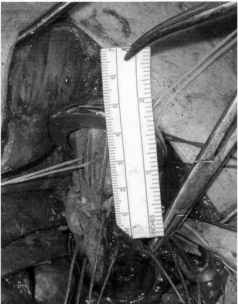
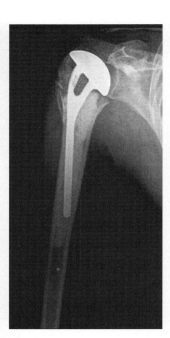

Figure 4-30 Picture of the technique measuring of pectoralis major insertion.

that this distance is a reliable and accurate measurement that can be used for hemiarthoplasty reconstruction when other landmarks are lost due to proximal humerus fracture (79).

ROTATOR CUFF TEARS

Rotator cuff tears occurring after shoulder arthroplasty are common. Postoperative tearing of the rotator cuff occurs in approximately 2% to 4% of patients with total shoulder arthroplasty (1,5,6,15). Although this has been considered a common occurrence following shoulder arthroplasty, associated pain has not been reported in many series (21, 80–82). Although tearing of the subscapularis tendon typically mandates immediate operative repair, there is no consensus on treatment (operative versus nonoperative) of nonsubscapularis rotator cuff tears. Operative intervention for rotator cuff tears (without or without involvement of the subscapularis) has demonstrated limited success, often with recurrent tearing and little improvement in motion or function (23,26,30,56,80,81,83,84).

AUTHORS' SURGICAL TECHNIQUE FOR ROTATOR CUFF TEARS

The first priority is prevention by anatomic reconstruction and avoidance of oversized components. Next is early open operative repair for postoperative subscapularis tears with transossosseous suture techniques. Massive tears with supe-

rior migration of the prosthesis are best dealt with by conversion to reverse-type prosthesis arthroplasty.

PERIPROSTHETIC FRACTURES

Periprosthetic fractures can be divided into two groups: intraoperative and postoperative fractures. Extensive review of the literature by several authors (5,6) has shown a prevalence of periprosthetic fractures ranging from 2% to 3%, accounting for approximately 20% of all complications associated with total shoulder arthroplasty (15,41,85–87). Analysis of the literature finds that approximately 86% of the injuries represent humeral shaft or tuberosity fractures (5,6,18,26,29,56,60,81,88,89), whereas 12% of cases involve fractures of the glenoid (5,6,56,81,90). The division of fracture complications into the intraoperative and postoperative time period finds that intraoperative fractures account for approximately 62% of all periprosthetic fracture cases (6). Due to the fact that several of the articles in the existing literature fail to describe the exact mechanism of injury, subsequent management, and final outcome of many of cases of periprosthetic fracture, detailed analysis is very difficult.

INTRAOPERATIVE FRACTURES

The majority of intraoperative fractures appear to be avoidable and typically represent operative error (5,56,86, 87,91). Examples of operative errors are aggressive manipulation of the arm during glenoid exposure, inadvertent

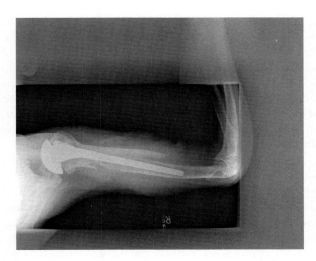

Figure 4-31 X-ray of humerus fracture after insertion of TSR prosthesis.

reaming, and overzealous impaction. Aggressive external rotation of the shoulder during glenoid exposure produces a large torisonal stress on the humeral shaft, which can fracture both osteoperotic and normal bone. The proximal aspect of the humerus is at risk for fracture during insertion of the medullary reamers or trial prosthesis if the adequate exposure of the humerus is not obtained (Fig. 4-31). In addition to a thorough soft-tissue release, adequate humerus exposure requires extension of the arm off of the operating table. Inaccurate humeral head resection can be another cause of intraoperative fracture, along with an errant entry point into the medullary canal of the humerus, which risks perforation distally either in the metaphysic or shaft. Several authors (6,15) have also stressed the importance of hand-reaming the humeral medullary canal as opposed to power instruments. Power reaming risks the removal of too much cancellous bone and increase the risk for fracture, especially in osteoportic bone.

Intraoperative fractures of the glenoid can also occur during shoulder arthroplasty (56,81,92). Overly aggressive reaming and/or nonconcentric reaming as a result of insufficient glenoid exposure can result in glenoid fracture.

AUTHORS PREFERRED TREATMENT FOR INTRAOPERATIVE PERIPROSTHETIC FRACTURES

The true key to the treatment of intraoperative periprosthetic fractures is avoidance through meticulous technique. However, if fractures do occur, we strongly believe that they require immediate stabilization whenever possible. Immediate rigid fixation allows for postoperative rehabilitation without additional protection or immobilization (93).

For humeral shaft fractures, the type of fixation depends upon fracture location, fracture pattern, and implant stability. Immediate treatment with open reduction and internal fixation by conversion to long-stem prosthesis in conjunction with simple cerclage wiring, or retention of the originally intended component with cerclage wiring, has been advocated by several authors (1,5,6,85,91,94). For fractures occurring distal to the prosthesis, or for fractures occurring in the proximal portion of the humerus with distal extension beyond the tip of the prosthesis, several authors recommend the use of a long-stem humeral component (5,6,85,93,95). When conversion to long-stem prosthesis with cerclage wiring is employed, the prosthesis should extend at least two cortical diameters beyond the most distal extent of the fracture in order to ensure construct stability (6,15). For humeral fractures occurring proximal to the tip of the humeral prosthesis, simple cerclage wiring of the proximal humerus and implantation of a standard-size prosthesis is appropriate (5,6). Autogeneous bone grafting, obtained from the resected humeral head and placed around the metaphyseal portion of the proximal humerus after insertion of prosthesis, has also been advocated by authors (6). For very distal humeral shaft fractures, plate fixation may be preferred (5). Plate fixation can additionally be used to reduce and stabilized periprosthetic fractures, which occur close to the humeral implant, in an effort to avoid having to remove the prosthesis. Unfortunately, plate fixation around a prosthesis is not as secure as cables and struts (1,6,15,93). In turn, failure of fixation at the fracture site can lead to nonunion.

The knowledge of the potential complications of glenoid resurfacing should help surgeons prevent and avoid them because, just like intraoperative humerus fractures, the majority of intraoperative glenoid complications can be attributed to poor surgical technique (96). An example of typical scenarios that can result in intraoperative glenoid fracture is misplacement of the drill bit outside of the medullary canal leading to perforation of the cortex. This can occur in situations where there is significant asymmetric glenoid wear. Removal of all peripheral osteophytes along with the use of a glenoid orientation guide can help avoid this complication (96). Glenoid fracture can also occur during insertion of the glenoid component if the direction not strictly inline with the glenoid bone stock; as a result, the abnormal lever arm may break the cortical bone of the glenoid neck. Glenoid resurfacing often has to be abandoned in these cases, because the remaining bone does not have enough support for the implant and the bone quality may preclude satisfactory component fixation. Finally, use of a glenoid implant with multiple pegs may lead to intraoperative fragmentation of the glenoid bone stock and subsequent fracture (97). Like many authors, we believe the majority of intraoperative glenoid fractures can be avoided by meticulous attention to principles of glenoid resurfacing including adequate exposure, proper glenoid preparation, and component orientation.

POSTOPERATIVE PERIPROSTHETIC FRACTURES

The prevalence of postoperative periprosthetic fractures has been reported to be between 0.61% and 2.4% (87,98,99). The overwhelming majority of postoperative periprosthetic fractures involve the humeral component. Common risk factors for periprosthetic fractures are cortical thinning due to osteolysis, reaming the medial cortex at the time of arthroplasty, and osteopenia (98,100).

The location and configuration of the fracture pattern have an important effect on outcome (Fig. 4-32). Postoperative humeral fractures can be classified on the basis of their location with respect to the distal tip of the humeral implant, according to the system of Wright and Cofield (94). Type A fractures are located at the tip of the stem and extend proximally, type B fractures lie at the tip of the prosthesis without extension or with only minimal extension proximally but can have a variable amount of extension distally, and type C fractures are located distal to the tip of the prosthesis.

Kumar and colleagues (100) concluded that fractures located distal to the tip of the prosthesis (type C fractures) are similar to closed fractures of the humeral shaft and can be treated nonoperatively. Previous studies (95,99) have also suggested that fractures distal to the tip of the prosthesis (type C fractures) may be treated successfully by nonoperative means.

Fractures which occur at the tip of the prosthesis (type A or type B) behave differently. The literature includes several reports (86,87,99) of failure of nonoperative management for fractures, which occurred about the tip of the prosthesis. Specific indications for surgical treatment include the presence of a loose humeral component, fracture through the bone and cement mantle, difficulty with fracture reduction secondary to an interposed prosthesis, and recent surgery on the contralateral extremity (98).

Kumar and the Mayo group (98) proposed a treatment algorithm for managing postarthroplasty periprosthetic humeral fractures. For a type C fracture with a well-fixed humeral component, a trial of nonoperative treatment should

be attempted if acceptable reduction can be obtained with an orthosis. Nonoperative treatment may also be considered for a well-aligned type B fracture with a well-fixed humeral component. However, operative treatment should be considered if the fracture has not progressed towards union in 3 months. The authors also recommend the use of iliac crest autogenous bone grafting at the time of treatment of the periprosthetic fracture, and feel this is a good alternative to revision when the prosthesis is well-fixed.

Revision with cemented long-stem fixation and supplementation with iliac crest bone grafting is recommended for type B fractures associated with a loose humeral component (98). Cortical strut allograft or plate fixation with cerclage wiring and screws to provide adjunctive fixation for a long-stem prosthesis has been reported in the literature (101) regarding periprosthetic fractures, but the techniques have not been described in the shoulder arthroplasty literature.

Based on their findings, Kumar et al. (98) do not believe operative treatment is indicated for type A fractures, unless the humeral component is loose. Type A fractures often are associated with a loose humeral component due to the substantial overlap between the length between the length of the periprosthetic fracture and that of the stem. Kumar and colleagues (98) recommend operative treatment for all loose components, whereby revision entails conversion to a cemented long-stem prosthesis typically supplemented with autogenous bone grafting. In order to obtain secure fixation, supplementary fixation with an allograft or with a plate, screws, and cables may be required.

AUTHORS' SURGICAL TREATMENT OF POSTOPERATIVE FRACTURES

Our treatment for postoperative fractures is very similar to the recommendations put forth by Kumar et al. (98). Our treatment decisions are based upon the stability of the prosthesis and the location of the fracture relative to the prosthesis. We believe a trial of nonoperative treatment is indicated for a fracture where the majority of the implant proximal to the tip of the prosthesis is well-fixed. However, surgery is required in any situation where the fracture is associated with a loose prosthesis. Stabilization in this setting requires conversion to a long-stem prosthesis (possibly cemented) extending at least two cortical diameters in length past the fracture site. In addition to long-stem prosthesis conversion, we use a sometimes use a method of fixation commonly employed in periprosthetic fractures occurring around the hip and knee, and used by some shoulder surgeons (2). This technique involves the use of allograft cortical struts prepared from the tibia or femur and fixed to the humeral shaft with multiple cables, in addition to the conversion to long-stem prosthesis. In addition to careful soft-tissue elevation and subperiosteal dissection around the fracture site, to avoid injury to the radial nerve, the surgeon must make sure that the cortical struts are placed well proximal and distal to the fracture site. We agree with the recom-

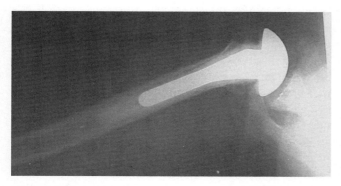

Figure 4-32 Radiograph demonstrating classification system for periprosthetic fractures. Classification of fractures: A, B, C.

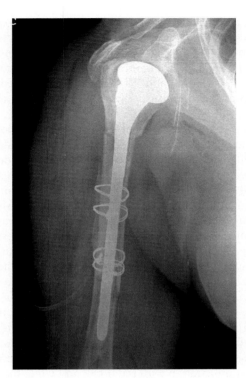

Figure 4-33 Radiograph of stabilization of periprosthetic fracture with long-stem component, allograft struts, and cerclage wires.

mendations of Norris and Gunther (2) that the fracture site should always be approached from the anterior aspect of the humerus away from the path of the radial nerve. Starting the subperiosteal dissection and elevation of the muscles and scar tissue at the site of the fracture or nonunion will allow adequate exposure without undue risk to the radial nerve.

Revision of a well-fixed humeral component is very difficult and risks significant iatrogenic injury to the humeral shaft. However, certain clinical scenarios that can occur with periprosthetic fractures mandate component removal regardless of solid fixation. These situations present when the periprosthetic fracture occurs in association with a humeral malpositioning, a loose glenoid, or glenohumeral arthritis. In these scenarios, the best course of action may be to revise the humeral component to a long-stem prosthesis with cerclage wire (Fig. 4-33). In case of a loose glenoid, a bone grafting may be needed; for glenohumeral arthritis, glenoid resurfacing may be employed.

INFECTION

Infection following shoulder arthroplasty continues to be a relatively rare occurrence compared to arthroplasty of the knee and hip (102). This has been attributed to an extensive soft-tissue envelope and rich vascular supply that is unfavorable to propagation of infection. The most comprehensive review of the literature on the incidence of infection following unconstrained TSA was reported by Cofield, with an incidence of only 5 in 1183 (0.4%) shoulders studied

(21,26,29,30,32,55,56,58,80,81,83,84,90,103). Neer (32) reported on only two infections in his series of 776 unconstrained total arthroplasties. A review of 20 patient series having undergone hemiarthoplasty of the shoulder revealed postoperative infection in only 5 of 498 (1%) shoulders studied (17,29,91,104–109,111–119).

The risk of infection following shoulder arthoplasty is enhanced by poor baseline protoplasm or chronic systemic illness. Most patients that develop infection have one or more chronic diseases that alter the host immune response or vascularity. These include diabetes mellitus, systemic lupus erythematosis, dialysis-induced renal dysfunction, blood dyscrasia, alcoholism, AIDS, malnutrition, malignancy, connective tissue disorders, or in the setting of revision surgery (120–124). Additional factors that may increase susceptibility to infection include systemic immunosuppressive agents such as chemotherapy, oral corticosteroids, and even multiple focal injections of steroid about the shoulder (125).

The most common offending organism is *Streptococcus aureus*, accounting for nearly 50% of shoulder infections, followed by coagulase-negative *Streptococcus epidermidis*, *Streptococcus spp.*, and gram-negative organisms for the remaining 10% to 30% depending on the series reviewed (102,120,121,124,126). Although rare, mixed infections can be present and should be entertained in revision settings or in the setting of failed initial treatment. *S. aureus* and *Pseudomonas aeruginosa* are most common in intravenous drug users (102,122,123).

The diagnosis of infection begins with a thorough history and physical examination. Patients may complain of subjective fevers and chills, as well as increasing pain in the shoulder that is present at rest, aggravated by motion, and often awakens them from sleep. Patients who are immunocompromised or immunosuppressed may lack these early symptoms, which leads to a delay in diagnosis. Clinical examination can be variable, but will often reveal a warm, erythematous joint that is tender to palpation and painful in passive and active motion. In acute cases, there may be persistent drainage from the incision; however, in most cases, the presentation is subtle and often missed (121,124,126).

Laboratory studies including a serum white blood cell count with differential, erythrocyte sedimentation rate (ESR) and C-reactive protein should be obtained initially in all cases of suspected infection. Flatow and coworkers (127) reported on the laboratory findings in 18 patients suffering infection following shoulder arthroplasty with an average ESR of 49 mm/hour and white blood cell count of 11/mm³. If laboratory studies are abnormal, radioisotope scanning and aspiration arthrogram can be helpful, although often inconsistent. Of the 18 patients in Flatow's series, eleven underwent radioisotope scans with variable results: seven positive, two false negative, and two equivocal. Of the seven shoulders that were aspirated, only two cultures yielded an identifiable organism. In summary, the diagnosis is largely made by history, examination, and the overall suspicion of the orthopedist because laboratory markers can be variable and inconsistent.

AUTHORS' PREFERRED TECHNIQUE FOR TREATMENT OF INFECTION FOLLOWING ARTHROPLASTY

As with prosthetic infection of the major weight-bearing joints, management of shoulder prosthetic infections should be catered to the timing of infection and the type of organism involved. Generally, gram-negative organisms are more resistant to eradication with administration of parenteral antibiotics without removal of components and cement. Patients with documented infection by a gram-positive organism during the initial 3 to 4 weeks following implantation may be managed by aggressive wound exploration, irrigation, debridement of nonviable tissue, exchange of the polyethylene, and retention of components. In chronic cases (>4 weeks), resection arthroplasty should be performed, including removal of all components and cement, aggressive debridement of infected soft tissue and bone, and administration of appropriate antibiotics under the guidance of an infectious disease specialist. Boileau, Walch, and coworkers (128) have shown that a multidisciplinary approach to the management of infection following shoulder arthroplasty improves outcomes and reduces patient morbidity. Mileti (129) reported on four patients who underwent successful reimplantation following prior resection arthroplasty with a mean follow-up of 7.4 years. The present authors advocate use of an antibiotic-impregnated cement spacer as described by Loebenberg and Zuckerman (130) for two reasons: it assists in maintaining appropriate soft tissue tension and maintaining bony architecture for later reimplantation, and it provides high localized levels of antibiotic to the surrounding tissues that may assist in clearance of the microorganism (131).

In general terms, treatment may include antibiotic administration (oral or parenteral), irrigation and debridement with retention of components, irrigation and debridement with exchange of modular components, resection arthroplasty, resection arthroplasty with placement of an antibiotic-impregnated cement spacer, arthrodesis, and amputation. The authors' treatment algorithm is based on the timing of infection (<4 weeks versus >4 weeks) and the type of organism involved (gram-positive versus gram-negative/polymicrobial). Any draining wound in the acute postoperative period should be explored operatively and managed aggressively. Patients with a susceptible gram-positive infection within 4 weeks of implantation may be managed with aggressive open irrigation and debridement followed by exchange of modular components including polyethylene. This is followed by 6 weeks of parenteral antibiotic administration with serial ESR and white blood cell monitoring to assess response to treatment. In the setting of gram-negative infection, although a trial of the above management can be attempted, in most cases resection arthroplasty with removal of all components, cement, and placement of an antibiotic-impregnated cement spacer is usually necessary (Fig. 4-34). This more aggressive approach is also performed by the authors in the setting of

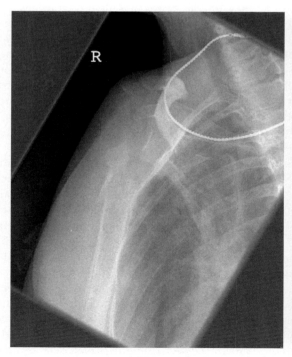
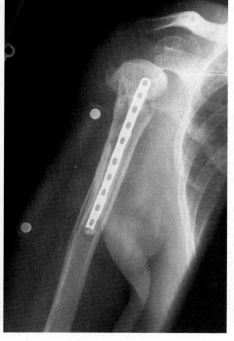

Figure 4-34 Radiographs of resection arthroplasty with and without antibiotic spacer.

infection occurring greater than 4 weeks following the index procedure. Following a 6-week course of antibiotics, a 2-week "grace" period off antibiotics is allowed, followed by repeat implantation if pathologic evaluation (frozen section) at the time of surgery does not yield the presence of persistent leukocytosis (>5 polymorphonuclear leukocytes/high-powered field). Studies in the hip and knee arthroplasty literature have shown, however, that the sensitivity, specificity, and positive predictive value of frozen sections can be inconsistent. A prospective series of 121 revision hip and knee total joint arthroplasties revealed a 67% sensitivity, 93% specificity, 67% positive predictive value, and 93% negative predictive value of frozen sections compared to intraoperative cultures (132).

NERVE INJURIES

Nerve injury following shoulder arthroplasty is a rare, but devastating, complication. In a meta-analysis examining 1183 total shoulder arthroplasties, seven (0.6%) patients suffered a nerve injury, with most affecting the axillary nerve (Fig. 4-35) (21,26,29,30,32,55,56,58,80,81, 83,84,90,103–110). The etiology is usually aggressive retraction of the deltoid or injury during soft-tissue release of the inferior joint capsule. With increasing use of peripheral anesthesia and interscalene blockade, it is important to differentiate surgical from anesthetic antecedent events. In ad-

dition, overzealous traction of the extremity or improper patient positioning should be avoided.

Most nerve injuries result from neuropraxia and resolve within the first 2 months following surgery. Electromyography (EMG) and nerve conduction velocity (NCV) studies can be obtained 6 weeks following surgery in cases where no clinical improvement is noted. The Sunderland classification, first described in 1951, places the injured nerve into one of six categories based on severity of injury and can assist the clinician in directing an appropriate treatment plan (133).

AUTHORS' PREFERRED METHOD OF TREATMENT OF NERVE INJURY FOLLOWING ARTHROPLASTY

Surgical exploration and attempted microsurgical repair should be performed in cases of severe axonotmesis or frank neurotmesis at 6 weeks, with no improvement by 12 weeks after the index surgery. In the setting of improvement, observation is warranted.

The authors routinely identify, isolate, and protect the axillary nerve during both primary and revision shoulder arthroplasty at the posterolateral aspect of the humerus. In addition, careful, gentle retraction of the conjoined tendon is performed in order to avoid stretching the musculocutaneous nerve. In the setting of a nerve injury that has not improved at 3 months following surgery based on EMG/NCV studies, the authors would advocate surgical exploration and attempted microsurgical repair.

IMPLANT FAILURE OR DISSOCIATION

Implant-related complications can occur by dissociation or failure of the polyethylene or metal component. With improvements in implant design, fixation methods, and the material properties of shoulder arthroplasty components, the frequency of implant fracture or failure has been supplanted by implant dissociation. Prior to the advent of modular components in shoulder arthroplasty almost 20 years ago, shoulder replacements would occasionally fail by dissociation of the polyethylene from the metal-backed glenoid component, fracture of the glenoid keel, fracture of the humeral component at the metaphysis, or, in rare cases, fracture or dislocation of polyethylene subacromial spacers (134–136).

Modular components have brought about their own share of complications despite the benefits of improved restoration of normal anatomy, soft-tissue balancing, and improved stability. There have been rare reports of dissociation of the humeral head from the morse taper of the humeral stem (137,138). According to Rockwood, these tend to occur in the acute setting within 6 weeks of the index

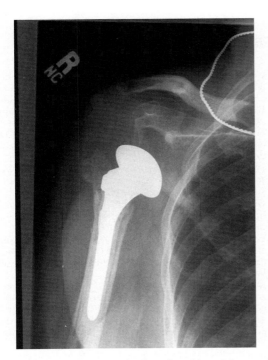

Figure 4-35 Radiograph of inferiorly subluxed humeral arthroplasty resulting from axillary nerve injury.

procedure and rarely result in dislocation of the glenohumeral joint (138).

DELTOID DYSFUNCTION

Injury to the deltoid muscle is an avoidable complication that can be devastating to the patient and functional outcome following shoulder replacement (Fig. 4-36). In the absence of axillary nerve injury described above, deltoid dysfunction is the result of surgical exposure or excessive retraction with resultant injury to the musculature. Neer was the first to report on deltoid dysfunction following his series of 194 total shoulder arthroplasties (139). He found a clear correlation between the type of surgical approach and the incidence of injury. In his initial series of total shoulder replacements, Neer performed a short deltopectoral approach with detachment of the anterior deltoid origin from the clavicle. Given the relative frequency of anterior deltoid weakness, he abandoned this approach for a superior approach that involved detachment of the middle deltoid. Not surprisingly, this was abandoned due to dysfunction of the middle deltoid and replaced by the deltopectoral approach used today, which does not violate the origin or insertion of the muscle. He concluded that deltoid weakness and resultant atrophy was a major instigating factor leading to failure of 92% of his failed total shoulder arthroplasties (140).

In the setting of deltoid disruption following arthroplasty, the best results are obtained when the injury is recognized early, all adhesions are released, and the deltoid is mobilized and repaired (141). Chronic deltoid detachments with an atrophic anterior deltoid have a greater than 50% risk of poor surgical outcome following treatment (142).

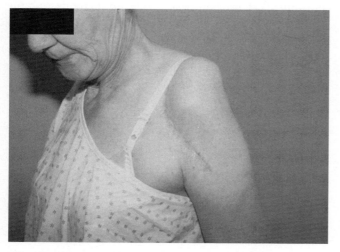

Figure 4-36 Photograph of deltoid injury after multiple shoulder surgeries.

CONCLUSION

Although the exact incidence of complications can vary depending on the initial diagnosis, several types of complications can occur with any shoulder arthroplasty such as: prosthetic loosening, glenohumeral instability, rotator cuff tears, periprosthetic fracture, infection, implant failure or dissociation, deltoid dysfunction, and neurovascular injury. In the normal glenohumeral joint, shoulder stability is achieved by a complex interplay of static and dynamic constraints (143–147). Stability and function rely on coordination of these components, including precise control of muscle firing patterns in the shoulder muscles and the integrity of the capsuloligamentous structures (143,148). Shoulder arthroplasty by its nature disrupts the complex interactions about the shoulder, and therefore increases the shoulder's propensity for instability and component failure. Precise soft-tissue balancing and component positioning are necessary to restore both the rotational and translational components of normal shoulder kinematics after arthroplasty. In addition to soft-tissue balancing, shoulder stability following arthroplasty is dependent upon obtaining correct glenoid version, correct humeral version, and maintaining subscapularis intergrity. The best treatment for a complication is avoidance. To increase the chances of a successful outcome the surgeon must have the correct indications, correct patient selection, accurate preoperative planning, precise dissection, proper component selection, proper implantation, secure soft-tissue repair, and sterile technique. With meticulous attention to detail, the majority of complications in shoulder arthroplasty can be avoided.

REFERENCES

1. Gunther SB, Norris TR. Shoulder arthroplasty: complications and revision. In Norris TR, ed. *Orthopaedic Knowledge Update: Shoulder and Elbow 2.* Rosemont, IL: American Shoulder and Elbow Surgeons, American Academy of Orthopaedic Surgeons, 2003:285–293.
2. Norris TR, Gunther SB. Revision shoulder surgery. In: Craig EV, ed. *Masters Techniques in Orthopaedic Surgery: The Shoulder.* Philadelphia: Lippincott Williams & Wilkins, 2004:621–641.
3. Jain N, Pietrobon R, Hocker S, et al. The relationship between surgeon and hospital volume and outcomes for shoulder arthroplasty. *J Bone Joint Surg Am* 2004;86:496–505.
4. Godeneche A, Boileau P, Favard L, et al. Prosthetic replacement in the treatment of osteoarthritis of the shoulder: early results of 268 cases. *J Shoulder Elb Surg* 2002;11:11–18.
5. Cofield R, Chang W, Sperling J. Complications of shoulder arthroplasty. In: Ianotti J, Williams G, eds. *Disorders of the Shoulder: Diagnosis and Management.* Philadelphia: Lippincott Williams & Wilkins, 1999:571–593.
6. Matsen FA III, Rockwood CA, Wirth MA, et al. Glenohumeral arthritis and its management. In: Matsen FA III, Rockwood CA, eds. *The Shoulder.* Philadelphia: WB Saunders, 1998:840–964.
7. Antuna SA, Sperling JW, Cofield RH, et al. Glenoid revision surgery after total shoulder arthroplasty. *J Shoulder Elbow Surg* 2001; 10:217–224.
8. Bonutti PM, Jacksins S, Matsen FA III. Component loosening in unconstrained shoulder arthroplasty. *Semin Arthroplasty* 1990;1: 124–128.

9. Boyd AD, Thomas WH, Sledge CB, et al. Failed shoulder arthroplasty. *Orthop Trans* 1990;14:255.

10. Cofield RH. Revision procedures for shoulder arthroplasty. In: Morrey BF, ed. *Reconstructive Surgery of the Joints.* New York: Churchill Livingston, 1996:789–799.

11. Hawkins RJ, Greis PE, Bonutti PM. Treatment of symptomatic glenoid loosening following unconstrained shoulder arthroplasty. *Orthopaedics* 1999;22:229–234.

12. Petersen SA, Hawkins RJ. Revision shoulder arthroplasty. In: Friedman RJ. *Arthroplasty of the Shoulder.* New York: Thieme Medical Publishers, 1994:234–241.

13. Seltzer DG. Revision shoulder arthroplasty. *Orthop Trans* 1996; 19:773.

14. Wirth MA, Rockwood CA. Complications of shoulder arthroplasty. *Clin Orthop* 1994;307:47–69.

15. Wirth MA, Rockwood CA Jr. Complications of total shoulder-replacement arthroplasty. *J Bone Joint Surg Am* 1996;78:603–616.

16. Wirth MA, Seltzer DG, Senes HR, et al. An analysis of failed humeral head and total shoulder arthroplasty (abstract). *J Shoulder Elb Surg* 1995;4:S13.

17. Arntz CT, Jackins SE, and Matsen FA III. Prosthetic replacement of the shoulder for the treatment of defects in the rotator cuff and the surface of the glenohumeral joint. *J Bone Joint Surg Am* 1993;75:485–491.

18. Franklin JL, Barrett WP, Jackins SE, et al. Glenoid loosening in total shoulder arthroplasty: association with rotator cuff deficiency. *J Arthroplasty* 1988;3:39–46.

19. Rodosky MW, Bigliani LU. Indications for glenoid resurfacing in shoulder arthroplasty. *J Shoulder Elbow Surg* 1996;5:231–248.

20. Brems J. The glenoid component in total shoulder arthroplasty. *J Arthroplasty* 1991;6:1–7.

21. Cofield RH. Total shoulder arthroplasty with Neer prosthesis. *J Bone Joint Surg Am* 1984;66:899–906.

22. Neer CSI, Watson KC, Stanton FJ. Recent experience in total shoulder replacement. *J Bone Joint Surg Am* 1982;64:1–13.

23. Wilde AH, Borden LS, Brems J. Experience with the Neer total shoulder replacement. In: Bateman JE and Welch RP, eds. *Surgery of the Shoulder.* St. Louis: Mosby, 1984:224–228.

24. Brems J. The glenoid component in total shoulder arthroplasty. *J Bone Joint Surg Am* 1993;2:47–54.

25. Kelly IG, Foster RS, Fisher WD. Neer total shoulder replacement in rheumatoid arthritis. *J Bone Joint Surg Br* 1987;69:723–726.

26. Barrett WP, Franklin JL, Jackins SE, et al. Total shoulder arthroplasty. *J Bone Joint Surg Am* 1987;69:865–872.

27. Torchia ME, Cofield RH, Settergren CR. Total shoulder arthroplasty with the Neer prosthesis: long-term results. *J Shoulder Elbow Surg* 1997;6:495–505.

28. Collins D, Tencer A, Sidles J, et al. Edge displacement and deformation of glenoid components in response to eccentric loading. The effect of preparation of the glenoid bone. *J Bone Joint Surg Am* 1992;74:501–507.

29. Boyd AD, Thomas WH, Scott RD, et al. Total shoulder arthroplasty versus hemiarthroplasty. *J Arthroplasty* 1990;5:329–336.

30. Brenner BC, Ferlic DC, Clayton ML, et al. Survivorship of unconstrained total shoulder arthroplasty. In Fourth International Conference on Surgery of the Shoulder. New York, 1989.

31. Cofield RH. Complications in total shoulder arthroplasty. In ICL No. 317. American Academy of Orthopaedic Surgeons Annual Meeting, San Francisco, CA, 1993.

32. Neer CSI, Watson KC, Stanton FJ. Recent experience in total shoulder replacement. *J Bone Joint Surg Am* 1982;64:319–337.

33. Barrett WP, Thornhill TS, Thomas BJ. Non-constrained total shoulder arthroplasty for patients with polyarticular rheumatoid arthritis. *J Arthroplasty* 1989;4:91–96.

34. Atkins RM, Langkamer VG, Perry MJ, et al. Bone-membrane interface in aseptic loosening of total joint arthroplasties. *J Arthroplasty* 1997;12:461–464.

35. Wirth MA, Agrawal CM, Mabrey JD. Isolation and characterization of polyethylene wear debris associated with osteolysis following total shoulder arthroplasty. *J Bone Joint Surg Am* 1999; 81:29–37.

36. Gunther SB, Graham J, Norris TR, et al. Retrieved glenoid components: a classification system for surface damage analysis. *J Arthroplasty* 2002;17:95–100.

37. Itamura JM, Papadakis SA, Roidis NT. Revision shoulder arthroplasty including bone deficiency. *Operative Tech Orthop* 2002;12:50–58.

38. Marra G, Yamaguchi K, Flatow EL. Failed total shoulder arthroplasty: revision and arthrodesis. In: Chapman MW, ed. *Chapman's Orthopaedic Surgery.* Philadelphia: Lippincott Williams & Wilkins, 2001.

39. Boyd AD, Aliabadi P, Thornhill TS. Postoperative proximal migration in total shoulder arthroplasty. *J Arthroplasty* 1991;6:31–37.

40. Moeckel BH, Dines DM, Warren RF, et al. Modular hemiarthroplasty for fractures of the proximal part of the humerus. *J Bone Joint Surg Am* 1992;74:884–889.

41. Miller SR, Bigliani LU. Complications of total shoulder replacement. In: Bigliani LU, ed. *Complications of Shoulder Surgery.* Baltimore: Williams & Wilkins, 1993:59–72.

42. Soghikian GW, Neviaser RJ. Complications of humeral head replacement. In: Bigliani LU, ed. *Complications of Shoulder Surgery.*, Baltimore: Williams & Wilkins, 1993:81–92.

43. Cofield RH, Edgerton BC. Total shoulder arthroplasty: complications and revision surgery. *Instr Course Lect* 1990;39:449–462.

44. Jahnke AHJ, Hawkins RJ. Instability after shoulder arthroplasty: causative factors and treatment options. *Semin Arthroplasty* 1995;6.

45. Wirth MA, Rockwood CA. Glenohumeral Instability following shoulder arthroplasty. Orlando, FL: American Academy of Orthopaedic Surgeons 62nd Annual Meeting, 1995.

46. Sanchez-Sotelo J, Sperling JW, Rowland CM, et al. Instability after shoulder arthroplasty: results of surgical treatment. *J Bone Joint Surg Am* 2003;85:622–631.

47. Matsen FA 3rd, Rockwood CA, Wirth MA, et al. Glenohumeral arthritis and its management. In: Matsen FA 3rd, ed. *Practical Evaluation and Management of the Shoulder.* Philadelphia: WB Saunders, 1994:851–852.

48. Cockx E, Claes T, Hoogmartens M, et al. The isoelastic prosthesis for the shoulder joint. *Acta Orthop Trans* 1983;49:275–285.

49. Faludi DD, Weiland AJ. Cementless total shoulder arthroplasty: preliminary experience with thirteen cases. *Orthopedics* 1983;6:431–438.

50. Gristina A, Romano RL, Kammire GC, et al. Total shoulder replacement. *Orthop Clin North Am* 1987;18:444–453.

51. McElwain JP, English E. The early results of porous-coated total shoulder arthroplasty. *Clin Orthop* 1987;218:217–224.

52. Moeckel BH, Altchek DW, Warren RF. Instability of the shoulder after arthroplasty. *J Bone Joint Surg Am* 1993;75:492–497.

53. Boyd AD, Thornhill TS, Thomas WH. Postoperative proximal migration in total shoulder replacement: Incidence and significance. New York: American Shoulder and Elbow Surgeons Annual Meeting, 1989.

54. Clayton ML, Ferlic DC, Jeffers PD. Prosthetic arthroplasty of the shoulder. *Clin Orthop* 1982;164:184.

55. Cofield RH, Stauffer RN. Total shoulder arthroplasty with a tissue-ingrowth glenoid component. *J Shoulder Elbow Surg* 1992;1:77–85.

56. Hawkins RJ, Bell RH, Jallay B. Total shoulder arthroplasty. *Clin Orthop* 1989;242:188–194.

57. Neer CSI, Morrison DS. Glenoid bone-grafting in total shoulder arthroplasty. *Clin Orthop* 1982;170:189–195.

58. Frich LH, Sojbjerg JO, Sneppen O. Shoulder arthroplasty with the Neer Mark-II prothesis. *Arch Orthop Trauma Surg* 1988;107:110–113.

59. Neer CSI, Kirby RM. Revision of humeral head and total shoulder arthroplasty. *Clin Orthop* 1982;170:189–195.

60. Pahle JA, Kvarnes L. Shoulder replacement arthroplasty. *Ann Chir Gynaecol* 1985;74(Suppl 198):85–89.

61. Matsoukis J, Tabib W, Guiffault P, et al. Shoulder arthroplasty for osteoarthritis after prior surgery for anterior instability: a report of 27 cases. *Rev Chir Orthop Reparatrice Appar Mot* 2003;89:580–592.

62. Matsoukis J, Tabib W, Guiffault P, et al. Shoulder arthroplasty in patients with a prior anterior shoulder dislocation. Results of a multicenter study. *J Bone Joint Surg Am* 2003;85:1417–1424.

63. Gerber A, Clavert P, Millett PJ, et al. Split pectoralis major and teres major tendon for reconstruction of irreparable tears of the subscapularis. *Tech Shoulder Elb Surg* 2004;5:5–12.

64. Wirth MA, Rockwood CA Jr. Complications of shoulder arthroplasty. *Clin Orthop* 1994;307:47–69.

65. Collins D, Tencer A, Sidles J, et al. Edge displacement and deformation of glenoid components in response to eccentric loading. *J Bone Joint Surg Am* 1992;74:501–507.

66. Pollack RG, Deliz ED, McIlveen SJ, et al. Prosthetic replacement in rotator cuff-deficient shoulders. *J Shoulder Elbow Surg* 1992;1:173–186.

67. Frich LH, Sojbjerg JO, Sneppen O. Shoulder arthroplasty in complex acute and chronic proximal humeral fractures. *J Bone Joint Surg Am* 1991;14:949–954.

68. Brems J. Management of osteoarthritis in the shoulder. In: Norris TR, ed. *Orthopaedic Knowledge Update: Shoulder and Elbow 2*. Rosemont, IL: American Academy of Orthopaedic Surgeons, 2003.

69. Sirveaux F, Favard L, Oudet D, et al. Grammont inverted total shoulder prosthesis in the treatment of glenohumeral arthritis with massive rupture of the rotator cuff. *J Bone Joint Surg Br* 2004;86:388–395.

70. Norris TR, Lipson SR. Management of unstable prosthetic shoulder arthroplasty. *Instr Course Lect* 1998;47:141–148.

71. Neer CSI. *Shoulder Reconstruction*. Philadelphia: WB Saunders, 1990.

72. Post M, Pollack RG. Operative treatment of degenerative and arthritic diseases of the glenohumeral joint. In: Post M. *The Shoulder: Operative Technique*. Philadelphia: Lippincott Williams & Wilkins, 1998:73–132.

73. Schenk T, Iannotti J. Prosthetic arthroplasty for the glenohumeral arthritis with and intact or repairable rotator cuff: indication, techniques, and results. In: Inannotti JW, ed. *Disorders of the Shoulder: Diagnosis and Mangement*. Philadelphia: Lippincott Williams & Wilkins, 1999:521–557.

74. Neer, CSI, Morrison DS. Glenoid bone grafting in total shoulder arthroplasty. *J Bone Joint Surg Am* 1988;70:1154–1162.

75. Cofield RH. Total shoulder replacement: managing bone deficiencies. In: Craig EV. *Master Techniques in Orthopaedic Surgery: The Shoulder*. Philadelphia, Lippincott Williams & Wilkins, 2004:549–575.

76. Friedman RJ, Hawthorn K, Genez BM. Evaluation of glenoid bone loss with computerized tomography for total shoulder arthroplasty. *Orthop Trans* 1991;15:749–753.

77. Fenlin JMJ. Total glenohumeral joint replacement. *Orthop Clin North Am* 1976;67:565–583.

78. Wirth MA, Rockwood CA. Glenohumeral instability following shoulder arthroplasty. *Orthop Trans* 1995;19:459.

79. Gerber A, Warner JJP, Clavert P, et al. Hemiarthroplasty for proximal humerus fracture: A new method to obtain correct humeral length. In *4th Biennial AAOS/ASES Shoulder and Elbow: Current Techniques and Controversies*. Monterey, CA: American Academy of Orthopaedic Surgeons and the American Shoulder and Elbow Surgeons, 2004.

80. Barrett WP, Thornhill TS, Thomas WH, et al. Nonconstrained total shoulder arthroplasty in rheumatoid arthritis. *J Arthroplasty* 1989;4:91–96.

81. Kelly IG, Foster RS, Fisher WD. Neer total shoulder replacement in rheumatoid arthritis. *J Bone Joint Surg Br* 1987;69:723–726.

82. Neer CSI. Replacement arthroplasty for glenohumeral arthritis. *J Bone Joint Surg Am* 1974;56:1–13.

83. Amstutz HC, Thomas BJ, Kabo JM, et al. The Dana total shoulder arthroplasty. *J Bone Joint Surg Am* 1988;70:1174–1182.

84. Figgie LH, Inglis AE, Figgie HE 3rd, et al. Custom total shoulder arthroplasty in inflammatory arthritis: preliminary results. *J Arthroplasty* 1991;7:1–6.

85. Wirth MA. Part I: periprosthetic fractures of the upper extremity. In: Rockwood CA, ed. *Fractures*. Philadelphia: J.B. Lippincott, 1996:540–576.

86. Bonutti PM, Hawkins RJ. Fracture of the humeral shaft associated with total replacement arthroplasty of the shoulder: a case report. *J Bone Joint Surg Am* 1992;74:617–618.

87. Boyd AD, Thornhill TS, Barnes CL. Fractures adjacent to the humeral prosthesis. *J Bone Joint Surg Am* 1992;74:1498–1504.

88. Averill RM, Sledge CB, Thomas WH. Neer total shoulder arthroplasty (abstract). *Orthop Trans* 1980;4:287.

89. Torchia ME, Cofield RH, Settergren CR. Total shoulder arthroplasty with the Neer prosthesis: long-term results. *Orthop Trans* 1995;18:1994–1995.

90. McCoy SR, Warren RF, Bade HA 3rd, et al. Total shoulder arthroplasty in rheumatoid arthritis. *J Arthroplasty* 1989;4:105–113.

91. Groh GI. Treatment of fractures adjacent to the humeral prosthesis. *Orthop Trans* 1994–1995;18:1072.

92. Krakauer JD, Cofield RH. Periprosthetic fractures in total shoulder replacement. *Operative Tech Orthop* 1994;4:243–252.

93. Cambell JT, Moore RS, Iannotti JP, et al. Periprosthetic humeral fractures—mechanisms of fracture and treatment options. *Orthop Trans* 1996;20:59–63.

94. Wright TW, Cofield RH. Humeral fractures after shoulder arthroplasty. *J Bone Joint Surg Am* 1995;78:1340–1346.

95. Campbell JT, Moore RS, Iannotti JP, et al. Periprosthetic humeral fractures: mechanisms of fracture and treatment options. *J Shoulder Elbow Surg* 1998;7:406–413.

96. Boileau P, Mole D, Walch G. Technique of glenoid resurfacing in shoulder arthroplasty. In: Walch G, Boileau P, eds. *Shoulder Arthroplasty*. Berlin: Springer, 2000.

97. Wirth MA, Basamania C, Rockwood CA. Fixation of the glenoid component. *Operative Tech Orthop* 1994;4:218–221.

98. Kumar S, Sperling JW, Haidukewych GH, et al. Periprosthetic humeral fractures after shoulder arthroplasty. *J Bone Joint Surg Am* 2004;86:680–689.

99. Worland RL, Kim DY, Arredondo J. Periprosthetic humeral fractures: management and classification. *J Shoulder Elbow Surg* 1999;8:590–594.

100. Cameron B, Iannotti JP. Periprosthetic fractures of the humerus and scapula: management and prevention. *Orthop Clin North Am* 1999;30:305–318.

101. Incavo SJ, Beard DM, Pupparo F, et al. One-stage revision of periprosthetic fractures around loose cemented total hip arthroplasty. *Am J Orthop* 1998;27:35–41.

102. Esterhai JL Jr, Gelb I. Adult septic arthritis. *Orthop Clin North Am* 1991;22:503–514.

103. Amstutz HC, Sew Hoy AL, Clarke IC. UCLA anatomic total shoulder arthroplasty. *Clin Orthop Relat Res* 1981;(155):7–20.

104. Bell SN, Gschwend N. Clinical experience with total arthroplasty and hemiarthroplasty of the shoulder using the Neer prosthesis. *Int Orthop* 1986;10:217–222.

105. Brostrom LA, Kronberg M, Wallensten R. Should the glenoid be replaced in shoulder arthroplasty with an unconstrained DANA or St. Georg prosthesis? *Ann Chir Gynaecol* 1992;81:54–57.

106. Fenlin JM Jr, Ramsey ML, Allardyce TJ, et al. Modular total shoulder replacement. Design rationale, indications, and results. *Clin Orthop* 1994;307:37–46.

107. Figgie HE 3rd, Inglis AE, Goldberg VM, et al. An analysis of factors affecting the long-term results of total shoulder arthroplasty in inflammatory arthritis. *J Arthroplasty* 1988:123–130.

108. Petersson CJ. Shoulder surgery in rheumatoid arthritis. *Acta Orthop Scand* 1986:222–226.

109. Roper BA, Paterson JMH, Day WH. The Roper-Day total shoulder replacement. *J Bone Joint Surg Br* 1990;72:694–697.

110. Vahvanen V, Hamalainen M, Paavolainen P. The Neer II replacement for rheumatoid arthritis of the shoulder. *Int Orthop* 1989:57–60.

111. Bodey WN, Yeoman PM. Prosthetic arthroplasty of the shoulder. *Acta Orthop Scand* 1983:900–903.

112. Cockx E, Claes T, Hoogmartens M, et al. The isoelastic prosthesis for the shoulder joint. *Acta Orthop Belg* 1983;49:275–285.

113. Cruess RL. Corticosteroid-induced osteonecrosis of the humeral head. *Orthop Clin North Am* 1985:789–796.

114. Hawkins RJ, Neer CS 2nd, Pianta RM, et al. Locked posterior dislocation of the shoulder. *J Bone Joint Surg Am* 1987;69:9–18.

115. Jonsson E, Brattstrom M, Lidgren L. Evaluation of the rheumatoid shoulder function after hemiarthroplasty and arthrodesis. *Scand J Rheumatol* 1988:17–26.

116. Jonsson E, Egund N, Kelly I, et al. Cup arthroplasty of the rheumatoid shoulder. *Acta Orthop Scand* 1986; 57:542–546.

117. Kay SP, Amstutz HC. Shoulder hemiarthroplasty at UCLA. *Clin Orthop* 1988:42–48.
118. Moeckel BH, Dines DM, Warren RF, et al. Modular hemiarthroplasty for fractures of the proximal part of the humerus. *J Bone Joint Surg Am* 1992;74:884–889.
119. Pritchett JW, Clark JM. Prosthetic replacement for chronic unreduced dislocations of the shoulder. *Clin Orthop* 1987:89–93.
120. Brennan PJ, DeGirolamo MP. Musculoskeletal infections in immunocompromised hosts. *Orthop Clin North Am* 1991:389–399.
121. Gelberman RH, Menon J, Austerlitz MS, et al. Pyogenic arthritis of the shoulder in adults. *J Bone Joint Surg Am* 1980;62:550–553.
122. Gristina AG, Naylor PT, Myrvik QN. Musculoskeletal infection, microbial adhesion, and antibiotic resistance. *Infect Dis Clin North Am* 1990:391–408.
123. Gristina AG, Naylor PT, Webb LX. Molecular mechanisms in musculoskeletal sepsis: the race for the surface. *Instr Course Lect* 1990:471–482.
124. Ward WG, Goldner RD. Shoulder pyarthrosis: a concomitant process. *Orthopedics* 1994:591–595.
125. Lichtman EA. Candida infection of a prosthetic shoulder joint. *Skeletal Radiol* 1983:176–177.
126. Leslie BM, Harris JM 3rd, Driscoll D. Septic arthritis of the shoulder in adults. *J Bone Joint Surg Am* 1989:1516–1522.
127. Codd TP, Yamaguchi K, Flatow EL. *Infected shoulder arthroplasties: treatment with staged reimplantations vs. resection arthroplasty.* Orlando, FL: Annual Meeting of the American Shoulder and Elbow Surgeons, 1995.
128. Coste JS, Reig S, Trojani C, et al. The management of infection in arthroplasty of the shoulder. *J Bone Joint Surg Br* 2004;86:65–69.
129. Mileti J, Sperling JW, Cofield RH. Reimplantation of a shoulder arthroplasty after a previous infected arthroplasty. *J Shoulder Elbow Surg* 2004:528–531.
130. Loebenberg MI, Zuckerman JD. An articulating interval spacer in the treatment of an infected total shoulder arthroplasty. *J Shoulder Elbow Surg* 2004:476–478.
131. Springer BD, Lee GC, Osmon D, et al. Systemic safety of high-dose antibiotic-loaded cement spacers after resection of an infected total knee arthroplasty. *Clin Orthop* 2004:47–51.
132. Banit DM, Kaufer H, Hartford JM. Intraoperative frozen section analysis in revision total joint arthroplasty. *Clin Orthop* 2002:230–238.
133. Sunderland S. Funicular suture and funicular exclusion in the repair of severed nerves. *Br J Surg* 1953:580–587.
134. Brenner BC, Ferlic DC, Clayton ML, et al. Survivorship of unconstrained total shoulder arthroplasty. *J Bone Joint Surg Am* 1989;71:1289–1296.
135. Driessnack RP, Ferlic DC, Wiedel JD. Dissociation of the glenoid component in the Macnab/English total shoulder arthroplasty. *J Arthroplasty* 1990:15–18.
136. Clayton ML, Ferlic DC, Jeffers PD. Prosthetic arthroplasties of the shoulder. *Clin Orthop* 1982:184–191.
137. Cooper RA, Brems JJ. Recurrent disassembly of a modular humeral prosthesis. A case report. *J Arthroplasty* 1991:375–377.
138. Blevins FT, Deng X, Torzilli PA, et al. Dissociation of modular humeral head components: a biomechanical and implant retrieval study. *J Shoulder Elbow Surg* 1997;6:113–124.
139. Neer CS 2nd, Watson KC, Stanton FJ. Recent experience in total shoulder replacement. *J Bone Joint Surg Am* 1982:319–337.
140. Neer CS 2nd, Kirby RM. Revision of humeral head and total shoulder arthroplasties. *Clin Orthop* 1982:189–195.
141. Warner JJ, Greis PE. The treatment of stiffness of the shoulder after repair of the rotator cuff. *Instr Course Lect* 1998:67–75.
142. Sher JS, Iannotti JP, Warner JJ, et al. Surgical treatment of postoperative deltoid origin disruption. *Clin Orthop* 1997;343:93–98.
143. McMahon PJ, Jobe FW, Pink MM, et al. Comparative electromyographic analysis of shoulder muscles during planar motions: anterior glenohumeral instability versus normal. *J Shoulder Elbow Surg* 1996;5:118–123.
144. Blaiser RB, Guldberg RE, Rothman ED. Anterior shoulder stability: contributions of rotator cuff forces and the capsular constraints in the cadaver model. *J Shoulder Elbow Surg* 1992;1:140–150.
145. Cain PR, Mutschler TA, Fu FH, et al. Anterior stability of the glenohumeral joint. A dynamic model. *Am J Sports Med* 1987;15:144–148.
146. O'Brien SJ, Schwartz RS, Warren RF, et al. Capsular restraints to anterior-posterior motion of the abducted shoulder: a biomechanical study. *J Shoulder Elbow Surg* 1995;4:298–308.
147. O'Connell PW, Nuber GW, Mileski RA, et al. The contribution of the glenohumeral ligaments to anterior stability of the shoulder joint. *Am J Sports Med* 1990;18:579–584.
148. McFarland EG, Edward G, Park HB, et al. Modification of the subscapularis splitting technique for anterior shoulder reconstructions. *Tech Shoulder Elbow Surg* 2003;4:18–23.

Complications of Fracture Management

5

Theodore F. Schlegel   *Patrick N. Siparsky*   *Richard J. Hawkins*

INTRODUCTION

This chapter focuses on identifying the potential complications that are encountered when caring for patients with fractures of the proximal humerus and clavicle. By becoming familiar with these potential problems, it is our hope that most of these adverse outcomes can be avoided. As has been stated so eloquently in the past, "An ounce of prevention is worth a pound of cure." This is particularly relevant when managing difficult fractures of the shoulder girdle. For operative treatment, it is the surgeon's obligation to discuss all the potential complications as part of an informed consent. If the unfortunate situation arises in which an undesirable outcome occurs, it is important to have an array of options to deal with these situations. It is our goal to provide strategies to avoid these situations and advice on what to do if they do happen.

COMPLICATIONS OF OPERATIVE MANAGEMENT IN SHOULDER GIRDLE FRACTURES: NONSPECIFIC TO FRACTURE TYPE

There have been many reported complications following open treatment of clavicle and displaced proximal humeral fractures. For discussion purposes, it is easiest to think of these in one of two ways: nonspecific complications that can occur regardless of the fracture pattern and location, including infection, neurovascular injuries, hardware failure, joint stiffness, and heterotopic ossification; or fracture-specific complications that are known to occur secondary

to the type of fracture and location, including problems such as malunions, nonunions, or avascular necrosis. Avascular necrosis is rarely seen in two- and three-part fractures, but is more likely to occur in four-part displaced proximal humeral fractures (1).

Infection

Infection is rare with open reduction and internal fixation (ORIF) of fractures involving the shoulder girdle. Fortunately, the shoulder girdle has adequate soft-tissue coverage with an extensive vascular supply to the tissues, decreasing the risk of infection. However, infection is still possible, and it is for this reason that care should be taken to maintain sterility, administer prophylactic antibiotics, and minimize excessive soft-tissue dissection. Obtaining homeostasis at the time of closure and appropriately draining the wound (particularly in proximal humeral fractures) is important in preventing hematoma formation, which increases the risk of infection.

If the infection occurs early in the postoperative period, the patient may present with a constellation of findings from increased pain, decreased motion, erythema, and skin temperature changes, as well as systemic complaints of fever/chills, loss of appetite, and fatigue. If an infection is suspected, then a thorough workup is warranted. This should include a panel of blood tests including a complete blood cell count with differential, erythrocyte sedimentation rate, and a C-reactive protein measurement. Although these tests may be suggestive of an infection, the combination of results are probably the most important when attempting to make the diagnosis. Imaging should include plain film radiographs to look for the possibility of a retained foreign body such as a surgical sponge or for any early loosening of surgically implanted hardware (Fig. 5-1). Other studies such as magnetic resonance imaging (MRI) with gadolinium can be helpful in difficult situations and may be useful in surgical planning, particularly if an abscess is identified. However, the difficulty of using an MRI comes with the imaging artifact that occurs with metal implants.

In cases of deep infection, it is necessary to address this problem early with a formal open irrigation and debridement. With proximal humerus fractures, arthroscopic treatment alone is usually not sufficient to treat these problems because the infection usually involves both the joint and more superficial structures. At the time of surgery, both aerobic and anaerobic cultures should be obtained. Early infection within the first 2 weeks is frequently the result of a *Staphylococcus aureus* infection (2). In more indolent cases with a later presentation, one should consider causes such as *Peptostrepococcus*. In this situation, it is often necessary to request the lab culture specifically for this organism. Positive results may take up to 7 days in certain circumstances.

Regardless of the suspected organism, the principals of a complete and thorough surgical debridement should be adhered to specifically. This includes a sharp resection of the skin edges back to healthy bleeding tissues, followed by a similar treatment of the deeper layers. Inspection of the joint should be completed, particularly in cases involving the proximal humerus where the joint has been previously violated. A pulsed lavage device using a bacteriostatic

solution such a bacitracin is recommended (3). The hardware should be retained in these situations if there is no gross loosening. The wound is closed over heavy drains, usually left in place for at least 48 hours or until there is minimal output. A heavy monofilament absorbable suture is recommended for closure, minimizing the risk of harboring residual bacteria with a braided-type stitch. For long-term function, it is important to try to preserve the integrity of the rotator cuff if possible by repairing the tissue. If the tissue is of poor quality or there is excessive tension on the repair, then it is better to avoid repair.

Neurovascular Injuries

Neurovascular injuries have been well documented following both clavicle and displaced proximal humeral fractures. With clavicle fractures, neurovascular compromise often is the result of abundant callus, malunion, or fracture displacement. The vascular structures that have been reported to be involved in compression syndromes include the carotid artery and subclavian vein and/or artery. The brachial plexus can be injured as a result of a neuropraxia or progressive compression affecting the medial cord, which often produces primarily ulnar nerve symptoms (4).

Complications can also occur from hardware placement or abnormal migration, particularly with intramedullary fixation devices. Injuries have been reportedly associated with Hagie pins migration to the aorta and subclavian artery (5). Hence, care must be taken in pin placement and observation of pin location postoperatively should be noted.

With displaced proximal humeral fractures, Stableforth (6) reported a 5% incidence of axillary artery compromise and a 6.2% incidence of brachial plexus injuries. Vascular injury is most often associated with penetrating or violent blunt trauma caused by the initial injury, but also occurs after ORIF (7). If a vascular disruption occurs, the lesion is usually found at the junction of the anterior humeral circumflex artery and axillary artery. The diagnosis is often difficult to make because peripheral pulses may be normal as a result of collateral circulation. Paraesthesis may be a helpful clinical finding. Because early diagnosis and repair are crucial to the outcome, angiography and exploration should be performed immediately when a vascular injury is suspected.

The axillary nerve is susceptible to injury following fractures and surgical treatment. The axillary nerve provides motor supply to the deltoid and teres major muscles with sensory distribution over the lateral aspect of the upper arm. Sensation over the lateral deltoid region is not a reliable means of determining if there is an axillary nerve injury. A more reliable means of testing the axillary nerve is palpating all three leaves of the deltoid muscle for contraction. Due to pain in an acute fracture, this is often difficult to

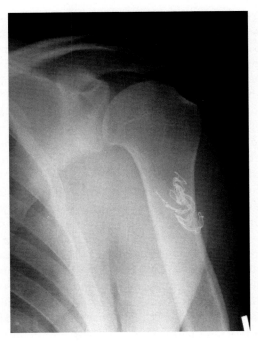

Figure 5-1 Postoperatively retained foreign body.

accurately assess. Immediate surgical intervention is considered in cases where there is felt to be the possibility of iatrogenic injury caused by a trauma from a suture around the nerve or entrapment of the nerve under the hardware. However, most of these injuries are secondary to a neuropraxia and improve with time.

Electromyelography should be performed if a nerve injury is suspected. This study should be obtained no earlier than 3 weeks after the injury where the results are more accurate, both for documentation and as a baseline for subsequent comparisons of recovery. If a complete axillary nerve injury does not improve within a 3-month period, surgical exploration should be considered.

Stiffness

Postoperative stiffness is not uncommon after surgical treatment of these complex fractures (Fig. 5-2). Factors contributing to the development of postsurgical stiffness include extensive soft-tissue trauma, delay in surgical intervention, necessary protection of comminuted bone fragments, and inability to aggressively institute active and passive motion until satisfactory early healing has occurred. Early passive range-of-motion exercises and careful patient selection minimize the likelihood of the development of stiffness.

If arthrofibrosis develops, surgical intervention can be considered if the patient fails to progress with an aggressive, well-supervised rehabilitation program. It is our preference to avoid operative treatment within the first 12 weeks following surgery for two reasons. First, despite instituting early patient restrictions, it is often possible to make gradual gains in motion with joint distraction techniques and terminal stretching programs. Careful documentation of

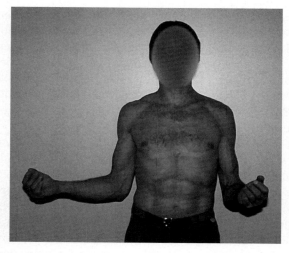

Figure 5-2 Clinical presentation of significant restriction of external rotation of the left shoulder.

motion measurements is critical in determining if progress is being made. Even if only small gains are seen, it is reasonable to continue with the program. Only after the patient plateaus is it necessary to consider surgical intervention. Second, because of the ongoing inflammatory healing cascade that is present during the first 3 months after surgery, it is better to delay an additional operation, which would create a second traumatic event and a further inflammatory process.

In our experience with patients who do not progress with therapy, it is critical to determine whether the loss of motion represents a functional disability. This may vary greatly between patients depending on their preinjury level of activity. Realistic goals should be set because the outcome of surgery may be unpredictable. Only after that time is it reasonable to consider surgical intervention. As opposed to idiopathic arthrofibrosis, postsurgical stiffness is rarely responsive to manipulation alone. This method of treatment is unpredictable and potentially fraught with problems.

If surgery is necessary, we prefer to administer arthroscopic capsular release. This is completed by placing the arthroscope through a standard posterior portal, followed by establishing an anterior working portal. As with other conditions of stiffness, it is important to resect the fibrotic scar from the rotator cuff interval. This can be achieved most effectively using a bipolar device rather than a mechanical shaver, which often creates more bleeding. This is then followed by separation of the middle glenohumeral ligament and capsule from the underlying subscapularis tendon. This tissue can then be divided halfway between the glenoid and humerus without disrupting the subscapularis tendon. By using the bipolar cautery device, there is a minimized chance of injury to the axillary nerve, particularly as the release is carried more inferiorly in the pouch.

It is also important to limit the resection only through the capsule and avoid plunging deep to prevent neurologic damage. Contraction of the deltoid during the capsular release should be carefully monitored. Even when an interscalene block is present, contraction of the deltoid can occur through direct electrical stimulation of the nerve. With a postsurgical contracture, the normal anatomic course of the nerve may be altered leading to close proximity of this structure particularly inferiorly. The release is then completed inferiorly. This is followed by switching the arthroscope to the anterior portal and using the posterior portal to complete the release posteriorly. A circumferential release enhances the likelihood of successful outcome. At this point, glenohumeral motion is assessed. If external rotation is still limited, it is then reasonable to consider releasing the subscapularis tendon. After this time, a gentle manipulation under anesthesia can be considered.

Postoperatively, it is helpful to have a long-acting interscalene block for pain control. This also allows for repeat therapeutic terminal stretching exercises to be performed with the supervision of a therapist. It may also be helpful to use a shoulder continuous passive motion (CPM) machine in these cases. A compressive cryotherapy unit will assist in reducing postoperative inflammation. During the first 2 weeks, supervised physical therapy should be completed at least three to five times per week. The patient will also be expected to perform terminal stretching exercises at home with three sets of 20, in all planes of motion, at least five times per day.

Heterotopic Ossification

Heterotopic ossification appears to be related to both forceful attempt at closed reduction and delay in open reduction beyond 1 week for fracture dislocations (Fig. 5-3). Inadequate irrigation to wash out bony fragments following ORIF may also increase the risk of heterotopic ossification. Exercises to maintain range of motion should be the mainstay of treatment. After 1 year, if a negative bone scan indicates quiescence, excision of the heterotopic bone with soft-tissue releases may be considered.

Wire Breakage and Hardware Complications

Although wire breakage can occur, particularly if the fracture fails to unite, it is not a common complication. Nevertheless, wire breakage has caused some surgeons to recommend very heavy nonabsorbable suture in this tension-band technique. This seems to be a sensible way to avoid this potential complication without compromising the fixation or result.

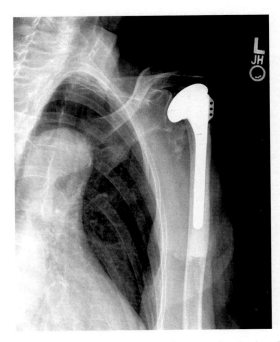

Figure 5-3 Heterotopic ossification following hemiarthroplasty.

COMPLICATIONS OF OPERATIVE MANAGEMENT FOR FRACTURES OF THE SHOULDER GIRDLE: SPECIFIC TO FRACTURE LOCATION AND PATTERN

Proximal Humeral Fractures

Two-Part Fractures

Malunion/Nonunion

Malunions and nonunions tend to occur in two-part fractures where the greater tuberosity segment remains displaced, typically superiorly or posteriorly. Subacromial decompression does not usually successfully treat the problem, and hence repositioning of the segment is necessary. In these situations, an osteotomy of the displaced fragment is necessary. With this technique, it is important to take a large enough bone fragment to achieve rigid fixation once the tuberosity is transposed to its normal anatomic position. Releases may be required to mobilize the fragment and take tension off the repair. The rotator cuff interval should be closed at the end of the procedure. Pain and limited range of motion are common indicators for surgical intervention (Fig. 5-4) (8).

Nonunion from displaced tuberosity fracture can occur, although it is rare. If a nonunion arises, treatment can be achieved employing a tension band wiring technique with bone grafting.

Three-Part Fractures

Malunion

In three-part fractures, it is unusual where a tension-band technique would result in malposition of the humeral head because the tuberosities are carefully reapproximated to each other and one tuberosity remains attached to the hu-

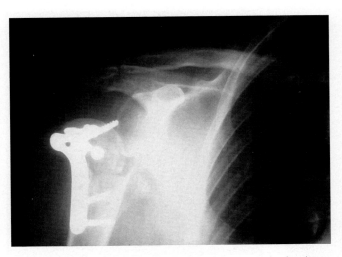

Figure 5-4 Humeral head collapse and intraarticular hardware following ORIF.

meral head. Mild degrees of abnormal angulation of the humeral head relative to the shaft may also occur. These are ordinarily not functionally a problem.

Nonunion

With secure internal fixation by tension-band method, nonunion is rarely seen. Alternate forms of fixation have been associated with a higher incidence of nonunion. This may be related to the extensive dissection required for other internal fixation devices, or it may be related to poor-quality bone inadequately supporting plates and screws. The possibility of nonunion is minimized by careful attention to intraoperative technique, making certain the fracture is well reduced, carefully controlling the direction and degree of arm movement in the early postoperative rehabilitation period. More frequently, nonunion results from displaced three-part fractures seen specifically with surgical neck fracture. In this situation, a second operation of internal fixation and bone grafting or prosthetic arthroplasty is usually required.

Avascular Necrosis

Although the three-part fracture by definition has one tuberosity remaining to give the humeral head blood supply, late avascular necrosis may occur (Fig. 5-5). This most frequently occurs when the lesser tuberosity remains with the humeral head. This potential complication can be minimized by careful patient selection. If doubt exists about adequacy of bone, adequacy of soft-tissue attachment to residual humeral head or tuberosity structures, or failure to obtain secure internal fixation, the surgeon should proceed directly to a primary prosthetic arthroplasty. Should late collapse of the humeral head from avascular necrosis occur, the degree of symptoms may not warrant further surgical

intervention. However, should the patient develop symptomatic avascular necrosis following a complex fracture of the proximal humerus, total shoulder replacement rather than hemiarthroplasty is probably the wisest choice.

Four-Part Fractures

The complications associated with treatment of four-part proximal humerus fractures are similar to those of three-part fractures, but with increasing severity and more frequent avascular necrosis and malunion (9).

Malunion

There is an increased likelihood of malunion in four-part humerus fractures due to the difficulty of soft-tissue balancing and maintenance of soft-tissue resection, especially after hemiarthroplasty. Malunion of the greater tuberosity can be a functional problem when the displaced fragment limits the subacromial space, causing impingement when the arm is in abduction. Osteotomy of the tuberosity is then performed as a salvage procedure, particularly in those cases with significant displacement (10). Careful dissection is required to avoid further complications with neurovascular structures near scar tissue, and a large enough fragment is necessary for rigid fixation (9).

Tuberosity Failure

Failure of fixation of the tuberosity can be a source of pain and functional disability following hemiarthroplasty. This can occur either from inadequate initial fixation of the fracture fragment or from aggressive physical therapy after surgery. These patients will frequently have persistent pain and present with symptoms consistent with those of rotator cuff tears. This can be an extremely challenging problem. These

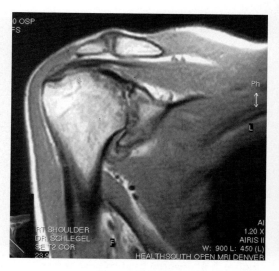 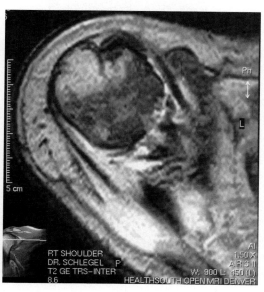

Figure 5-5 Coronal and axial views of avascular necrosis humeral head.

patients will frequently present with symptoms of pain and weakness. The diagnosis can often be made on plain film alone. Additional imaging using a computed tomography (CT) arthrogram can help by determining the position of the tuberosity and also may help with confirmation of the rotator cuff integrity. If there is tuberosity failure, an attempt at rerepair is reasonable, particularly if the symptoms are warranted. However, one should know that the outcome may be unpredictable. In our experience, up to half of the time it may not be possible to reattach the tuberosity or repair the torn rotator cuff.

Instability

Postsurgical instability in four-part fractures is not uncommon; however, there are different rates reported in the literature following hemiarthroplasty. Anterior-superior migration of the humeral head is thought to be the most frequent pattern of humeral head instability (10). Migration patterns are often associated with inadequate soft tissue, tuberosity failure, poor arthroplasty positioning, or neurologic injury. Extensive displacement of the head can lead to various functional limitations, and unfortunately the treatment for this still is difficult and often unsuccessful.

Prosthesis-Associated Complications

Prosthesis malpositioning can present as a common complication in proximal humerus fractures. It is important that the surgeon be competent and careful in selecting component sizes and eventual component alignment. Malposition can result in extensive complications, thus proper prosthetic height, angle, and fixation should always be thought of prior to surgery to avoid adverse outcomes. It has been suggested that using contralateral templating and intraoperative guides to assess version may be useful in avoiding undesirable complications (10).

Clavicle Fractures

Most acute fractures of the clavicle do not require surgical intervention to heal properly. However, when surgery is indicated, complications specific to this location include hardware problems, malunion/nonunions, and neurovascular compromise.

Hardware Problems

Hardware problems are seen commonly in repair of clavicle fractures (11). This is concerning because of the extensive neurovascular structures located near the injury site, especially with migration of wires, pins, and screws. More commonly, patients complain of contact pain, including difficulty carrying bags with straps that irritate the screw heads. This may also indicate failed fixation. Plating and screw fixation is often subject to failure from poor bone quality, such as in an elderly patient. Because of the standard superior position of the plate, patients frequently experience

discomfort. Therefore, patients should be counseled on the possibility of symptomatic hardware, which may require delayed removal of the plate following fracture union.

Malunion and Nonunions

The majority of clavicle fractures can be successfully treated nonoperatively (12). However, it is not uncommon for these fractures to heal with some angulation and/or shortening (Fig. 5-6). In these cases, it is less common for the patient to complain of a functional disability, but more frequently of a cosmetic issue. In many of these cases, it is possible to improve on the cosmetic appearance by simply contouring the bone at the malunion site. Functional disabilities more frequently occur as a result of nonunion. Nonunion typically occurs with fractures of the middle third of the clavicle with large fragment separation (1,12,13). Several different techniques have been developed for repairing this injury, including plating and pinning; however, there is currently no consensus on which repair is most effective. If a plate is used, anatomical reduction of the fracture fragments is nearly always possible, despite the potential for osteoporosis under the plate and fracture at the ends of the plate or near the screws (13). If a clavicle pin is employed, there is a theoretical possibility of not obtaining an anatomic reduction. In this situation, a limited exposure is used to perform a retrograde pinning technique, which could lead to malalignment. Even if there is some residual shortening or angulation, this will usually be well tolerated by most patients. Rarely does one require revision surgery in these cases because it is performed in specific cases only. It has been our preference to perform an open reduction and rigid plating of the nonunion. As has been previously described by Jupiter et al. (14), we prefer to place the plate on the superior surface, which is the tension side of the bone. We will make an incision slightly inferior to the clavicle to avoid problems with wound healing. It is important to achieve as much soft tissue coverage over the plate as possible at the time of closure. For atrophic non-

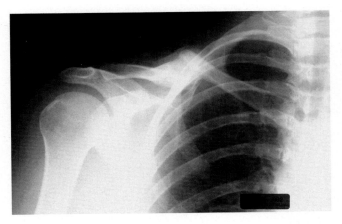

Figure 5-6 Nonunion clavicle with significant displacement.

unions, we always take down the psuedoarthrosis and bone graft the site.

Neurovascular Injury

Though relatively uncommon, neurovascular injury can occur in clavicle fracture. This is seen frequently if there is extensive callus formation or bony fragment separation (11,12). Callus formation on the inferior aspect of the clavicle can disrupt subclavian vessels, causing potentially serious complications. Similarly, the brachial plexus can suffer compressive type injury with clavicle fracture. This is most commonly recognized as ulnar nerve insufficiency or irritation. Careful examination should be done to expose potential neurovascular injury and action should be taken as quickly as possible to avoid potentially serious complications associated with neurovascular injury, including excessive bleeding or permanent neurological damage.

CONCLUSION

A proactive mindset is the best way to avoid complications. As surgeons, there are many things that we can control in our treatment of fractures occurring around the shoulder. Attention to aseptic techniques, prophylactic antibiotics, and careful handling of soft tissues can lessen the potential risk of infection. A detailed understanding of the pertinent anatomy will help avoid neurovascular injuries. A thorough understanding of the fracture pattern and treatment options will help maximize a successful treatment algorithm. Despite our best intentions, many of these problems may be out of our control. Even if we strive to avoid them, they are inevitable. When they occur, it is our hope that the information in this chapter will help lead to the best possible outcome. These situations can often be very stressful for both the patient and the treating physician. The key to a successful outcome is early identification of the problem and a well thought-out treatment plan. It is important to communicate with the patient and outline realistic expectations.

ACKNOWLEDGEMENTS

We are grateful for the assistance provided by Jenna Godfrey in preparing this manuscript.

REFERENCES

1. Schlegel T, Hawkins R. Operative treatment of three-part proximal humeral fractures. In: Craig EV, ed. *Master Techniques in Orthopaedic Surgery: The Shoulder*. Philadelphia: Lippincott Williams & Wilkins, 2004:413–426.
2. Canale ST, ed. *Campbell's Operative Orthopaedics*, 10th ed. St. Louis: Mosby, 2003.
3. Bhandari M, Adili A, Schemitsch EH. The efficacy of low-pressure lavage with different irrigating solutions to remove adherent bacteria from bone. *J Bone Joint Surg Am* 2001;83:412–419.
4. Schlegel T, Hawkins R. Fractures of the shoulder girdle. In: Hawkins R, Misamore G, eds. *Shoulder Injuries in the Athlete*. New York: Churchill Livingstone, 1996:219–241.
5. Sethi GK, Scott SM. Subclavian artery laceration due to migration of a Hagie pin. *Surgery* 1976;80:644–646.
6. Stableforth PG. Four-part fractures of the neck of the humerus. *J Bone Joint Surg Br* 1984;66:104–108.
7. Hagg O, Lundberg B. Aspects of prognostic factors of comminuted and dislocated proximal humeral fractures. In: Bateman J, Welsh R, eds. *Surgery of the Shoulder*. Philadelphia: BC Decker, 1984: 51–59.
8. Craig EV. Operative treatment of tuberosity fractures, mal-unions, and non-unions. In: Craig EV, ed. *Master Techniques in Orthopaedic Surgery: The Shoulder*. Philadelphia: Lippincott Williams & Wilkins, 2004:495–511.
9. Bigliani L. Fractures of the proximal humerus. In: Rockwood C, Matsen F, eds. *The Shoulder*. Philadelphia: WB Saunders, 1990: 278–334.
10. Lervick G, Bigliani L. Proximal humeral arthroplasty for acute fractures. In: Craig EV, ed. *Master Techniques in Orthopaedic Surgery: The Shoulder*. Philadelphia: Lippincott Williams & Wilkins, 2004: 427–448.
11. Kloen P, Helfet DL. Open reduction and internal fixation of fractures and non-unions of the clavicle. In: Craig EV, ed. *Master Techniques in Orthopaedic Surgery: The Shoulder*. Philadelphia: Lippincott Williams & Wilkins, 2004:385–411.
12. Schlegel T, Hawkins R. Management of distal clavicle fractures. *Oper Tech Sports Med* 1997;5:93–99.
13. Boehme D. Non-union of fractures of the mid-shaft of the clavicle. Treatment with a modified Hagie intramedullary pin and autogenous bone-grafting. *J Bone Joint Surg Am* 1991;73:1219–1226.
14. Jupiter JB, Leffert RD. Non-union of the clavicle. Associated complications and surgical management. *J Bone Joint Surg Am* 1987; 69:753–760.

Complications of Surgery to the Acromioclavicular and Sternoclavicular Joints

6

Jonathan P. Braman   **Evan L. Flatow**

The preponderance of shoulder pathology involves the glenohumeral joint and the subacromial articulation. However, the acromioclavicular (AC) and the sternoclavicular (SC) joints also provide sources of disability from degenerative and traumatic conditions. These conditions often coincide with pathology found in other regions of the shoulder, and consequently their treatment is often simultaneously performed with other shoulder procedures. Even so, there are complications associated with surgery of the joints on the ends of the clavicle in isolation of other concomitant shoulder pathology.

AC JOINT ANATOMY

The AC joint bridges the clavicle and the acromion of the scapula with a diarthrodial joint covered with fibrocartilage. A meniscoid intra-articular cartilage in the joint degenerates over time and its function is not well understood. The inclination of this joint varies from near vertical to an approximately 50-degree inclination downward medially (1,2).

Bony congruency is inadequate for intrinsic stability, so ligamentous and capsular structures provide support. The coracoclavicular ligaments (trapezoid laterally and conoid medially) prevent caudad migration of the shoulder in relation to the clavicle and deformation with axial compression. Acromioclavicular ligaments provide stability in the anteroposterior direction (2–4). Additional stability is added by the blending of the trapezial and deltoid fascia on the surface of the clavicle and joint capsule (5).

AC JOINT PATHOLOGY AND SURGICAL TREATMENT

AC joint disorders manifest as instability of the joint or pain in the location of the joint. Instability issues are usually related to traumatic insults, such as a direct load on the point of the shoulder. Painful conditions, on the other hand, can be the result of primary osteoarthritis, posttraumatic osteoarthritis, or distal clavicle osteolysis.

COMPLICATIONS OF AC JOINT STABILIZATION

Surgical indications for instability of the clavicle have been debated and many techniques of stabilization have been

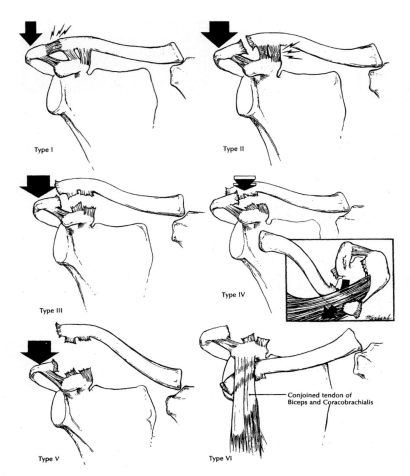

Type I

Type II

Type III

Type IV

Type V

Type VI

Conjoined tendon of
Biceps and Coracobrachialis

Figure 6-1 Rockwood's classification of acromioclavicular joint dislocations.

described (6–14). Rockwood's six-type classification is by far the most widely used (Fig. 6-1) (15). A thorough review of the indications for surgery on the unstable acromioclavicular articulation is outside the scope of this chapter; however, symptomatic instability of the clavicle, especially those in the posterior direction (Type IV) or with severe displacement (Types V and VI) can require surgical stabilization (Fig. 6-2). Whichever surgery is performed on the AC joint to restore stability, several recognized complications can occur (16,17). These complications take many forms, but most common are loss of reduction, continued symptoms, new-onset arthritis, and migration of hardware.

Loss of reduction has been reported to be as high as 44% following AC joint reconstruction (11). Reoccurrence can occur regardless of which technique is used (Fig. 6-3). Many different methods have been attempted to reduce this rate. Transarticular AC pinning has been shown to have high rates of loss of reduction and dangerous pin migration (Fig. 6-4) (8,18–22). Taft et al. (8) had 4 of 26 patients with loss of reduction and six patients with AC joint arthritis at an average follow-up of 9.5 years. Two of the six with arthritis required distal clavicle excision. In Larsen's series (20), they noted 9 out of 39 patients had at least slight pain, two of whom required distal clavicle excision. Three patients had poor range of motion.

Bosworth screw fixation, first described by Bosworth in 1949 (23), is a method of screw fixation between the clavicle and the coracoid designed to reduce and hold the clavicle in anatomic position. A variation on this device was evaluated by Tsou (10) using a percutaneous cannulated

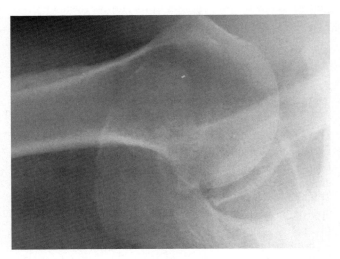

Figure 6-2 Posterior (type IV) dislocations of the acromioclavicular joint can be symptomatic and require stabilization.

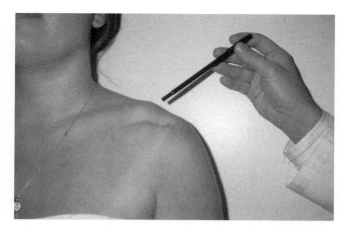

Figure 6-3 Recurrence of clinical deformity is a frequently seen complication after stabilization procedures regardless of which surgical technique is used.

device to facilitate insertion. In Tsou's series, 5 of 53 patients had postoperative AC joint pain, 15 of 53 patients had loss of reduction, and the technique required staged removal. He reported an overall 32% "technical complication" rate (17 of 53 patients). Taft et al. (8) reported 11 of 26 coracoclavicular screw patients with loss of reduction in his series.

Ferris et al. (9) reported on the results of 20 coracoid transfers in their series. This is a dynamic transfer in which the coracoid with attached muscles is transferred to the clavicle to act as a clavicle depressor. A variation of this transfer was originally described by Vargas in 1942 (24). Ferris et al. (9) had 9 of 20 patients with residual pain, two superficial infections, two frozen shoulders requiring manipulation, and a 100% clinical "deformity" at the AC joint, which the authors attributed to a combination of "soft-tissue swelling and residual subluxation of the acrom-

ioclavicular joint." Additionally, one patient reported subjective weakness. Lastly, their procedure required a second surgery to remove the AC staple approximately 6 weeks after the index procedure.

Increasing the strength of the stabilizing device also failed to reduce the rate of loss of fixation. Use of a hook plate as reported by Sim (13) failed to prevent subluxation (4 of 20 displaced) while necessitating a second operation with significant dissection to remove the plate and allow resumption of normal activities with the shoulder. They also reported a high infection rate.

By far the most common reconstructions for AC separations are variations of the Weaver-Dunn procedure. They originally described their technique for reconstruction of the coracoclavicular ligaments in 1972 (7). This procedure uses the coracoacromial ligament as a prosthetic to restore clavicular alignment. They noted 4 of 15 patients with at least partial recurrence of the deformity, one of which required reoperation. Attempts to reduce the recurrence rate by augmenting ligamentous reconstruction with fascial loops, nonbiodegradable suture, or tape have still failed to eliminate recurrence of the deformity completely. Modification of their technique by Stam and Dawson (11) using a Dacron ligament showed similar results with 9 of 20 non-anatomic reductions and 8/20 patients with at least occasional pain. Weinstein et al. (25) reported on a series using nonabsorbable suture and had 9 of 44 patients with loss of reduction. Morrison and Lemos (12) reported much better results at 2 years follow-up with slightly different tunnel placement in the clavicle and a different artificial graft. In their series, 2 of 14 patients had poor results acutely; one was a frozen shoulder that responded well to manipulation and the other was a patient with rupture of his graft who did well with revision surgery. Loss of reduction, osteolysis, coracoid fracture, and reaction to synthetic materials have also been reported (Fig. 6-5).

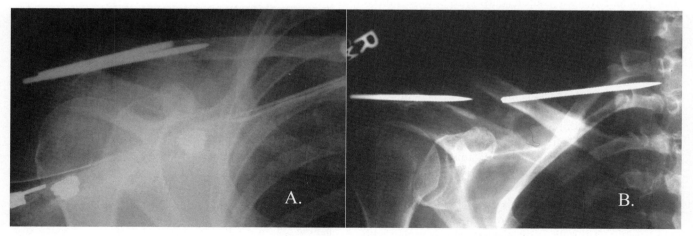

Figure 6-4 Migration of pins is an often reported complication of AC and SC joint pinning. **A:** Immediate postoperative radiograph showing anatomic restoration of AC relationships. **B:** Follow-up film showing loss of reduction and medial migration of one of the threaded pins. This can occur whether pins are smooth or threaded as in this case.

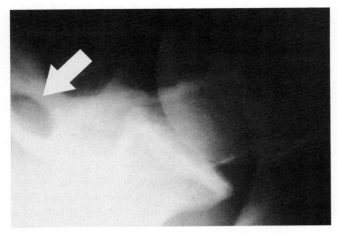

Figure 6-5 Osteolysis surrounding a drill-hole in the base of the coracoid (*arrow*), which had held a synthetic loop for reduction. The patient had skin changes as well. Such osteolysis can progress to the point of coracoid fracture.

Paavolainen et al. (26) combined a direct repair of the acromioclavicular and coracoclavicular ligaments with a AC joint transfixion screw. Their results demonstrated subluxation or dislocation in 7 of 36 patients. Additionally, they had 12 of 36 patients who showed distal clavicular osteolysis in addition to four who showed AC arthosis. Consequently, some surgeons prefer routine resection of the distal clavicle at the time of repair of AC dislocations to avoid the complication of later AC pain.

With the incorporation of hardware or ligature, additional complications have been seen such as failure of hardware placement, coracoid fracture (27), hardware failure and migration (28–30), and increased risk of infection (27).

Irrespective of which technique is used, there is a chance for loss of reduction and complications. In a series by the senior author (25), there were 11 acromioclavicular open reduction and internal fixation (ORIF) procedures without distal clavicle resection (DCR). In that series, two patients developed AC joint pain and one of those underwent eventual DCR. Consequently, the senior author feels that if the injury is acute (<6 weeks) and the injury is reducible, then simple ORIF with repair of the coracoclavicular ligaments with repair of the AC capsule and CC loop is adequate. If, however, the injury is more than 6 weeks of age, he would advocate DCR in addition.

For primary reconstructions of the AC joint, the senior author prefers restoration of the CC ligaments with primary repair if possible, as well as augmentation with no. 5 nonabsorbable ligature around the coracoid and passed into drillholes in the clavicle. This is augmented with autogenous hamstring graft, which also passes around the coracoid base via drill hole in the clavicle. This, coupled with meticulous reattachment of the deltoid to the acromion and closure of the deltotrapezial raphe, reduces the risk of loss of reduction.

COMPLICATIONS OF DISTAL CLAVICLE RESECTION

Painful lesions of the AC joint are either the result of degeneration of the AC fibrocartilage lining leading to spur formation or age-related narrowing of the joint. This degeneration occurs in a significant percentage of patients, and in the vast majority of the population is asymptomatic. Symptoms may arise from spur formation and impingement of the spurs on the rotator cuff, or more commonly, from direct compressive loads causing localizable pain in the region of the AC joint (31). Symptoms in the AC joint are not directly related to the severity of their radiographic appearance.

In addition to degenerative arthritis, symptoms may arise from distal clavicle osteolysis. This process has been described as posttraumatic sequelae from intra-articular fractures (type III) of the clavicle and grade I or II AC separations. Additionally, it can be seen in repetitive microtrauma (weightlifters), rheumatoid arthritis, and hyperparathyroidism. Regardless of the cause of AC joint degenerative lesions, the treatment of choice is DCR.

Distal clavicle resection has been described from the open and arthroscopic techniques. Both techniques have been shown to be effective at resecting the appropriate amount of distal clavicle (32–38). Complications from AC joint surgery, whether open or arthroscopic, can occur. Complications of open techniques include deltoid and trapezial detachment, peri-incisional numbness, poor cosmesis, and wound and skin complications (33). Overresection can also lead to instability of the clavicle if there is elimination of the trapezoid and conoid ligaments, which maintain coracoclavicular alignment (Fig. 6-6).

With either technique, symptoms can continue postoperatively. This is often related to inadequate resection of clavicle, but can occur even with sufficient resection (33).

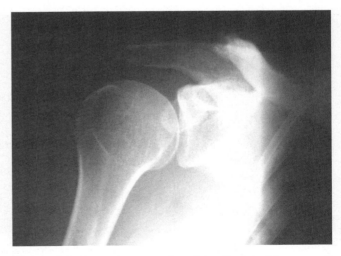

Figure 6-6 Overzealous resection of the distal clavicle can result in AC joint instability. Such instability can be especially deforming if the coracoclavicular ligaments are disrupted as in this case.

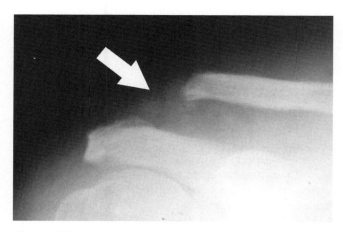

Figure 6-7 Regrowth of bone can occur in the area of distal clavicle resection. Such bone can cause recurrence of symptoms.

Some patients may have a symptom-free period prior to "regrowth" of bone in the region of their resection (Fig. 6-7). Rates of continued symptoms in the literature are between 7% and 25% depending on the series (32,34,35, 39,40). Risk factors for continued symptoms are diagnostic error, inadequate resection of bone, iatrogenic or unrecognized instability of the clavicle, and psychiatric or substance abuse comorbidity.

Results of strength testing have been mixed. Although many authors have reported weakness associated with distal clavicular excision (DCE), Cook et al. (41) reported no loss of strength except in slow-speed Cybex testing. Higher-speed testing showed no difference between operative and nonoperative sides. Some of the patients in this series reported loss of maximal bench press strength subjectively. Other, less common complications reported in the literature include infection and wound complications.

Many authors have commented on techniques for adequate resection of the distal clavicle. As noted previously, underresection is a significant cause of recurrent symptoms. However, overzealous resection can cause the clavicle to become unstable. In order to reduce the likelihood of instability and still obtain adequate resection, the senior author uses several techniques. First, he measures his resection of the distal clavicle with a tool of known length. In our practice, we use an 8-mm rasp. When this rasp fits easily in the AC joint through the entire resected area, there has been adequate bony resection. It is also important to verify that the resection is even. All bone, including the posterosuperior bone, must be adequately visualized and the adequacy of resection verified. Consequently, it is important to view the resection from more than one plane, and be willing to switch portals into the anterior accessory AC portal with the scope to verify that adequate bone has been removed. To prevent overresection of bone and subsequent instability, the author preserves the entirety of the superior capsular restraints to the AC joint and as much of the anterior and posterior ligaments as possible. Additonally, care is taken

to resect the 8-mm rasp width, but not much more. As long as these points are followed, the likelihood of postoperative AC instability is low. In the rare case of overresection with clavicular instability, treatment would only be initiated if the patient were symptomatic. See below for the senior author's technique.

STERNOCLAVICULAR JOINT ANATOMY

Pathology at the medial aspect of the clavicle is much less common. Like the lateral aspect this can be the result of instability or of degenerative processes.

The anatomy of the SC joint is quite different than that of the AC joint. It is a diarthrodial joint that contains a meniscus, which is rarely incomplete. Less than 50% of the clavicle articulates with the sternum, and the remainder of the medial end of the clavicle forms parts of the sternal notch. This inherent lack of stability from osseous structures requires stability to be provided by the ligaments which cover the anterior and posterior surfaces of the two joint capsules as well as providing interclavicular connection. Various condensations have been described as the sternocostal ligament, the sternoclavicular capsule and ligaments, and the interclavicular ligament (2,4). Spencer et al. (42,43) demonstrated with a sectioning study that the posterior capsule is a much more significant anterior and posterior restraint than the anterior capsule. Costoclavicular and interclavicular ligament sectioning did little to increase anteroposterior translation.

STERNOCLAVICULAR JOINT PATHOLOGY AND SURGICAL TREATMENT

Sternoclavicular instability is almost always the result of high-energy trauma. In a review of the literature, Wirth and Rockwood (44) found that 40% resulted from motor vehicle crashes, 21% from sports-related injuries, and the remainder from associated falls, trauma, and industry-related injuries. These injuries are most often anterior displacements and can usually be treated nonoperatively as they rarely cause symptoms. Previous reports of operative treatment (45,46) have not been able to improve on the reports of nonoperative management, which yielded 7 of 10 good results (47,48). When degeneration occurs at the SC joint secondary to instability, medial clavicle resection can provide adequate relief. Operative treatment through medial clavicle resection with or without reconstruction can lead to worsening instability and cause further morbidity.

Posterior dislocations, on the other hand, have the potential to cause life-threatening complications. Due to the proximity of the great vessels, the trachea, and the lung, there are many possible sources of significant morbidity in this area. Consequently, most authors recommend an attempt at closed reduction. If this is unsuccessful, then open reduction, with a thoracic surgeon available, is the next step (48–52). Similar to AC joint stabilization, there have been many different procedures described to stabilize the SC joint following reduction. These use autogenous grafts and nonabsorbable suture constructs as well as direct repair of any available structures. Due to the mobility of the joint, arthrodesis is avoided. Migration of pins from the SC joint is well documented, so hardware fixation (especially with smooth or threaded pins) is to be avoided (53). Spencer and Kuhn (42) have biomechanically evaluated reconstruction techniques and found semitendinosus figure-of-eight to be superior initially to other techniques.

Degenerative conditions of the SC joint can also present without instability. In this setting, medial clavicle excision with preservation of the anatomic structures can provide adequate results (Fig. 6-8). Omer reported a series of 15 patients with symptoms related to the SC joint (54). In that series, there were two with osteomyelitis, two with pin fracture and recurrence of the deformity, and one with migration of the pin into the mediastinum. Of those treated with reconstruction of the capsule and ligamentous structures, two recurred and one developed arthritis.

Regardless of the indication for surgery on the SC joint, the ramifications of complications can be severe. The proximity of the great vessels and the trachea, as well as the brachial plexus, combined with the infrequency with which orthopaedic surgeons operate in this area, make any surgery a serious undertaking. Additionally, although the risk of infection is probably not higher than in other regions of the body, Wohlgethan et al. (55) reported a 20% abscess formation rate with their series of (nonpostsurgical) infections. This carries with it a risk of retrosternal and mediasti-

nal seeding and abscess propagation and requires aggressive debridement (56).

As a result of these data, the senior author does not operate on anterior sternoclavicular dislocations. In the setting of posterior SC dislocation, the author only operates on those which have symptomatic compression of the mediastinal structures. When this is the case, an attempt at closed reduction with a towel clip is attempted. If this is unsuccessful, ORIF is performed with the assistance of a thoracic surgeon as needed. Reconstruction is by preservation of the capsular ligaments as much as possible, and reconstruction using heavy nonabsorbable suture as described below.

PEARLS

Surgery of the articulations of the clavicle requires stable and reliable reconstruction. As these are the only true articulations supporting the weight of the upper arm, it is imperative to create durable suspension.

The single most important aspect of operating on a symptomatic AC joint is to verify that the AC joint is indeed the source of the painful symptoms. As alluded to above, there can be quite dramatic spurring of the AC joint in the asymptomatic patient, and some symptomatic AC joints have little radiographic abnormality. Consequently, injection of the AC joint with local anesthetic with steroid can be a diagnostic as well as a therapeutic adjunct. Differential injections of the AC joint and the subacromial space can help to approximate how much contribution each of these often coexisting pathologies contribute to the overall picture of pain in the shoulder region.

When considering an operation on an unstable AC joint, consider nonoperative management prior to indication for surgery. The senior author only operates acutely on Type IV, V, and VI AC separations. In certain active individuals, he will operate on a Type III after a thorough discussion of the risks of surgery and the emphasis that most Type III dislocations that are treated nonoperatively will do well. Additionally, this discussion emphasizes the fact that delayed reconstructions for Type III dislocations have equivalent results to those treated acutely (25).

When treating a failed AC reconstruction or facing clavicular instability from overresection of the distal clavicle (and concomitant injury to the CC ligaments), it is imperative to verify that symptoms are from the AC joint. Additional shoulder girdle pathology causing subacromial symptoms will not be improved by restoration of AC alignment. Differential injections can be even more valuable in the revision setting. Once the decision has been made to proceed with reconstruction, the selected technique must restore anatomic alignment and durable fixation. In this setting, the senior author prefers secure coracoclavicular fixation with heavy nonabsorbable sutures and reconstruction of the coracoclavicular ligaments. In the revision setting, this

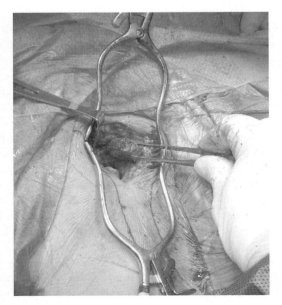

Figure 6-8 Resection of the medial 10 to 15 mm of clavicle can provide symptomatic relief in patients with arthritis of the SC joint.

often entails allograft hamstring graft passed through a drillhole in the clavicle and looped around the coracoid. Additionally, if possible, repair of the CC ligaments and coracoacromial ligament transfer are helpful in reducing the risk of loss of fixation. Finally, the repair is backed up with a CC screw for 8 weeks. This screw is removed at an outpatient procedure at 8 weeks (Fig. 6-9). It is also important to support the weight of the arm for 6 weeks, during which no exercises are performed.

Glenohumeral stiffness is rare after acromioclavicular surgery, but loss of coracoclavicular fixation from too-early use of the arm is all too common. Although it has been described that suture can "saw through" the clavicle or the coracoid, this has not been the experience of the senior author, perhaps because of the "belt and suspenders" technique of the hamstring graft and the suture.

When operating on the sternoclavicular joint, the authors prefer to have a thoracic surgeon scrubbed to assist. In the setting of acute SC joint pathology, there has been little time for adhesions to form, but the anatomy is still altered by the displacement of the clavicle. Furthermore, in the setting of chronic pathology, adhesions formed between the posterior aspect of the clavicle and the mediastinal structures can cause significant difficulty with dissection. For these reasons, we try to use the same thoracic surgeon for all procedures as the combination of abnormal anatomy and some adhesions can make less experienced colleagues uncomfortable.

Lastly, reconstruction of the medial suspensory structures is imperative. All attempts are made to preserve the posterior capsular structures. This is facilitated by resection of only 10 to 15 mm of medial clavicle, and passing no. 5 nonabsorbable sutures from the lateral sternum through

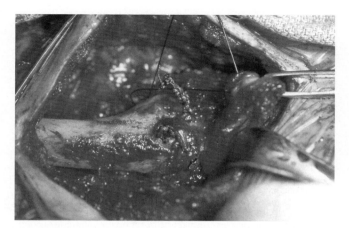

Figure 6-10 Reconstruction of the medial clavicular stabilizers with durable nonabsorbable sutures reduces the likelihood of instability. Additional augmentation by fascial or tendon grafts is advocated by some authors.

a dorsal drillhole on the medial clavicle. Additional stability is provided by a plication of the capsular structures involving a suture passed through the cartilaginous portion of the first rib (Fig. 6-10). Patients are immobilized for 6 weeks in a sling lest painful laxity develop at the reconstructed SC articulation.

In summary, complications of the acromioclavicular and sternoclavicular articulations are unavoidable, but these complications can be reduced by following several principles. Certainty of diagnosis, although difficult to obtain, greatly reduces the risk of continued symptoms postoperatively. Durable reconstruction of these joints prevents symptomatic instability postoperatively. Lastly, familiarity with the surgical anatomy and the procedures reduces complications further. All of these techniques will help to reduce complications during surgery on the ends of the clavicle.

REFERENCES

1. Depalma AF. Surgical anatomy of acromioclavicular and sternoclavicular joints. *Surg Clin North Am* 1963;43:1541–1550.
2. Flatow EL. The biomechanics of the acromioclavicular, sternoclavicular, and scapulothoracic joints. *Instr Course Lect* 1993;42: 237–245.
3. Branch TP, Burdette HL, Shahriari AS, et al. The role of the acromioclavicular ligaments and the effect of distal clavicle resection. *Am J Sports Med* 1996;24:293–297.
4. Renfree KJ, Wright TW. Anatomy and biomechanics of the acromioclavicular and sternoclavicular joints. *Clin Sports Med* 2003;22: 219–237.
5. Debski RE, Parsons IM 4th, Woo SL, et al. Effect of capsular injury on acromioclavicular joint mechanics. *J Bone Joint Surg Am* 2001; 83:1344–1351.
6. Phemister D. The treatment of dislocation of the acromioclavicular joint by open reduction and threaded-wire fixation. *J Bone Joint Surg Am* 1942;4:166–168.
7. Weaver JK, Dunn HK. Treatment of acromioclavicular injuries, especially complete acromioclavicular separation. *J Bone Joint Surg Am* 1972;54:1187–1194.

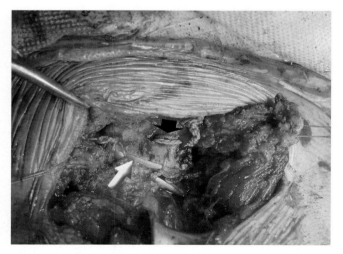

Figure 6-9 Reconstruction of a dislocated AC joint demonstrating the hamstring loop through a hole in the clavicle (*white arrow*) and backed up by heavy nonabsorbable sutures (*black arrow*). This should be followed by meticulous deltoid reattachment to the acromion via bone tunnels, and anatomic restoration of the deltotrapezial raphe.

8. Taft TN, Wilson FC, Oglesby JW. Dislocation of the acromioclavicular joint. An end-result study. *J Bone Joint Surg Am* 1987;69: 1045–1051.

9. Ferris BD, Bhamra M, Paton DF. Coracoid process transfer for acromioclavicular dislocations. A report of 20 cases. *Clin Orthop* 1989;242:184–194.

10. Tsou PM. Percutaneous cannulated screw coracoclavicular fixation for acute acromioclavicular dislocations. *Clin Orthop* 1989;243: 112–121.

11. Stam L, Dawson I. Complete acromioclavicular dislocations: treatment with a Dacron ligament. *Injury* 1991;22:173–176.

12. Morrison DS, Lemos MJ. Acromioclavicular separation. Reconstruction using synthetic loop augmentation. *Am J Sports Med* 1995;23:105–110.

13. Sim E, Schwarz N, Hocker K, et al. Repair of complete acromioclavicular separations using the acromioclavicular-hook plate. *Clin Orthop* 1995;314:134–142.

14. Jones HP, Lemos MJ, Schepsis AA. Salvage of failed acromioclavicular joint reconstruction using autogenous semitendinosus tendon from the knee. Surgical technique and case report. *Am J Sports Med* 2001;29:234–237.

15. Rockwood CA. Fractures and dislocations of the shoulder. In: Rockwood CA, Green DP, eds. *Fractures in Adults,* 2nd ed. Philadelphia: JB Lippincott, 1978:860–910.

16. Kwon YW, Iannotti JP. Operative treatment of acromioclavicular joint injuries and results. *Clin Sports Med* 2003;22:291–300.

17. Rudzki JR, Matava MJ, Paletta GA Jr. Complications of treatment of acromioclavicular and sternoclavicular joint injuries. *Clin Sports Med* 2003;22:387–405.

18. Baker D. Acute complete acromioclavicular separation: report of 51 cases. *JAMA* 1965;192:105–108.

19. Larsen E, Bjerg-Nielsen A. Acromioclavicular lesions. Clinical and radiological follow-up study of lesions of the acromioclavicular joint. *Ugeskr Laeger* 1979;141:2310–2312.

20. Larsen E, Bjerg-Nielsen A, Christensen P. Conservative or surgical treatment of acromioclavicular dislocation. A prospective, controlled, randomized study. *J Bone Joint Surg Am* 1986;68:552–555.

21. Larsen E, Hede A. Treatment of acute acromioclavicular dislocation. Three different methods of treatment prospectively studied. *Acta Orthop Belg* 1987;53:480–484.

22. Larsen E, Petersen V. Operative treatment of chronic acromioclavicular dislocation. *Injury* 1987;18:55–56.

23. Bosworth B. Complete acromioclavicular dislocation. *New Engl J Med* 1949;241:221–225.

24. Vargas L. Repair of complete acromioclavicular dislocation, utilizing the short head of the biceps. *J Bone Joint Surg Am* 1942;24: 772–773.

25. Weinstein DM, McCann PD, McIlveen SJ, et al. Surgical treatment of complete acromioclavicular dislocations. *Am J Sports Med* 1995; 23:324–331.

26. Paavolainen P, Bjorkenheim JM, Paukku P, et al. Surgical treatment of acromioclavicular dislocation: a review of 39 patients. *Injury* 1983;14:415–420.

27. Moneim MS, Balduini FC. Coracoid fracture as a complication of surgical treatment by coracoclavicular tape fixation. A case report. *Clin Orthop* 1982;168:133–135.

28. Mazet R. Migration of a Kirschner wire from the shoulder region into the lung: a report of two cases. *J Bone Joint Surg Am* 1943; 25:477–479.

29. Norrell H Jr., Llewellyn RC. Migration of a threaded Steinmann pin from an acromioclavicular joint into the spinal canal. A case report. *J Bone Joint Surg Am* 1965;47: 1024–1026.

30. Sethi GK, Scott SM. Subclavian artery laceration due to migration of a Hagie pin. *Surgery* 1976;80:644–646.

31. Chen AL, Rokito AS, Zuckerman JD. The role of the acromioclavicular joint in impingement syndrome. *Clin Sports Med* 2003;22: 343–357.

32. Petersson CJ. Resection of the lateral end of the clavicle. A 3 to 30-year follow-up. *Acta Orthop Scand* 1983;54:904–907.

33. Flatow EL, Cordasco FA, Bigliani LU. Arthroscopic resection of the outer end of the clavicle from a superior approach: a critical, quantitative, radiographic assessment of bone removal. *Arthroscopy* 1992;8:55–64.

34. Bigliani LU, Nicholson GP, Flatow EL. Arthroscopic resection of the distal clavicle. *Orthop Clin North Am* 1993;24:133–141.

35. Gartsman GM. Arthroscopic resection of the acromioclavicular joint. *Am J Sports Med* 1993;21:71–77.

36. Flatow EL, Duralde XA, Nicholson GP, et al. Arthroscopic resection of the distal clavicle with a superior approach. *J Shoulder Elbow Surg* 1995;4:41–50.

37. Nuber GW, Bowen MK. Acromioclavicular joint injuries and distal clavicle fractures. *J Am Acad Orthop Surg* 1997;5:11–18.

38. Nuber GW, Bowen MK. Arthroscopic treatment of acromioclavicular joint injuries and results. *Clin Sports Med* 2003;22: 301–317.

39. Snyder SJ, Banas MP, Karzel RP. The arthroscopic Mumford procedure: an analysis of results. *Arthroscopy* 1995;11:157–164.

40. Zawadsky M, Marra G, Wiater JM, et al. Osteolysis of the distal clavicle: long-term results of arthroscopic resection. *Arthroscopy* 2000;16:600–605.

41. Cook FF, Tibone JE. The Mumford procedure in athletes. An objective analysis of function. *Am J Sports Med* 1988;16:97–100.

42. Spencer EE Jr, Kuhn JE. Biomechanical analysis of reconstructions for sternoclavicular joint instability. *J Bone Joint Surg Am* 2004; 86:98–105.

43. Spencer EE, Kuhn JE, Huston LJ, et al. Ligamentous restraints to anterior and posterior translation of the sternoclavicular joint. *J Shoulder Elbow Surg* 2002;11:43–47.

44. Wirth MA, Rockwood CA Jr. Acute and chronic traumatic injuries of the sternoclavicular joint. *J Am Acad Orthop Surg* 1996;4: 268–278.

45. Eskola A. Sternoclavicular dislocation. A plea for open treatment. *Acta Orthop Scand* 1986;57:227–228.

46. Eskola A, Vainionpaa S, Vastamaki M, et al. Operation for old sternoclavicular dislocation. Results in 12 cases. *J Bone Joint Surg Br* 1989;71:63–65.

47. de Jong KP, Sukul DM. Anterior sternoclavicular dislocation: a long-term follow-up study. *J Orthop Trauma* 1990;4:420–423.

48. Bicos J, Nicholson GP. Treatment and results of sternoclavicular joint injuries. *Clin Sports Med* 2003;22:359–370.

49. Mehta JC, Sachdev A, Collins JJ. Retrosternal dislocation of the clavicle. *Injury* 1973;5:79–83.

50. Brinker MR, Bartz RL, Reardon PR, et al. A method for open reduction and internal fixation of the unstable posterior sternoclavicular joint dislocation. *J Orthop Trauma* 1997;11:378–381.

51. Rockwood CA Jr, Groh GI, Wirth MA, et al. Resection arthroplasty of the sternoclavicular joint. *J Bone Joint Surg Am* 1997;79: 387–393.

52. Yeh GL, Williams GR Jr. Conservative management of sternoclavicular injuries. *Orthop Clin North Am* 2000;31:189–203.

53. Lyons FA, Rockwood CA Jr. Migration of pins used in operations on the shoulder. *J Bone Joint Surg Am* 1990;72:1262–1267.

54. Omer GE. Osteotomy of the clavicle in surgical reduction of anterior sternoclavicular dislocation. *J Trauma* 1967;7:584–590.

55. Wohlgethan JR, Newberg AH, Reed JI. The risk of abscess from sternoclavicular septic arthritis. *J Rheumatol* 1988;15:1302–1306.

56. Salvatore JE. Sternoclavicular joint dislocation. *Clin Orthop* 1968; 58:51–55.

Neurologic Injury

Robert H. Cofield   Scott P. Steinmann

INTRODUCTION

There are four nerves immediately in the vicinity of shoulder surgery: the axillary, the suprascapular, the musculocutaneous and the subscapular, with extensions of the brachial plexus extending very close to the surgical field. Thus, there is great opportunity for neurologic compromise during a surgical procedure. It is important to have adequate exposure so one does not become confused about location in a surgical field that may well be altered by previous injury or earlier surgery. Hemostasis is a critical component of the ability to visualize the tissue as well. In this era, minimally invasive surgery sometimes is considered important but may compromise the extent of surgical exposure. Of course, one should not do so at the risk of damage to internal structures, particularly the nerves with their variable ability to recover.

Careful preoperative assessment is critical. There are many situations where nerve injuries exist preoperatively in association with injuries or various pathologic conditions such as advanced rotator cuff tearing with muscle retraction (1). If there is uncertainty about whether or not a nerve injury exists, relative to the history and physical examination, adjunctive assessment can be useful. Often the muscles are well visualized on magnetic resonance imaging (MRI), and this will give a strong clue about nerve injury with the presence of muscle atrophy and fatty infiltration. An electromyelogram (EMG) is an important part of assessment should one be substantively concerned about preexisting nerve injury.

These days, interscalene block anesthesia is often an accompaniment of shoulder surgery and is an important advance in lessening the need for general anesthesia and measurably improving pain relief postoperatively. Although nerve injury associated with interscalene block anesthesia is uncommon, it has been recognized to occur (2).

Series reporting experience with postoperative nerve injuries are rather uncommon, and series from referral centers may in fact represent a concentration of worst case examples, stilted toward poorer outcomes following such injuries (3,4). These reports indicate there is clearly a risk that is present for nerve injury during surgery. The nerves should be carefully respected during surgical procedures.

Surgeons take pride in being well grounded in anatomy and the application of anatomy to surgery. Several articles are published each year by surgeons further detailing anatomic relationships of nerves to the operative field. We will describe a number of studies that have recently been published, which better define the positions of the axillary, suprascapular, musculocutaneous, and subscapular nerves about the shoulder.

Burkhead, recognizing that many surgical approaches split the deltoid muscle and put the axillary nerve at risk, carefully studied the course of the axillary nerve within the deltoid muscle (Fig. 7-1) (5). The distance of the axillary nerve from the acromion was a mean of 5.5 cm at the posterior corner of the acromion, 5.8 cm at the midportion of the acromion, 5.7 cm at the anterolateral corner of the acromion, and 5.8 cm distal to the acromioclavicular joint. However, there was some variation with the ranges in the four locations: 3.1 to 7.3 cm, 4.3 to 7.4 cm, 4.1 to 7.1 cm, and 4.6 to 7.7 cm, respectively. Shorter distances are present in women and particularly those with shorter arm lengths. The authors further recognized that abducting the shoulder to 90 degrees decreases the distance from the nerve to the edge of the acromion by nearly 30%. An additional detailed study of the course of the axillary nerve was performed by Duparc (6) who recommended considering the position of the axillary nerve in five segments: from its origin to the inferior border of the subscapularis, from the subscapularis to the anterolateral border of the tendon of the long head of the triceps, from the triceps to the posteromedial part of the surgical neck, from the humerus to the entry into the deltoid, and, as Burkhead studied, the anterior muscular distribution of the nerve in the deltoid.

Recently, there has been a heightened interest in safe

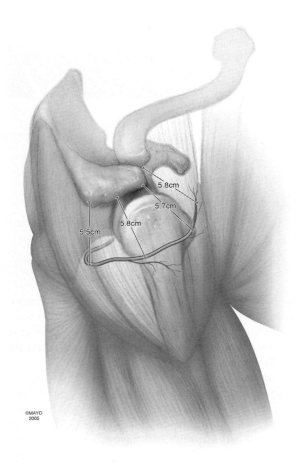

Figure 7-1 Location of the axillary nerve on the undersurface of the deltoid muscle. The numbers refer to average distances of the nerve from various aspects of the acromion process (5).

of the nerve across the operative field beneath the glenohumeral joint.

A moderate amount of attention has been directed toward the course of the suprascapular nerve and effects on the nerve by muscle retraction or rotator cuff muscle advancement. The suprascapular nerve, of course, lies on the undersurface of the supraspinatus and infraspinatus muscle tendon units. In a dissection of 52 shoulders by Shishido (10), the distance from the superior glenoid rim to the suprascapular nerve at the suprascapular notch averaged 2.9 cm (range 2.3 to 3.5 cm) and the distance from the posterior–superior rim of the glenoid to the suprascapular nerve at the base of the scapular spine averaged 1.8 cm (range 1.2 to 2.4 cm) (Fig. 7-2). Thus, when dissecting the shoulder capsule on the inferior aspect of the rotator cuff to allow for musculotendinous advancement, a sharp dissection should not occur much greater than 1 cm medial to the glenoid rim to avoid direct contact with the nerve.

Greiner et al. (11) evaluated the vulnerability of the suprascapular nerve to muscle advancement. This neurovascular pedicle was tethered both at the suprascapular notch and by the periosteum of the supraspinous fossa. They noted the branches of the nerve were placed under tension when advancing the muscle more than 1 cm lateralward. In a study by Albritton et al. (1), they assessed tension in the reverse direction, noting that medial retraction of the supraspinatus muscle substantively changed the course of the nerve. This created increased tension on the nerve, to the point of the nerve being quite tight in all specimens at 2 to 3 cm of medial retraction. This again points out how the nerve has multiple points where it can be tethered and

zones for operating on the shoulder capsule during instability surgery. It is recognized that the axillary nerve is held to the shoulder capsule with loose aerolar tissue between the 5 and 7 o'clock position (considering the superior aspect of the glenoid as the 12 o'clock position) (7). The closest point between the axillary nerve and the glenoid rim is at the 6 o'clock position, where the average distance between the axillary nerve and the glenoid rim as defined by Price (8) was 12.4 mm. The average distance of the axillary nerve from the capsule throughout its course was 2.5 mm. It is also recognized that the position of the axillary nerve changes with the position of the arm. With shoulder abduction, external rotation, and perpendicular traction, the axillary nerve moves somewhat away from the glenoid. Clearly, knowing the position of the axillary nerve during surgery is of eminent importance. A tug test has been described (9) during which the axillary nerve is gently palpated on the anterior aspect of the subscapularis and simultaneously palpated as it courses from the posterior aspect of the neck of the humerus to the deltoid muscle. By gently balloting the nerve in each area, one can sense the course

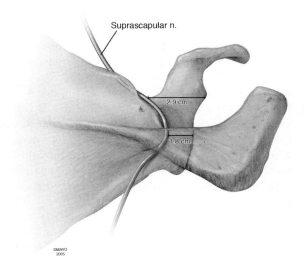

Figure 7-2 Location of the suprascapular nerve below the surfaces of the supraspinatus and infraspinatus muscles as the nerve courses across the top and posterior aspect of the scapula. The distances represented are average distances of the nerve from the glenoid rim (10).

also reminds us to carefully evaluate for nerve compromise before surgery is undertaken.

The musculocutaneous nerve has long been recognized to be at risk during surgery because it deviates laterally from the main nerve trunk to enter the coracobrachialis, to traverse the coracobrachialis, and then course between the brachialis and the biceps brachii. Flatow et al. (12) studied the anatomy of the nerve in 93 anatomic shoulder specimens. Small branches of the nerve to the coracobrachialis proximal to the main trunk entered the muscle an average of 3.1 cm below the coracoid. Some of these twigs entered as close as 1.7 cm below the coracoid. The important main trunk of the musculocutaneous nerve entered the coracobrachialis on its posterior surface an average of 5.6 cm below the coracoid, with a range from 3.1 to 8.2 cm (Fig. 7-3). Interestingly, in seven of these shoulders the main trunk of the musculocutaneous nerve passed over the coracobrachialis, sending it multiple small nerve branches. The authors mention a frequently cited range of 5 to 8 cm below the coracoid for the level of nerve penetration. However, given their data, this would not necessarily represent a safe zone for all people as the main trunk of the nerve entered the undersurface of the coracobrachialis as close as 3.1 cm below the coracoid in some individuals.

Subscapularis muscle release is common in reconstructive shoulder surgery for a number of reasons, and dissection on the anterior aspect of the muscle surface may in fact damage its innervation. In 1994, McCann et al. (13) performed an anatomic study of the subscapular nerves with a guide to electromyographic analysis. They examined 50 shoulders from 36 human cadavers, and 82% of the specimens revealed three independent nerves to the subscapularis with the remainder of the specimens having two or four nerves. The entry points of the nerves into the subscapularis were found to follow a line parallel to the vertebral border of the scapula and inferior from the medial surface of the base of the coracoid (Fig. 7-4). Similar studies were performed by Checchia (14) and Yung (15). In the first study (14), the entry of the nerves into the muscle was noted to be quite close to the surgical field, as close as 1 cm medial to the glenoid border. The mean distance though of the main upper subscapularis nerve from the border of the glenoid was 3.9 cm with the shoulder in internal rotation, 3.3 cm with the shoulder in neutral rotation, and 2.5 cm with the shoulder in external rotation. Interestingly, the authors also identified that the size of the patient did not appreciably alter the distance of the nerves to the subscapularis from the border of the glenoid.

Yung et al. (15) examined 11 cadaveric shoulders and felt that the palpable anterior border of the glenoid rim deep to subscapularis, along with the medial border of the conjoined tendon, could serve as guides to the subscapularis nerve insertion points. In this study, all the nerve branches were no closer than 1.5 cm medial to these land-

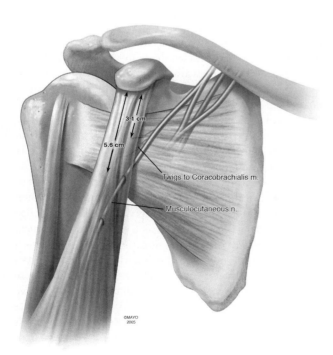

Figure 7-3 Course of the musculocutaneous nerve as it passes under and through the coracobrachialis muscle. The distances indicated on the illustration are averages from the highest twig of the musculocutaneous nerve entering the coracobrachialis and the average distance from the tip of the coracoid to the main muscle branch entering the coracobrachialis (12).

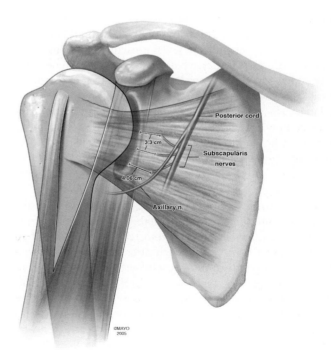

Figure 7-4 Locations of the subscapularis nerve branches in reference to the glenoid rim. The distances are averages (14,15).

marks for all positions of humeral rotation with the arm at the side. It was noted that the lower subscapular nerve was immediately posterior to the axillary nerve. During a standard anterior approach, potential injury to the subscapularis innervation was thought to be minimized by locating and protecting the axillary nerve because it serves as a useful guide to the insertion point of the lower subscapularis nerve, which is the nerve closest to the surgical field.

All these above studies stress the importance of understanding the anatomy of the shoulder and carefully recognizing the locations of the vulnerable nerves in the area of dissection. With ample exposure and careful hemostasis, one can, with this knowledge, almost always prevent direct injury to the nerves by retraction or dissection; however, it seems that many of these nerves and the brachial plexus and its other extensions are particularly vulnerable to contusion or stretching as a result of shoulder surgery. This seems particularly true when the glenohumeral relationship is altered during surgery, as might occur with the treatment of shoulder instability, prosthetic shoulder arthroplasty, or in the care of fracture patients.

After surgery, it is critical to evaluate for the function of the musculotendonitis units innervated by the nerves about the shoulder. This can be done (following recovery from interscalene nerve block) by assessing hand function and by assessing isometric muscle contracture of the biceps, triceps, and deltoid muscles.

INCIDENCE

Richards et al. (3) reported on eight patients who were referred with nerve injuries after Putti-Platt and Brisow procedures. These patients had seven musculocutaneous nerve injuries, two axillary nerve palsies, and two partial radioulnar and median nerve palsies. In exploring these patients surgically, they identified structural injuries to these nerves related to laceration or suturing. With their experience, one can see how they would recommend exploration in those patients who do not have a rapid and complete neurologic recovery. However, this is a sample of patients with nerve injury and does not represent a compilation of people undergoing surgery for anterior shoulder instability.

On our review of the neurologic complications of surgery for anterior shoulder instability in 282 patients undergoing surgery for recurrent instability, 23 (8.2%) had some form of neurologic deficit after surgery (16). Seven had only sensory disturbances, whereas 16 had sensory and motor neuropathies. Eight had multiple deficits representing a diffuse brachial plexopathy and eight had a more defined deficit in one or two cords or peripheral nerves. In all patients, there was some indication of early recovery of nerve function within days of surgery, particularly the sensory deficits. Seven of the eight patients with diffuse plexopathy recovered fully, and one patient had residual dysesthesias in the thumb and index finger. In the group

with more focal nerve lesions, the most common structures involved were distributions of the posterior and lateral cords. The musculocutaneous nerve was the most commonly involved peripheral nerve. Complete resolution of the neurologic deficit occurred in five of the eight patients. One patient had persistent moderate biceps weakness. One patient had dysesthesias in the small and ring fingers. The remaining patient was lost to follow-up. In the group of seven with poorly localized sensory deficits, the majority had dysesthesias in the thumb or distal forearm regions. Complete resolution occurred in six patients, with one patient having some persistent numbness along the medial aspect of the forearm and thumb. In summary, 82% had complete recovery from the neurologic deficits, one patient had the residual biceps weakness, and the remainder had some dysesthesias remaining in the hand. Of patient and surgical factors analyzed, older age and the presence of a Bankart lesion were associated with a statistically higher likelihood of developing a nerve injury, but the p values were just barely less than 0.05. There were no other variables related to the development of a nerve injury. The development of a recurrent instability was slightly higher and the Rowe score was slightly lower in those patients developing nerve injuries, but these differences were not significant at a statistical level.

Similar reviews were performed by other authors. O'Driscoll and Evans (17) reported no neurologic injuries in 204 staple capsulorrhaphies. Rowe (18) reported one axillary nerve injury in a long-term outcome study of 162 Bankart repairs. Cameron (19) described two transient musculocutaneous nerve injuries in 32 Bristow type procedures. Thus, in surgery for anterior shoulder instability, it is clear that nerve injuries are possible. They can be related to nerve laceration or suturing, but in general the injuries seem to be traction- or compression-related and most commonly involve elements of the posterior and lateral cords. Of the isolated peripheral nerve injuries, the musculocutaneous nerve is most frequently involved with the axillary a distant second in terms of frequency of involvement. The risk factors identified by Ho (16) are not under control of the surgeon, but there is the general admonition that when performing anterior shoulder surgery, detailed knowledge of the anatomy is important as is a sequence of surgical maneuvers: careful patient positioning, gentle retraction during exposure, and identification of peripheral nerves within the surgical field would all seem useful. In those studies canvassing procedures rather than specifically nerve injuries, early surgical exploration seemed to be of little value; however, if a well-defined isolated nerve injury is present and does not recover, exploration might prove beneficial as will be outlined below.

Nerve injury after rotator cuff repair is much less common than following repair for instability. Zanotti (20) reviewed 104 rotator cuff repairs, including 10 patients who underwent mobilization and repair of a massive rotator cuff tear. On electromyographic evaluation, one of these shoulders had an iatrogenic suprascapular nerve palsy. It was questioned whether persistent postoperative weakness after surgery for massive rotator cuff tears might on occasion be due to neurologic injury from aggressive tissue mobilization that is needed to perform the repair.

Mansat (21) specifically reviewed the complications of rotator cuff repair in 116 shoulders. There were three nerve injuries. A laceration of a small branch of the axillary nerve anteriorly that was sutured; no clinical consequence could be identified. There was compression of the radial nerve postoperatively associated with wearing an abduction splint. The patient recovered following adjustment of the splint. The third patient had paresthesias in the ulnar nerve, which resolved in 1 week. Thus again, the occurrence of nerve injury following rotator cuff repair seems unusual unless it is associated with significant dissection along the superior and posterior aspects of the glenoid as a part of the mobilization process.

Concerning rotator cuff tearing, it is important to recall, as Brown et al. (22) reminded us, that patients with injury and rotator cuff tearing can also have nerve injuries. It is important to consider this and evaluate for it before surgery is done.

Arguably the most extensive surgical procedure about the shoulder would be prosthetic shoulder arthroplasty. The risk of neurologic complication associated with glenohumeral arthroplasty seems to be quite low, based on reports of clinical series or meta-analyses (23,24). Yet again we must recognize that injury does occur and attention to preventing nerve injuries is critical. The most detailed report on nerve injuries associated with this procedure was by Lynch (25). Out of 417 shoulder arthroplasties analyzed, 17 patients with 18 operated shoulders did have a neurologic deficit after surgery. In 12 patients with 13 operated shoulders, the deficit affected the brachial plexus, with the upper and middle trunks most commonly involved. Three patients were thought to have had an idiopathic brachioplexopathy and one patient had intensification of preexisting dysesthesias in the lower trunk (medial cord distribution). One patient had a median neuropathy at the wrist. Of these involved patients, six had nerve injuries that temporarily (within the first 6 weeks) interfered with rehabilitation and four additional patients had nerve involvement that interfered not only significantly with rehabilitation but also with general use of the extremity. Two patients were lost to follow-up; one died of unrelated causes and a second patient sought medical care elsewhere. Of those 16 with complete follow-up, recovery was rated as good in 11 and fair in 5 patients. Maximum improvement from the neurological injury was achieved in less than 3 months in eight shoulders, in 3 to 6 months in four shoulders, and in 6 to 12 months in one shoulder. The clinical outcome of the shoulder arthroplasty at a minimum of 2 years of follow-up was graded as excellent or satisfactory in all but one shoulder in this patient group.

There were several factors associated with nerve injury and prosthetic shoulder arthroplasty. This included the use of the long deltopectoral approach rather than the anteromedial approach, a shorter operative time, and also the use of methotrexate. The presumed mechanism of injury in this patient group was traction on the plexus during the operation. Williams (26) monitored peripheral nerve function during shoulder arthroplasty in 30 patients. Fifteen patients had some nerve dysfunction during the monitoring at surgery; in 12 patients, this occurred when the arm was abducted, extended, and externally rotated. Repositioning the extremity and retractors resulted in return of the nerve signal in 11 patients. The nerves infected included predominantly a mixed plexopathy, followed by axillary, ulnar, and radial. Factors associated with an increased incidence of nerve dysfunction included previous shoulder surgery and limited preoperative passive external rotation. They rightfully concluded that the incidence of nerve injury during shoulder arthroplasty is likely to be greater than reported, and that the arm should be maintained in extreme positions for preparation of the humerus and the glenoid for as short a period of time as possible. They are contemplating continued use of interoperative nerve monitoring for patients undergoing revision procedures or who have substantively limited preoperative external rotation.

Clearly, nerve injuries occur with traumatic fractures or fracture dislocations about the shoulder, and careful preoperative assessment is important but can be quite difficult in this group requiring early manipulation or surgery. This has engendered some uncertainty about whether or not the nerve injuries pre-existed operative treatment for these problems or occurred during surgery. Probably almost all existed prior to surgical treatment, but this is not known with precision. Recently there has been a focused analysis of complications of operatively treated proximal humeral fractures at our institution. In this review of 116 shoulders undergoing operative treatment (93 for osteosynthesis and 23 for humeral head replacement), no intraoperative nerve injuries could be identified. So we must conclude that in this distorted operative field when one uses gentleness and care in performing osteosynthesis or humeral head replacement, the probability of iatrogenic nerve injury during surgery is quite likely low. However, as we have outlined for earlier problems, the probability will not be nonexistent.

CLASSIFICATION OF NERVE INJURY

Before contemplating surgical treatment of a nerve injury around the shoulder, it is helpful to understand the patterns of nerve injury. Nerve injuries have been described historically using the Seddon and Sunderland classification (27). The Seddon classification describes three possibilities for a nerve injury: neuropraxia, axonotmesis, or neurotmesis. A neuropraxia is felt to be present when there is a conduction block at the site of nerve injury but no obvious visual injury to the nerve. There is potentially a demyelinating injury but Wallerian degeneration will not take place past the zone of injury. When the conduction block has resolved, nerve function will begin to normalize. The recovery time from the neuropraxia may be only hours if there is a traction neuropathy, or potentially a few months depending on the severity of the injury to the myelin covering. Typically, physical examination will not show a Tinel's sign in these patients. Electrodiagnostic evaluation will tend to show a loss of conduction across the zone of injury; there will, however, be normal conduction distal to the area of injury (28).

In axonotmesis, the nerve fibers have physically been disrupted. However, the epineurium and the perineurium remain intact. Wallerian degeneration will occur distal to the zone of injury, but regeneration is still possible due to the intact nerve sheath and typically occurs at a rate of 1 to 4 mm per day. In a neurotmesis, the nerve itself is physically disrupted and because of this, axonal continuity is severely disrupted. In such a nerve injury, surgical intervention is required in order to obtain any meaningful functional outcome.

ELECTRODIAGNOSTIC STUDIES AND SURGICAL EXPLORATION, TECHNIQUES AND OUTCOME

Electrodiagnostic studies are quite helpful during the preoperative and intraoperative planning period. Electrodiagnostic studies can help confirm the diagnosis and give information on the location of the injury and define the type of axonal loss that may exist. Additionally, electrodiagnostic studies can help define a neuropraxia from a neurotmesis. Electrodiagnostic studies, therefore, are an important part of the initial evaluation period but are not a substitute for an appropriate physical examination of the shoulder patient. Together with an adequate history and physical examination, an electrodiagnostic study can be used to decide whether to proceed with operative intervention.

A baseline electromyographic study and nerve conduction study is best performed within 3 to 4 weeks after potential injury to a shoulder nerve. At this point, Wallerian degeneration has occurred. Follow-up serial electrodiagnostic studies performed with a repeat physical examination every 2 to 3 months will help document potential ongoing reinnervation. Denervation patterns on electromyography can be seen as early as 10 to 14 days after injury in proximally innervated muscles and 3 to 6 months postinjury in more distal muscles. A loss of motor unit potential recruitment can be demonstrated immediately after weakness is noted from a lower motor neuron injury. The detection of active motor units with voluntary effort and occasional fibrillations at rest is a good prognostic indicator compared with an absence of motor units and many fibrillations. The electromyography can also distinguish between a preganglionic and a postganglionic lesion by needle examination of very proximally innervated muscles, such as the cervical paraspinal, rhomboids, and the serratus anterior.

Typically, nerve conduction studies are also performed at the time of electromyography. The sensory nerve axon potential is an important part of helping to determine if a potential nerve lesion is preganglionic or postganglionic. Typically, sensory nerve axon potentials are preserved in lesions that are proximal to the dorsal root ganglion. Because the sensory nerve cell body is intact and contained within the dorsal root ganglion, a nerve conduction study will show that the sensory nerve axon potential is normal and the motor conduction is absent, when clinically the patient may demonstrate no sensation in the associated dermatomal pattern. Sensory axon potentials are absent in a postganglionic lesion.

Electromyographic studies can show evidence of early recovery in muscles. These electrical findings may occur before clinically apparent recovery begins to be noticed. An improvement in the electromyographic study does not necessarily equal a similar clinically relevant recovery. A positive improvement in the electromyographic study indicates that an unknown number of nerve fibers has reached the muscle target and re-established a motor endplate connection.

Intraoperative electrodiagnostic studies are a very helpful part of guiding decision-making. Typically, the use of nerve axon potentials and somatosensory evoked potentials are used commonly. The use of nerve axon potentials will allow the operating surgeon to directly test across an area of suspected nerve lesion and determine a reinnervation pattern, typically before electromyographic tests may become positive. The ability to detect a nerve axon potential across a nerve lesion at surgery indicates some preservation of axons and regeneration. The presence of a nerve axon potential across a zone of potential injury indicates the viability of thousands of axons and is a good indication of potential recovery. Patients that have preserved nerve axon potentials noted at the time of surgical exploration tend to gain some clinically useful recovery. Intraoperative somatosensory evoked potentials will help establish the existence of potential continuity in the nerve between the peripheral nervous system and the central nervous system through the dorsal root. A positive response during somatosensory evoked potential indicates integrity and continuity of a few hundred intact nerve fibers. The testing itself does not test the ventral root itself but its status is inferred from the state of the sensory nerve rootlets, although at times there is not always correlation between dorsal and ventral root avulsions. The use of electrodiagnostic techniques at surgery requires the combined teamwork of both the shoulder surgeon and the physician performing the electrical studies to correctly interpret the results.

A nerve injury around the shoulder that may have resulted from a sharp (knife) object should be explored early within several days if there is an extremely high level of suspicion. Patients who have a defined nerve injury but have an increasing loss of function over several days of observation should also undergo early exploration. If a patient does have an increase in deficit in a particular nerve or nerve region over a several day period, this may indicate a vascular injury from a pseudoaneurysm or expanding hemoatoma. If a neurotmetic nerve injury is felt to be associated with blunt trauma, this should be explored after several weeks have passed when injury at the ends of the nerve has demarcated. A nerve that was noted to be injured at the time of a vascular repair should be sutured down under tension and definitive treatment should be performed several weeks later. Maintaining the length of the nerve while demarcation of the nerve ending takes place will help shorten the length of any potential graft.

At the time of surgery, the surgeon should develop a preoperative plan based on review of the patient's clinical examination and electrophysiologic examinations and studies. The operating surgeon should determine a list of what is working around the shoulder and what is not. This will allow a tabulation of what is potentially available for transfer and a determination of what is needed most. The operating surgeon must learn to establish realistic goals during consultation with the patient and their family based on the type of injury and the timing of surgical intervention.

A traditional surgical approach to nerve injuries about the shoulder or the brachial plexus is typically through a supraclavicular or infraclavicular incision depending on the level of the suspected injury (Fig. 7-5). If a combined supraclavicular and infraclavicular approach is determined to be warranted, two explorations with two separate incisions are perhaps most helpful. A transverse supraclavicular incision rather than the traditional zig-zag incision can be performed for the supraclavicular region and a separate extended deltopectoral approach can be incorporated for exploration of the infraclavicular area.

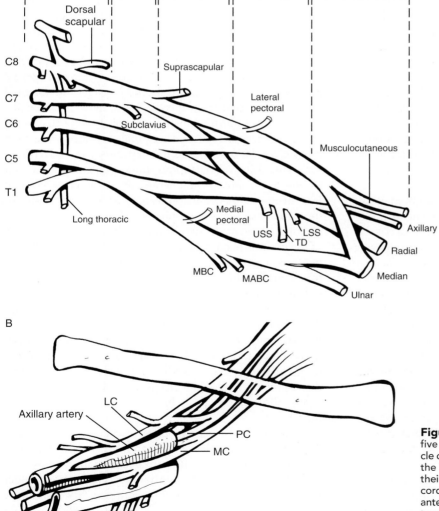

Figure 7-5 Anatomy of the brachial plexus. **A:** The five major segments of the brachial plexus. The clavicle overlies the divisions. **B:** The relationship between the axillary artery and the cords that are named for their anatomic relationship to the artery. LC, lateral cord; LSS, lower subscapular nerve; MABC, medial antebrachiocutaneous nerve; MBC, medial brachiocutaneous nerve; MC, medial cord; PC, posterior cord; TD, thoracodorsal; USS, upper subscapular nerve.

With a deltopectoral approach to the coracoid, detachment of the coracobrachialis and pectoralis minor from the coracoid will allow excellent visualization of the brachial plexus in close proximity to the glenohumeral joint. Typically, these muscles can be detached with a bovie cautery approximately 1 cm distal to their origin on the coracoid and tagged for later repair. At the end of the procedure, these can be simply sutured back to the coracoid stump with nonabsorbable sutures.

In the past, clavicular osteotomy was recommended for complete exposure of the plexus and nerve branches to the shoulder; however, this is not currently recommended. By simply placing a clamp on the clavicle with superior retraction or inferior retraction, examination and exposure of nerve elements behind the clavicle can be facilitated. In the rare instance where clavicular osteotomy is thought to be the best option, typically the clavicle is preplated with use of a compression plate.

Good exposure of the proximal nerve origins of shoulder muscles from the brachial plexus permits intraoperative electrophysiologic monitoring. Unfortunately, direct visualization at the time of surgery or palpation of the shoulder nerve itself does not accurately determine a nerve's histologic appearance or any potential for recovery. It is therefore best to use intraoperative electrodiagnostic techniques at the time of exploration to draw inferences and conclusions about the status of the nerve in question. Direct nerve repair involving suture repair of two nerve endings is often not possible, except in the rare instance of an acute sharp injury which is treated urgently. Over days to weeks, even after a sharp injury, nerves tend to retract and it is quite difficult to reapproximate the nerve endings without significant traction or trauma to the proximal or distal aspects of the nerves themselves.

The standard approach to an exposed injured nerve around the shoulder should be neurolysis of a nerve injury that shows a regenerating nerve axon potential and consideration of grafting of a lesion that does not conduct a nerve axon potential. If two ends of a disrupted nerve are encountered, typically the stumps of the nerve are sectioned back under visual observation until good fascicular structure is identified under either loop magnification or microscopic examination. The best option at this point would be interpositional grafting of the gap in the injured nerve. Grafts should ideally be sutured in place without any undue tension. If a nerve is grafted under tension, shoulder motion may allow for rupture in the postoperative period, which typically would go undetected until several months have passed. In fact, the repairs should ideally be performed with the arm somewhat abducted and externally rotated to be sure that any shoulder nerve is not being repaired under undue tension.

Donor nerve grafts traditionally include the sural nerve, which can be harvested from both legs. Occasionally, however, cutaneous nerves in the forearm or arm may be used. Typically several small sutures, usually 9-0 or 10-0 sutures, are used to coapt the ends of a primary repair or a nerve grafting repair; this construct is then reinforced with the use of fibrin glue. At the end of any shoulder nerve repair, the limb should be put through arc of motion while the wound is observed to be sure that there is no undue tension on the repaired nerve. Postoperatively the shoulder is placed in an immobilizer or sling for a period of 3 weeks to allow the sutured graft to begin the healing process. After 3 weeks, pendulum exercises may begin to the shoulder and active motion is initiated with the help of a therapist. If there is neuropathy involving the elbow or wrist, resting splints can help to immobilize the paralyzed wrist. Electrical stimulation can be used in the postinjury and postoperative period, although there is little hard clinical data to validate this technique. Patients are typically seen back in follow-up every 3 to 6 months and examined for signs of clinical recovery.

Nerve transfer (neurotization) is an indispensable technique that exchanges a nonfunctioning nerve with a dispensable working nerve. Nerve transfer is quite helpful to achieve a more rapid or predictable recovery of a distal target muscle and to enable function of a free-muscle transfer. Nerve transfers can provide a source of axons, which allow surgeons to reconstruct muscles and potentially improve outcome. Ideally, nerves selected for transfer should contain a large number of motor axons and preferably be synergistic with the proposed function. When considering a nerve transfer, the surgeon should consider the potential disadvantages of using a specific donor nerve. Historically, popular nerve transfers include use of the intercostals for powering biceps function. The spinal accessory nerve, after it has given off branches to the trapezius, can be sacrificed for reanimating of the suprascapular nerve or with a graft to power the musculocutaneous nerve. Other nerves that have been used as nerve donors include the cervical plexus, thoracodorsal nerve, and branches of the pectoralis major.

Some of the newer nerve transfers have included the use of the phrenic nerve and the contralateral C-7. The phrenic nerve is a particularly powerful nerve as it is primarily purely motor fibers and has been used extensively for reinnervation. The use of the contralateral C-7 is a relatively new procedure but allows for a very large number of donor axons to permit distal reinnervation. Newer techniques for deltoid reanimation include use of fascicles from an intact radial nerve to be directly transferred to the distal stump of the axillary nerve. In addition, transfer of ulnar or median nerve fascicles to the biceps motor branch will significantly shorten the time for reinnervation of a biceps muscle.

Shoulder fusion as an option in nerve injuries about the shoulder is used less now than in the past. Potentially, voluntary control even with partial reanimation tends to be more favorable than a fused shoulder. However, shoulder fusion is usually a reliable procedure in failed shoulder reconstruction or in patients with painful instability from paralysis of the deltoid or rotator cuff. In the adult, shoulder fusion is probably preferable to tendon transfers. When performing a shoulder fusion, a functioning trapezius, serratus anterior, levator scapulae, and rhomboid are required. The ideal position for shoulder fusion is debated. However, from a general standpoint, at the time of surgery the hand should be able to reach the mouth and the arm should be abducted enough for axillary bathing. The arm should also be internally rotated to allow for care of the opposite axillary region.

Recovery after surgery on nerves governing shoulder function depends on many factors including the pattern of injury, age of the patient, the patient's cooperation with rehabilitation and the time interval between injury and surgery. Functional outcome is usually seen best in incomplete lesions or neuromas that contain a functioning nerve axon potential at the time of surgical exploration. As a general rule, injuries to the upper portions of the brachial plexus tend to fare better than the lower portions of the brachial plexus. These latter elements do not respond well to nerve reconstructive surgery. Infraclavicular lesions to shoulder target muscles tend to do better than supraclavicular injuries. The best results after surgery can be achieved in those patients who undergo surgery before 6 months and those patients less than 50 years of age. As a general rule, when performing sural nerve grafting, a shorter distance for grafting allows for better results. Nerve transfers (neurotization) offer ability to speed up the recovery process and can potentially offer a better result than a nerve grafting procedure. The best results occur when a nerve can primarily be repaired directly; however, this is an uncommon situation. Nerve reconstruction beyond 12 months is not often a successful procedure and is even less successful in the elderly patient. As a general rule, 6 months should be the target time point to perform any surgical reconstruction of shoulder neuropathy. Waiting until 12 months has passed will result in much less optimal results and is not recommended. Overall, nerve reconstruction performed at 6 months or less tends to achieve a more functional result than tendon transfer or joint fusion.

PEARLS

- There can be pre-existing nerve injuries. Careful preoperative evaluation is essential.
- Detailed knowledge of neuroanatomy of the shoulder is important.
- Intraoperative nerve injuries about the shoulder are uncommon but are most commonly seen following repairs for anterior shoulder instability or surgery that includes prosthetic arthroplasty.
- The time period in which arms are in extreme positions during surgery should be as short as possible.

- Intraoperative nerve monitoring may prove useful in selected patients.
- Postoperative arm protection and rehabilitation should continue as best as practically possible in the presence of a nerve injury, as nerve recovery is likely and the outcome of the surgical procedure should not be compromised.

REFERENCES

1. Albritton MJ, Graham RD, Richards RS II, et al. An anatomic study of the effects on the suprascapular nerve due to retraction of the supraspinatus muscle after rotator cuff tear. *J Shoulder Elbow Surg* 2003;12:497–500.
2. Boardman ND 3rd, Cofield RH. Neurologic complications of shoulder surgery. *Clin Orthop* 1999;368:44–53.
3. Richards RR, Hudson AR, Bertoia JT, et al. Injury to the brachial plexus during Putti-Platt and Bristow procedures. *Am J Sports Med* 1987;15:374–380.
4. McIlveen SJ, Duralde XA, D'Alessandro DF, et al. Isolated nerve injuries about the shoulder. *Clin Orthop* 1994;306:54–63.
5. Burkhead WZ Jr, Scheinberg RR, Box G. Surgical anatomy of the axillary nerve. *J Shoulder Elbow Surg* 1992;1:31–36.
6. Duparc F, Bocquet G, Simonet J, et al. Anatomical basis of the variable aspects of injuries of the axillary nerve (excluding the terminal branches in the deltoid muscle). *Surg Rad Anatomy* 1997;19:127–132.
7. Uno A, Bain GI, Mehta J. Arthroscopic relationship of the axillary nerve to the shoulder joint capsule: an anatomic study. *J Shoulder Elbow Surg* 1999;8:226–230.
8. Price MR, Tillett ED, Acland RD, et al. Determining the relationship of the axillary nerve to the shoulder joint capsule from an arthroscopic perspective. *J Bone Joint Surg Am* 2004;86:2135–2142.
9. Flatow EL, Bigliani LU. Tips of the trade. Locating and protecting the axillary nerve in shoulder surgery: the tug test. *Orthop Rev* 1992;21:503–505.
10. Shishido H, Kikuchi S. Injury of the suprascapular nerve in shoulder surgery: an anatomic study. *J Shoulder Elbow Surg* 2001;10:372–376.
11. Greiner A, Golser K, Wambacher M, et al. The course of the suprascapular nerve in the supraspinatus fossa and its vulnerability in muscle advancement. *J Shoulder Elbow Surg* 2003;12:256–259.
12. Flatow EL, Bigliani LU, April EW. An anatomic study of the musculocutaneous nerve and its relationship to the coracoid process. *Clin Orthop* 1989;244:166–171.
13. McCann PD, Cordasco FA, Ticker JB, et al. An anatomic study of the subscapularis nerves. A guide for electromyographic analysis of the subscapularis muscle. *J Shoulder Elbow Surg* 1994;3:94-99.
14. Checchia SL, Doneux P, Martins MG, et al. Subscapularis muscle enervation: the effect of arm position. *J Shoulder Elbow Surg* 1996;5:214–218.
15. Yung SW, Lazarus MD, Harryman DT II. Practical guidelines to safe surgery about the subscapularis. *J Shoulder Elbow Surg* 1996;5:467–470.
16. Ho E, Cofield RH, Balm MR, et al. Neurologic complications of surgery for anterior shoulder instability. *J Shoulder Elbow Surg* 1999;8:266–270.
17. O'Driscoll SW, Evans DC. Long-term results of staple capsulorrhaphy for anterior instability of the shoulder. *J Bone Joint Surg Am* 1993;75:249–258.
18. Rowe CR, Patel D, Southmayd WW. The Bankart procedure: a long-term end-result study. *J Bone Joint Surg Am* 1978;60:1–16.
19. Cameron JC, Hall H, Courtney BG. The Bristow procedure for recurrent anterior dislocation of the shoulder. *J Bone Joint Surg Br* 1985;67:327.

20. Zanotti RM, Carpenter JE, Blasier RB, et al. The low incidence of suprascapular nerve injury after primary repair of massive rotator cuff tears. *J Shoulder Elbow Surg* 1997;6:258–264.
21. Mansat P, Cofield RH, Kersten TE, et al. Complications of rotator cuff repair. *Orthop Clinics NA* 1997;28:205–213.
22. Brown TD, Newton PM, Steinmann SP, et al. Rotator cuff tears and associated nerve injuries. *Orthopedics* 2000;23:329–332.
23. Wirth MA, Rockwood JR CA. Complications of shoulder arthroplasty. *Clin Orthop* 1994;307:47–69.
24. Wirth MA, Rockwood JR CA. Complications of total shoulder-replacement arthroplasty. *J Bone Joint Surg Am* 1996;78:603–616.
25. Lynch NM, Cofield RH, Silbert PL, et al. Neurologic complications after total shoulder arthroplasty. *J Shoulder Elbow Surg* 1996;5:53–61.
26. Williams GR, Rogers K, Ramsey M, et al. Monitoring of peripheral nerve function during shoulder arthroplasty using continuous intraoperative nerve monitoring. *ASES Abstracts*, Session VIII. New York: October 2, 2004:90.
27. Seddon HJ. Three types of nerve injury. *Brain* 1943;66:238–288.
28. Mackinnon SES. Nerve grafts. In: Goldwyn RM, Cohen MN, eds. *The Unfavorable Result in Plastic Surgery*. Philadelphia: Lippincott Williams & Wilkins, 2001:134–160.

Frozen Shoulder

8

Laith M. Jazrawi   *Andrew S. Rokito*   *Joseph D. Zuckerman*

INTRODUCTION

In 1934, Codman (1) coined the term *frozen shoulder* and described it as a "condition difficult to define, difficult to treat, and difficult to explain from the point of view of pathology." Adhesive capsulitis has continued to be one of the most poorly understood disorders of shoulder, posing significant challenges to the clinician. Much of the problem stems from the fact that it has not been easy to define or clearly differentiate from conditions with similar symptoms and findings but with distinctly different causes.

CLASSIFICATION AND DEFINITION

Numerous classification systems have been proposed, with a loosely woven common thread of the presence or absence of trauma (2–6). Reeves (5) used the subgroupings "idiopathic frozen shoulder" and "posttraumatic stiff shoulder" and related his arthrographic findings to the clinical descriptions provided by Jones and Lovett (7). Lundberg (8) classified patients with this condition into two groups: primary or secondary frozen shoulders. Primary frozen shoulder represents the idiopathic condition; secondary frozen shoulder is associated with a known intrinsic, extrinsic, or systemic abnormality. Although this is a worthwhile distinction, it is probably inappropriate to group all intrinsic, extrinsic, and systemic causes as secondary frozen shoulder. Extrinsic conditions such as cervical spine and intrathoracic disorders and systemic conditions such as diabetes mellitus should be considered together. Intrinsic disorders such as rotator cuff injury should be considered separately because they represent a known underlying primary disorder that results in the clinical picture of frozen shoulder (9). This schema is shown in Figure 8-1.

In addition to numerous classifications, the definition of frozen shoulder has varied greatly in the literature. In the late 19th century, Duplay in France (10) and, soon after, Putnam in North America (11) described "scapulohumeral periarthritis," which encompassed a broad spectrum of pathologic conditions causing similar symptoms of painful shoulder stiffness and dysfunction. In 1945, Neviaser (12) proposed the term "adhesive capsulitis," which he believed better described the underlying pathology. He identified a "chronic inflammatory process involving the capsule of the shoulder causing a thickening and contracture of this structure which secondarily becomes adherent to the humeral head." Today, this term is often used synonymously with frozen shoulder and, unfortunately, is also commonly used as an incorrect synonym for stiffness occurring secondary to an inciting event.

The senior author polled members of the American Shoulder and Elbow Surgeons (ASES) to ensure the best consensus on the definition of frozen shoulder, defining it as "a condition of uncertain etiology characterized by significant restriction of both active and passive shoulder motion that occurs in the absence of a known intrinsic shoulder disorder."

EPIDEMIOLOGY

Although the exact prevalence and incidence of frozen shoulder are unknown, most studies report the cumulative risk for at least one episode to be 2% (8). It is most frequently found in patients between the fourth and sixth decades of life, and it is more common in women than men (13). The nondominant extremity seems to be more commonly involved, with most reported cases describing an affected left side (8,14,15). Bilateral involvement occurs in 6% to 50% of cases, although only 14% of these bilateral cases manifest simultaneously (8,13,16–18). When a history of bilateral involvement is identified, the possibility

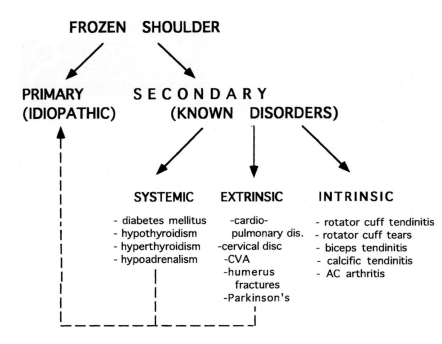

Figure 8-1 Proposed pathways for the development of frozen shoulder syndrome. (Reprinted from Warner JJP, Iannotti JP, Flatow EL, eds. *Complex and Revision Problems in Shoulder Surgery*, 2nd ed. Philadelphia: Lippincott Williams & Wilkins, 2005:206, with permission.)

of a constitutional predisposition should be explored (8,19,20).

PATHOGENESIS

Different pathologic mechanisms have been proposed to explain the cause of frozen shoulder, but all remain largely theoretic. The most common theories are reviewed here. Many plausible pathogenic mechanisms have been proposed during the last 60 years, yet none of the factors occasionally isolated and associated with the pathogenesis of frozen shoulder have been consistently found (Table 8-1) (21).

Several investigators have proposed an autoimmune basis for frozen shoulder (16,17,22–24). Although some clinicians have reported a high incidence of human leukocyte antigen (HLA) B27 in patients with frozen shoulder (22), others have not confirmed this association (25–28). In later studies, serum immunoglobulin (Ig) A levels were found to be significantly lower in patients with frozen shoulder, and immune complex and C-reactive protein levels were increased (16,17,23). In general, however, sufficient evidence to support an immunologic theory has been lacking.

A biochemical basis for frozen shoulder has also been proposed. In his analysis of the capsule in patients with frozen shoulder, Lundberg (8,29) found an increase in glycosaminoglycan and a decrease in glycoprotein content. These biochemical changes in the capsule, however, are consistent with the process of fibrosis, and they may represent the effect of frozen shoulder rather than its cause.

Neurologic dysfunction has been postulated to be a cause of frozen shoulder. In 1959, Kopell (30) proposed suprascapular compression neuropathy as a possible cause of frozen shoulder, but electromyography and nerve conduction studies have not supported this theory. Others have suggested that frozen shoulder is a result of autonomic dysfunction and represents a form of reflex sympathetic dystrophy (20). However, sufficient evidence to support these hypotheses has not been provided.

Various endocrine disorders are associated with frozen shoulder. Patients with diabetes mellitus in particular manifest a much greater incidence of frozen shoulder than nondiabetic controls. Bridgman (31) found that the incidence of frozen shoulder in 800 diabetic patients was 10.8%, compared with 2.3% in 600 nondiabetic controls. Another study identified abnormal glucose tolerance test results for 28% of patients with frozen shoulder, compared with 12% in age- and sex-matched controls with other rheumatologic conditions (32). Frozen shoulder has also been reported to occur with increased incidence among patients with thyroid disorders (33,34) as well as those with hypoadrenalism (35) or corticotropin deficiency (36).

Trivial trauma has been postulated to be an important factor, particularly when it is followed by a period of immobilization (37,38). This does seem to be the sequence of events in some patients who develop frozen shoulder (20). However, most patients who sustain minimal trauma, even when combined with a period of immobilization, do not develop frozen shoulder. This has led some investigators to conclude that there are some patients who possess a "constitutional predisposition" for the development of frozen shoulder. Support for this theory is provided by the significant incidence of bilateral frozen shoulders (8,18,22,39,40).

TABLE 8-1

PROPOSED PATHOGENIC MECHANISMS FOR PRIMARY FROZEN SHOULDER

Mechanism	Disorder	Pathology	Etiology Excluded By
Autoimmune	Collagen-vascular disorders	Type IV reaction (to infarcted cuff tendon)	Absence of immune complexes and autoantibodies, no other affected joints
Inflammatory	Infectious arthritis	Vital, bacterial, or fungal infection	Absence of prodromal illness and systemic symptoms
Crystal arthropathy	Calcium pyrophosphate dihydrate disease and gout	Crystal deposition	Absence of recurrences, crystals, and inflammatory phases
Reactive arthropathy	Spondyloarthritides and ankylosing spondylitis	Seronegative arthritis	No systemic manifestations, normal joint fluid, no blood markers
Hemarthrosis	Hemoglobinopathies and trauma	Chemical irritation (hemosiderin)	No capsulitis or fibrositis with hemoglobinopathies
Paralytic	Suprascapular nerve palsy	Compression neuropathy	Absence of electromyelogram or conduction abnormalities
Algodystrophy	Autonomic neuropathy	Neuropatic disturbance and hypervascularity	No sensory or vascular deficiency, stellate ganglion block not helpful
Degenerative	Rotator cuff tendon and degeneration/infarctoin	Microvascular infarction	Absence of tendon inflammation of infarction
Traumatic	Trauma and immobilization	Injury synovitis and tissue contracture	Brief shoulder stiffness after prolonged casting in the majority
Psychogenic	Hysteria and hypochondriasis	Depression, dependence, and chronic pain disorder	Similar Minnesota Multiphasic Personality Inventory between patients and controls
Fibrogenic	Cytokine induction of fibroplasia	Tissue contracture in response to cytokines, inflammatory cell products, and platelet-derived growth factor.	Represents only one phase of the disease

From Harryma DT II. Shoulders: frozen and stiff. *Instr Course Lect* 1993;42:247–257.

The role of psychologic factors has been considered in the development of frozen shoulder. Some investigators have suggested that a certain personality structure, coupled with untoward life events and inappropriate responses to stress, may serve as a predisposing or precipitating factor for the development of frozen shoulder (20,41–43). Other studies, however, have found no evidence for a characteristic personality disorder (39,40).

It appears that the precise cause for the development of frozen shoulder remains largely unknown. The condition probably results from the proper combination of host factors (i.e., predisposition) and extrinsic factors (e.g., trauma, hormonal changes, collagen-vascular disease, diabetes mellitus).

PATHOLOGY

Several investigators have described the pathologic findings associated with frozen shoulder in an attempt to offer an explanation for the observed macroscopic capsular changes (1,8,44–51). Neviaser (48) coined the term adhesive capsulitis to describe an "avascular, tense capsular markedly adherent to the humeral head and associated with a decreased joint volume and synovial fluid." The histologic changes were consistent with chronic inflammation, fibrosis, and perivascular infiltration in the subsynovial layer, with the synovial layer remaining uninvolved (48).

Based on intraoperative findings of gross contracture of the rotator cuff, Macnab (44) postulated that the primary lesion was in the cuff itself, with subsequent contracture in the capsule and coracohumeral ligament. He confirmed a region of constant hypovascularity in the supraspinatus tendon, called the *critical zone* by Codman (1), and theorized that this was responsible for the initial cuff degeneration (50). Ozaki and associates (49) described the role of contracture of the coracohumeral ligament and the rotator interval in the pathogenesis of frozen shoulder. These investigators found fibrosis, hyalinization, and fibrinoid degeneration in these structures. Neer (47,52) also reported the importance of the coracohumeral ligament contracture, but he stressed that it was unlikely that any one anatomic structure or pathologic process was responsible for causing the entire symptom complex associated with frozen shoulder.

An association between clinical frozen shoulder and Dupuytren's contracture has been identified by multiple authors dating back to 1936 (53). Biopsy samples of the rotator interval and coracohumeral ligament in patients with idiopathic frozen shoulder have demonstrated active fibroblastic proliferation amidst thick nodular bands of collagen accompanied by some transformation to a smooth muscle phenotype (myofibroblasts) very similar to the fibrotic changes seen in Dupytren's disease of the hand (54). These findings reflect at least one phase (i.e., freezing phase) of frozen shoulder (55).

Rodeo and associates (56) compared capsular tissue samples from patients with adhesive capsulitis and controls to determine specific cytokines involved in the inflammatory and fibroblastic response. Transforming growth factor (TGF)-β, platelet-derived growth factor (PDGF), and hepatocyte growth factor (HGF) are involved in the early inflammatory stages of adhesive capsulitis. PDGF is a mitogenic agent that causes fibroblastic cell proliferation and TGF-β increases extracellular matrix, both being potential precursors of capsular fibrosis. These findings are supported by Suzuki et al. (57) who found that PDGF-AB, HGF, and insulin-like growth factor type I all stimulated the migration of fibroblasts. Hannafin et al. (58) hypothesized that the hypervascular synovitis seen in adhesive capsulitis, via cell-mediated pathways, provokes a progressive fibroblastic response in the adjacent capsule resulting in diffuse capsular fibroplasia, thickening, and contracture. Recently, matrix metalloproteinases (MMPs), a family of naturally occurring proteinases, have been implicated as a contributing factor in the pathogenesis of frozen shoulder because they play a key role in controlling collagen matrix remodeling (59,60). Results from these studies suggest that although abnormalities in MMP expression are present in patients with frozen shoulder, a causal relationship cannot be established.

STAGING

Three distinct but overlapping phases with a variable clinical course of variable duration have been defined:

1. Painful phase characterized by insidious onset of diffuse pain lasting 2 to 9 months.
2. Stiffening or freezing phase characterized by progressive motion restriction lasting 4 to 12 months.
3. Thawing phase characterized by gradual resolution of pain and stiffness lasting up to 42 months.

Hannafin et al. (61) modified the traditional staging scheme incorporating clinical presentation, arthroscopic finding, and histological appearance of the capsular specimens:

1. Stage 1: Painful Phase

   - Duration: 0 to 3 months
   - Pain with active and passive range of motion (ROM)
   - With or without limitation of forward elevation (FE), abduction (Abd), internal rotation (IR), external rotation (ER)

   - Exam under anesthesia (EUA) or after glenohumeral (GH) injection: normal or minimal loss of motion
   - Arthroscopic findings: diffuse GH synovitis, most pronounced in the anterosuperior capsule

2. Stage 2: Freezing Phase

   - Duration: 3 to 9 months or more
   - Chronic pain with active and passive ROM
   - Significant limitation of FE, Abd, IR, ER
   - EUA or after GH injection: ROM under anesthesia/injection = ROM awake/no injection
   - Arthroscopic findings: diffuse pedunculated synovitis (tight capsule with rubbery or dense feel on insertion if the arthroscope)
   - Pathologic changes: hypertrophic, hypervascular synovitis with perivascular and subsynovial scar, fibroplasias and scar formation in underlying capsule

3. Stage 3: Frozen Phase

   - Duration: 9 to 14 months
   - Minimal pain except at end ROM
   - Significant limitation of ROM with rigid "end feel"
   - EUA or after GH injection: ROM under anesthesia/injection = ROM awake/no injection
   - Arthroscopic findings: no hypervascularity seen, remnants of fibrotic synovium can be seen. The capsule feels thick on insertion of the arthroscope with diminished capsular volume

4. Stage 4: Thawing Phase

   - Duration: 15 to 24 months
   - Minimal pain
   - Progressive improvement in ROM
   - EUA/arthroscopy: Data not available

SECONDARY FROZEN SHOULDER

Frozen shoulder associated with a known underlying disorder is considered to be secondary; this group includes intrinsic, extrinsic, or systemic disorders. Intrinsic shoulder abnormalities include rotator cuff tendonitis, rotator cuff tears, tendonitis of the long head of the biceps tendon, calcific tendonitis, and acromioclavicular (AC) arthritis. Extrinsic disorders, which represent pathologic conditions remote from the shoulder region, include: ischemic heart disease and myocardial infarction (40,62); pulmonary disorders including tuberculosis (63), chronic bronchitis, emphysema (64), and tumors (65); cervical disc disease and radiculopathy (13,40,66); cerebral vascular hemorrhage (67,68); previous coronary artery bypass graft surgery (69); previous breast surgery; lesions of the middle humerus (70); and central nervous system disorders such as Parkinson's disease (71). Systemic disorders represent generalized medical conditions that are known to occur in association with frozen shoulder. Such conditions include diabetes mellitus, hypothyroidism, hyperthyroidism, and hypoadrenalism.

POSTSURGICAL STIFFNESS

Surgical procedures in the shoulder are widely recognized as a cause of shoulder stiffness. These include: capsular procedures (i.e., capsulorrhaphies, open inferior capsular shifts), rotator cuff repairs (open and arthroscopic), labral repairs, and proximal humerus fractures. Surgical procedures in the vicinity of the shoulder include axillary node and cervical neck dissection, cardiac catherization in the axilla, coronary artery bypass grafting with sternotomy, and thoracotomy. Differentiation between primary adhesive capsulitis and postsurgical stiffness is usually made by the history. Primary adhesive capsulitis results in more global restriction of motion, whereas postsurgical stiffness can result in more selective restriction depending on which structures were tightened.

CLINICAL PRESENTATION

Patient History

Because frozen shoulder represents a symptom complex rather than a specific diagnostic entity, a careful clinical history is crucial in making the diagnosis. Patients with this condition report a gradual loss of function associated with vague discomfort about the shoulder after minimal or no trauma at all. These symptoms, which often are worse at night, usually begin insidiously. Overhead and behind-the-back activities become especially difficult to perform as motion is diminished. These symptoms closely resemble those found in patients with rotator cuff problems, thereby requiring a careful physical examination to consider frozen shoulder as the primary condition or one that is secondary to a specific shoulder problem.

Physical Examination

Physical examination of the cervical spine, opposite shoulder, and trunk should always be performed to exclude any associated abnormality. The clinical hallmark is the limitation of active and passive range of glenohumeral motion. The degree of motion, including FE in the scapular plane, ER at 0 degrees adduction, and IR relative to the spinous process must be documented accurately. Pain (depending on the stage) may be absent when the shoulder is moved within its free range (47). A firm endpoint is appreciated, with pain at the extremes of motion. There has been little consensus about the degree of restriction of shoulder motion needed to make a diagnosis of frozen shoulder (16,17). In general, ER, abduction, and IR are the motions that are most affected, with mild restriction in ER as the most sensitive early indicator (68). Unless there is associated rotator cuff tendonitis, strength tested in the midrange is usually unaffected.

LABORATORY AND IMAGING STUDIES

Routine hematologic testing should include a complete blood cell count, chemistry profile, rheumatoid factor test, and serology, even though the results are usually normal. The erythrocyte sedimentation rate is elevated in as many as 20% of patients (16,17). Except for osteopenia associated with disuse, radiographic findings are usually negative. Significant findings, however, may aid in the identification of an underlying intrinsic disorder, and a complete set of radiographs consisting of anteroposterior (in neutral, internal, and external rotation), supraspinatus outlet, and axillary views should be obtained.

Technetium bone scanning has been used in the evaluation of frozen shoulder. Findings of increased uptake, although nonspecific, are probably secondary to hypervascularity. Such studies have not been shown to have any correlation with disease symptoms, duration, or prognosis (17,72).

Arthrography (18,27,73–78) for the diagnosis of frozen shoulder is of historic interest. Typical findings associated with frozen shoulder include a reduced joint volume (5 to 10 mL), obliteration of the axillary recess and subscapularis bursa, and absence of contrast in the biceps tendon sheath (67,73,79). Such findings, however, have not been shown to have any predictive value in terms of disease severity or prognosis (72,77,80). The use of magnetic resonance imaging (MRI) in the diagnosis of frozen shoulder is equivocal with some studies documenting increased capsular thickness and synovial enhancement (81). MRI is most useful in ruling out associated intrinsic shoulder abnormalities (i.e., rotator cuff tendonitis, rotator cuff tears, tendonitis of the long head of the biceps tendon and calcific tendonitis, glenohumeral arthrosis, and AC arthrosis).

NATURAL HISTORY

Classically, frozen shoulder has been described as a self-limited, benign condition lasting 12 to 18 months (8,46,82,83). Several clinicians, however, have provided conflicting evidence about restoration of motion and function. Clark and associates (84) found 42% of patients studied had persistent limited range of motion 6 years after clinical presentation. Binder (72) found that 40% of patients followed for an average of 3 years failed to regain equivalent range of motion when compared with a control group. Shaffer and associates (85) found 50% of nonoperatively managed patients to be symptomatic at an average follow-up time of 7 years, with a measurable restriction of motion in 60% of cases. Although early presentation seems to be associated with a more favorable outcome, manual labor and dominant arm involvement have been implicated as poor prognostic factors (16,23,84).

In general, the natural history of frozen shoulder is uncertain and additional randomized, prospective studies are needed. However, despite persistent symptoms and restrictions at follow-up, most patients are minimally impaired. Recurrences are rare and the presence of diabetes mellitus portends a more protracted course.

TREATMENT

Nonoperative Treatment

The overall goal in the treatment of patients with frozen shoulder is to relieve pain and restore motion and function. Ideally, efforts should be directed toward prevention by identifying the patients at risk and initiating early intervention. This is best accomplished by emphasizing early motion in potential secondary cases (after trauma and surgery) whenever possible. Unfortunately, most patients present with an already painful, stiff shoulder. The clinician must design a treatment plan that is individualized and based on the severity and chronicity of the patient's symptoms, as well as previous therapeutic efforts.

Pain Management

The first objective in the treatment of patients with frozen shoulder is pain relief. This is essential because it permits patients to more readily participate in an exercise program aimed at restoring motion. The routine use of narcotics should be avoided as they carry a risk of dependency. Nonsteroidal anti-inflammatory medications are effective in controlling some of the symptoms, although there have been no controlled studies to document their efficacy compared with placebo (86–88). Oral corticosteroids have also been recommended for the treatment of frozen shoulder, but there exists little evidence to support their routine use (89–93).

Local intra-articular and subacromial corticosteroid injections have been used to relieve pain and, less frequently, to improve motion in patients with frozen shoulders (93–101). Opinions differ as to which is preferred, with no good evidence to support one over the other. They may be particularly helpful in the early phase of the condition, when pain prevents the patient from actively participating in rehabilitation. Although steroid injections have been reported to be beneficial, their use should be limited because of the potentially deleterious effects on connective tissue, and should also be used cautiously in diabetic patients who must monitor their blood sugars closely.

In 1941, Wertheim and Rovenstine (102) were the first to report on the use of suprascapular nerve blockade for relief of shoulder pain. In more recent reports from the anesthesiology literature, other authors have recommended a suprascapular block with a local anesthetic and steroid to relieve pain (103,104). Jones and Chattopadhyay (105) compared suprascapular nerve blockade with intra-articular corticosteroid injection and found quicker return

of comfort and function in the nerve block group (105). Most of these studies are confounded by concomitant use of therapy and oral pain medications. However, these results are encouraging.

Physical Therapy

Patients with frozen shoulders should be placed on an exercise program with the aim of maintaining and regaining range of motion. Each patient should begin an active and active-assisted range of motion program combined with gentle passive (i.e., stretching) exercises. These exercises, which should be performed four to five times per day, should include motion in four directions: forward elevation, external and internal rotation, and cross-body adduction (106). They can be performed standing or sitting, but are most readily performed supine.

Local modalities consisting of heat at the start of the exercise session and ice at its conclusion may be helpful to increase flexibility and reduce inflammation, respectively. Using the opposite extremity, the affected limb is stretched to its range limit, held in place for a count of three to four, and then brought to a resting position. Forward elevation of the shoulder is performed with the extremity kept close to the sagittal plane as it is grasped behind the elbow and pushed upward in a gradual fashion. A pulley can also be used to accomplish this motion (Fig. 8-2A–B). Similarly, cross-body adduction is performed as the affected extremity is pulled across the chest by the contralateral shoulder (Fig. 8-2C). This maneuver assists in stretching the posterior portion of the capsule. External rotation is accomplished supine and with the elbow close to the body; a stick held in both hands is used to rotate the affected extremity away from the body. Alternatively, this motion can be performed with the affected extremity placed against a door jam as the body is twisted in the opposite direction (Fig. 8-2D–E). Internal rotation can be performed by pulling the wrist of the affected extremity up the back with the opposite extremity or with a towel. This motion can also be accomplished by grasping a door handle behind the back while performing a deep knee bend (Fig. 8-2F–H). Whenever possible, the therapy program should be performed under the supervision of a physical therapist on weekly basis. Patients should be instructed that the success or failure of the therapy depends in large measure on their compliance in performing the exercises as directed.

Capsular Distention

The method of capsular distention, referred to as *distention arthrography* or *brisement*, has been advocated as a means of expanding the contracted capsule (74–78,107). This procedure involves injecting fluid into the glenohumeral joint in sufficient volume to generate pressures high enough to cause capsular disruption, which is evidenced by a significant decrease in the pressure necessary to continue injection. Although the reported results have been favora-

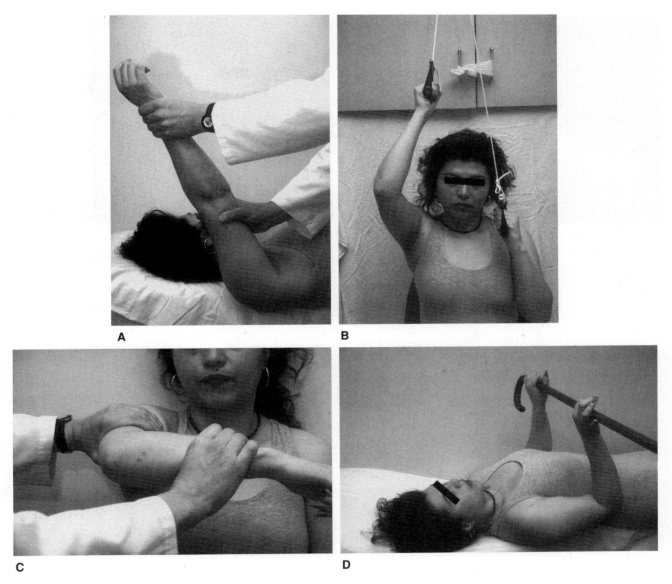

Figure 8-2 Stretching exercises. **A,B:** Forward elevation. **C:** Cross-body adduction. *(continues)*

ble, they have been difficult to interpret because this procedure often is combined with other procedures such as manipulation or cortisone injections, and experience has been limited (18,75,77,78). Currently there are few, if any, indications for this as an isolated procedure.

Operative Treatment

Manipulation Under Anesthesia

Historically, manipulation under anesthesia was considered for patients who had not improved despite compliance with a structured, supervised exercise program for a period of at least 3 to 6 months. This procedure has been a successful method of improving the range of motion of frozen shoulders that have not responded to a rehabilita-

tion program (108–114). However, currently it is usually not performed as an isolated procedure, but rather is done in combination arthroscopic evaluation and capsular releases. When utilized either alone or in combination with another procedure, it should be performed in a gentle, controlled manner to avoid complications. Complications that can occur include humeral fracture, glenohumeral dislocation, rotator cuff tears, and radial nerve injuries. Although there are numerous warnings in the literature about the potential for fractures and rotator cuff tears, the actual documentations of these events is scant. Reported complications of manipulation include subscapularis and rotator cuff rupture (115), surgical neck and humeral shaft fracture (116), glenohumeral dislocation (117,118) and complete brachial plexus palsy (119). Manipulation is contraindicated in patients with severe osteopenia and neurogenic

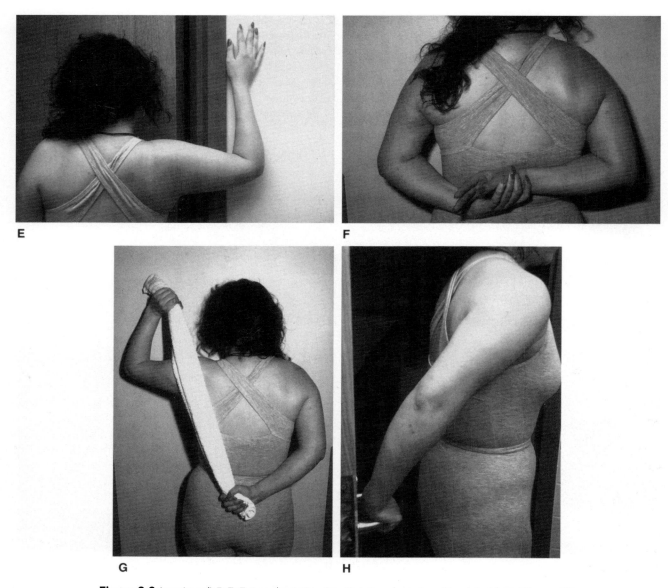

Figure 8-2 *(continued)* **D,E:** External rotation. **F to H:** Internal rotation. (Reprinted from Warner JJP, Iannotti JP, Flatow EL, eds. *Complex and Revision Problems in Shoulder Surgery*, 2nd ed. Philadelphia: Lippincott Williams & Wilkins, 2005:214–215, with permission.)

disorders because these disorders are probably more prone to proximal humeral fracture with manipulation. Long-term insulin dependent diabetes is a relative contraindication secondary to poorer results with manipulation (120).

Technique

Manipulation can be performed under general or regional (i.e., interscalene block) anesthesia. The advantage of regional anesthesia, our preferred technique, is that it allows direct observation of the recovered motion by the patient and more effective and immediate institution of passive ROM therapy.

The patient is placed supine along the edge of the operating table. The scapula is stabilized along its axillary border, allowing more isolated glenohumeral movement of the in-

volved extremity. Passive ROM is measured for both shoulders and documented. Although there is no consensus on the order of manipulation, we perform manipulation into forward elevation first as this produces less torque on the proximal humerus than some of the other manipulation maneuvers. The humerus is grasped close to the axilla to diminish the lever arm effect. With gradual upward manipulation, there is usually a palpable and audible release of adhesions. This maneuver usually results in rupture of the inferior axillary portion of the capsule (30,121). The arm is then stretched across the patient's chest into adduction to stretch the posterior capsule. The arm is then manipulated into abduction in the scapular plane to further stretch the inferior capsule. In 90 degrees of scapular plane abduction, external rotation is performed to stretch the anteroinferior capsule. Any remaining anterior capsular adhesions are released by slowly adducting the externally rotated arm toward the patient's side. With the arm held in scapular plane abduction, internal rotation is performed, further releasing the posterior capsule. While maintaining internal rotation, the arm is lowered to the patient's side with the elbow extended, and the forearm is pronated to complete the posterior capsular release. All rotational maneuvers must be performed carefully because of the risk of fracture.

Postmanipulation Treatment

Postmanipulation rehabilitation is of paramount importance in maintaining the motion gained. Immediately after manipulation, the patient is met in the recovery room by the therapist, who initiates the therapeutic exercise program. It is particularly helpful if regional anesthesia was used, because a long-acting block permits exercise without discomfort. Continuous passive motion machines have also been used after manipulation, but there have been no long-term, controlled studies to verify their efficacy. Patients can be discharged the same day, but frequently we arrange for them to return within the next 1 or 2 days for another interscalene block to facilitate therapy during the early postoperative period.

Results

Overall results in the literature demonstrate that 26% to 81% patients undergoing manipulation are significantly better at 3 months; 70% are better at 6 months (122–124). These conclusions are clouded by heterogeneity of patient populations, duration of premanipulation symptoms, inclusion criteria, and clinical stage. Results of manipulation in the diabetic population are less promising, with early return of stiffness and difficulty getting full motion with manipulation alone (125,126). However, data is conflicting in this population as well with Andersen (122) finding no difference in outcome following manipulation in a population of diabetics versus nondiabetics with idiopathic adhesive capsulitis.

Arthroscopy and Controlled Manipulation

The earliest report of using arthroscopic equipment to perform a partial arthroscopic surgical release of a contracted articular capsule was by Conti in France in 1979 (127). Arthroscopy provides the surgeon with diagnostic information (e.g., labral tears, partial- or full-thickness rotator cuff tears) that is not identified during the clinical evaluation (76,128). Arthroscopy has also been used as a means of capsular distention (33,35,76). The potential benefit of this procedure is difficult to evaluate, because it is usually combined with manipulation or other forms of treatment (35,128). Arthroscopy can also be used to debride intraarticular lesions (128) but this is probably of limited importance in the treatment of frozen shoulder. Perhaps the most significant potential benefit of arthroscopy in the treatment

of frozen shoulder is the possibility of releasing contracted structures. It is usually performed in association with some type of manipulation. This procedure allows precise, selective capsular release, thereby avoiding the potential morbidity associated with an open procedure. It has the advantage of allowing for more immediate, aggressive active and passive range of motion than after an open release.

The primary indication for arthroscopic capsular release is failure to improve despite compliance with a controlled, supervised exercise program for a period of at least 3 to 6 months. Arthroscopic releases have also been used in patients with postoperative stiffness, such as after rotator cuff repair. In these patients, a selective capsular release can be performed, lessening the chance of iatrogenic retear of the rotator cuff. This procedure should be avoided in patients who are sensitive to significant fluid shifts, have severe osteopenia, or have extensive extraarticular adhesions. These are usually patients who have sustained significant trauma or extensive prior surgery (106,129). The latter patients should be treated with an open release.

Technique

Before starting arthroscopy, 1 mL of 1:1000 injectable epinephrine is added to each 3 L bag of saline. As with manipulation under anesthesia, it is preferable to perform this procedure under regional anesthesia so passive ROM therapy can be started immediately in the recovery room. The procedure is performed with the patient in the beach chair or lateral decubitus position. ROM for both shoulders is carefully documented to determine degree and pattern of restriction. We prefer to start with a very gentle manipulation to determine if full or near-full ROM can be easily achieved. The decision to perform the manipulation before versus after release is generally based on the surgeon's preference. Our approach emphasizes the use of very gentle manipulation before the arthroscopy. Following arthroscopic releases, a second manipulation should be performed to take advantage of the capsular releases to increase the range of passive motion. If full motion is easily achieved with the manipulation, the arthroscopic procedure may be aborted, unless there is a specific need to evaluate the intraarticular or subacromial structures. Advantages of initial manipulation are the possibility of avoiding surgical intervention, and easier scope introduction and maneuverability. Disadvantages of manipulation are capsular rupture, fluid extravasation, soft tissue distension, and difficulty visualizing and potentially completing the procedure. The capsule can be addressed either via selective partial capsular release, predominantly addressing contracted rotator interval and anterior capsule, with variable attention to inferior, posterior capsule or via global capsular release (including the inferior and posterior capsule).

The arthroscope is inserted through a standard posterior viewing portal and carefully slid intra-articularly over the humeral head; more inferior passage is difficult because of inadequate joint distention. There is usually a synovitis

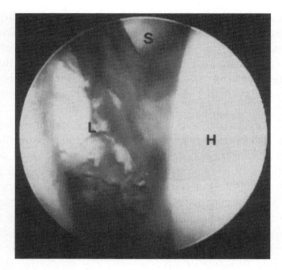

Figure 8-3 Arthroscopic view from a standard posterior portal, with the humeral head (*H*) to the right, demonstrating the thickened, inflamed perilabral anterior glenohumeral ligaments (*L*) overlying the subscapularis tendon (*S*). (Reprinted from Warner JJP, Iannotti JP, Gerber C, eds. *Complex and Revision Problems in Shoulder Surgery*, 1st ed. Philadelphia: Lippincott Williams & Wilkins, 1997:126, with permission.)

interval where a variety of instruments can be passed to begin the release, which is generally performed in the mid-capsule. Electrocautery can be used to incise the thickened, inflamed rotator interval capsule and coracohumeral ligament, as well as the anterior glenohumeral ligaments (Fig. 8-3). Capsular release forceps are also useful to release the capsule (Fig. 8-4A–B). The release proceeds from superior to inferior, including the inferior axillary portion of the capsule. The capsule is divided 1 cm from the glenoid rim until muscle fibers are seen. The arm is frequently manipulated during the procedure using the same maneuvers described previously to assess the adequacy of the release. A restriction in cross-body adduction and internal rotation generally indicates the need for posterior capsular release. In these cases, the viewing and working portals are switched, and a posterior capsular release is performed in a similar fashion. Although most authors proceed with an anterior release first (or exclusively), some begin with a posterior capsular release (130), which can greatly improve anterior access and limit fluid extravasation initially by the intact rotator cuff musculature posteriorly, which is not the case after releasing the anterior rotator interval capsule. Care is taken to preserve the lateralmost RI tissue, which provides important support to the biceps tendon. The subscapularis tendon and recess is debrided of all adhesions to ensure physiologic gliding throughout motion. In addition, during inferior release, caution must be exercised in the axilla recess regardless of the instrument used, as penetration beyond the external limit of the capsule carries great risk. The axillary nerve lies 1.7 cm lateral to the glenoid rim at this level. Some authors prefer manipulation to complete

present with the rotator interval nearly always involved, with variable involvement of other parts of joint depending upon severity/stage of the disease. In addition to the decreased capsular volume, there is a thickened, stiff capsule that is most dramatic in the rotator interval and inferior capsule, as well as obliteration of the subscapularis recess. A working portal is established anteriorly through the rotator

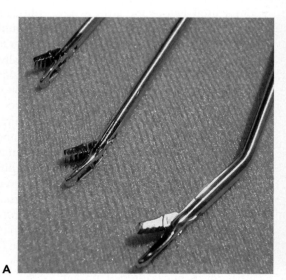

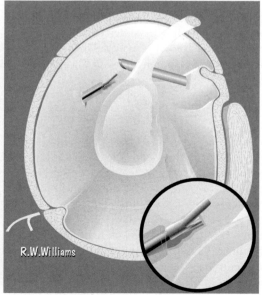

A   B

Figure 8-4 **A:** The Harryman style capsular release forceps (Dyonics, Smith & Nephew, Andover, MA) are useful to release the contracture of adhesive capsulitis. **B:** The Harryman forceps removing a 6-mm segment of capsule. (Reprinted from Snyder SJ: *Shoulder Arthroscopy*. Philadelphia: Lippincott Williams & Wilkins, 2003:70, with permission.)

inferior capsular release rather than direct surgical release. A subacromial release of bursal adhesions can also be accomplished. However, we do not perform an acromioplasty to avoid producing more adhesions. The goal is to obtain motion that is symmetric with the contralateral side.

Postoperative Treatment

Immediately after arthroscopic release, the patient should be met in the recovery room by the therapist to initiate the exercise program. A repeat manipulation can be performed later the same day if a long-acting block has been administered or the following day if an indwelling catheter has been placed. Continuous passive motion can also be used. An unrestricted stretching and strengthening program can be started immediately. Some authors have recommended a pain pump (131) but little data exists regarding their use.

Results/Complications

Potential complications of arthroscopic release include neurovascular risk (132). Cadaveric dissections with circumferential release 1 cm lateral to the glenoid rim revealed average 7 mm from release site to the axillary nerve, 8 mm to the pos-

terior circumflex humeral artery, and 16 mm to the brachial artery. However, in the literature only two cases are reported: one axillary neuropraxia and one diffuse brachial plexopathy, both resolved at 6 months (131). Operative instability has also been reported. Pearsall (133) reported 3% of patients had some subjective sense of instability, but no clinical instability was observed. Ogilvie Harris (134) also reported that 3 of 17 patients undergoing capsular release experienced mild anterior instability with apprehension on full abduction an external rotation. However, none went on to experience episodes of subluxation or dislocation. Although swelling occurs in all patients and can appear rather dramatic, no cases of compartment syndrome have been reported. At our institution, a diabetic patient undergoing manipulation for adhesive capsulitis suffered a bony Bankart which healed uneventfully with no long term sequelae (Fig. 8-5A–C). Most follow-up studies show good/excellent results in pain relief, functional improvement, and restoration of motion. However, most series include stiff shoulders of varied etiology and none are randomized, controlled studies. As with manipulation, diabetic patients appear to have a worse outcome, with more severe disease leading to a higher recurrence rate (Tables 8-2 and 8-3).

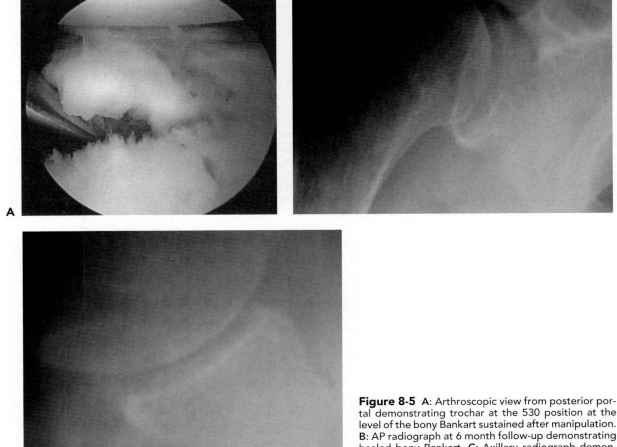

Figure 8-5 A: Arthroscopic view from posterior portal demonstrating trochar at the 530 position at the level of the bony Bankart sustained after manipulation. B: AP radiograph at 6 month follow-up demonstrating healed bony Bankart. C: Axillary radiograph demonstrating healed Bankart lesion.

TABLE 8-2

OUTCOME FOLLOWING PARTIAL OR SELECTIVE ARTHROSCOPIC CAPSULAR RELEASE

Year	Author	Patients	Follow-up (range)	Outcome	Failures
1995	Segmuller	24	13.5 months (6 to 20)	87% good/excellent, 88% very satisfied, 76% returned to normal or near normal shoulder function.	50% still had some restriction in IR. 3 patients were disappointed with procedure. 2 patients, both diabetics, reported no improvement. It is possible that adhesive capsulitis associated with diabetes is more resistant to operative treatment caution is urged in the treatment of the condition. Similarly, the proper timing for arthroscopic intervention remains poorly understood.
1995	Ogilvie-Harris	20	2 to 5 years	16 of 20 no pain, 4 had mild pain, more had mild or severe pain. 17 of 20 normal ROM in abduction. 16 of 20 normal ER. 17 of 20 no functional deficit.	Patients with diabetes mellitus did worse initially but outcome was similar.
1997	Ogilvie-Harris	17		13/17 statistically significantly improved in pain. ER, ABD, function. 13/17 had no pain, full ROM, and full function.	One poor result for no improvement, 3 with residual abnormality. Only patient had IR to the same segment vs. opposite side. 14 were within two segments.
1996	Warner	23	39 (24 to 64) months	CM score improved by 48 (13 to 77) ROM within 7 degrees.	
1999	Beaufils	25	21 months	13 satisfied, 5 satisfied, 5 improved, 3 unchanged.	None
1999	Pearsall	43	5 months. Final survey at 22 months for 35/43 patients	Postoperatively all patients showed substantial gains in shoulder ROM as well as diminished shoulder pain. 83% indicated that their shoulder was normal or had only mild pain.	
2000	Pearsall	35	22 months	No real outcome data comparing pre- to postoperative, or much discussion on results. No overt complication. Questionnaire scores of questionable value.	None reported.
2000	Perlmutter	32		Constant murley score 24 to 55. ASES pain score 8.2 to 3.1. ASES activity score 5.9 to 17.4.	
2000	Heis, Osbahr, Speer	17		HSS rating improved significantly in pain, ER, elevation, and function. 10/15 good to excellent results. Less NIDDM pain than IDDM comparable motion and function.	Only 2 of the 15 had no pain, full function and full range of motion compared with opposite side. Three patients reported moderate to severe pain, 8 had mild loss of ER, 7 had mild loss of elevation.
2002	Yamaguchi	20	22.4 (12 to 37) months	Near complete restoration of ROM without pain in 95%. 19/20 satisfied with initial surgical procedure and had significant range of motion.	One patient with recurrent stiffness/pain requiring repeat procedure.
2003	Nicholson		3 years	For just idiopathic, significant improvement in all categories (ASES, VAS, ROM). Time in formal physical therapy averaged 2.3 months (2–20 weeks); time to attain final pain free range to motion averaged 2.8 (1–6) months.	22% of all patients developed increased pain and plateaued in their motion progress bet- 3 to 6 weeks postoperatively. Flare proved transient, and by 6 to 8 weeks all were doing better. No identifiable factor to explain this transient decrease.

From AAOS Arthroscopic and Open Techniques in Shoulder Surgery. *AAOS* February 8, 2004:225.

TABLE 8-3
OUTCOME FOLLOWING PANCAPSULAR ARTHROSCOPIC CAPSULAR RELEASE

Year	Author	Patients	Follow-up (range)	Outcome	Failures
1997	Harryman	30	33 (12 to 56) months	73% recovered excellent function within 3 months and 88% by 6 months.For majority of patients motion recovered to within 5% to 10% of opposite side.	Three developed recurrent refractory stiffness. Three long-term diabetics did not improve significantly by initial release. 9/30 required repeat manipulation after the first 3 weeks. Five of 14 with diabetes required repeat manipulation.
2000	Watson	73	1 year	Improvement in all parameters achieved, with pain taking an average of 2.24 weeks to diminish and ROM improving to within 10% of other side at average of 5.5 weeks. Patients discharged with full ROM and without pain at an average of 8.9 weeks.	Some mild reaggravation of most patients (70%) pain within the postoperative period (mean 4.5 weeks). Pain usually settled with appropriate massage within a 2-week period. In 37% of cases, a cortisone injection was required as part of the postoperative management. 11% of patients have recurrence of pain or stiffness at an average of 3.5 months (2 to 4.5). Most pain was localized to biceps tendon. Average time to settle was 2.5 weeks. Despite overall good results it is interesting to note that at discharge, despite alleviation of pain and restoration of range of motion, some patients still had some significant functional limitation, usually in loaded shoulder activities, such as throwing a ball or lifting overhead.
2001	Jerosch Jara	28	22 (6 to 48) months	CM score improved mean 41 points (28 to 62). ROM improved significantly all planes. Subjective remarkably less pain vs. those treated with closed manipulation.	
2002	Massoud	11	29 months	Most obtained maximum relief of pain and functional recovery in 3 months.	

From AAOS Arthroscopic and Open Techniques in Shoulder Surgery. *AAOS* February 8, 2004:225.

Open Release

Open surgical release is reserved for patients who fulfill one or more of the following criteria:

1. Attempted manipulation or arthroscopic release that was unsuccessful in regaining range of motion.
2. Posttraumatic or postsurgical causes of shoulder stiffness where there are extensive extra-articular adhesions present or subscapularis involvement is present (i.e., stiffness after open inferior capsular shift).

Our main indication for an open surgical release is significant extra-articular adhesions or contracture that cannot be completely managed by an arthroscopic release. This is often seen in patients with posttraumatic or postoperative stiff shoulder. In general, the goal of the procedure is to release adhesions and contracted structures so that the range of motion can be increased, while maintaining glenohumeral stability (Fig. 8-6).

Open releases generally have been successful, but experience has been limited (49,135). The major advantage of this procedure is that it affords the surgeon the opportunity to accurately locate and release contracted structures intra-articularly and extra-articularly under direct vision. The major disadvantages of an open release are postoperative pain, which can interfere with initiating early motion, and the necessity to limit external rotation in an effort to protect a subscapularis repair if release and/or lengthening were necessary. Surgically, it can be difficult to achieve a complete release because access to the posterior capsule can be difficult.

Technique

When performing an open release, it is critical to identify tissues that are contracted and determine how their release should increase range of motion. The structures released include subacromial and subdeltoid bursal adhesions (49,135), the coracohumeral ligament and rotator interval

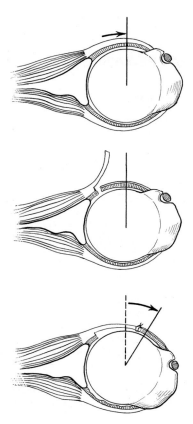

Figure 8-6 Contracted subscapularis and anterior capsule (top) limits external rotation. This condition is treated by incising the subscapularis from the lesser tuberosity laterally (middle) and suturing medially (bottom). This operation results in a substantial lengthening of these structures, and in general, each centimeter of length gained increases external rotation by approximately 20 degrees. (Reprinted from Warner JJP, Iannotti JP, Flatow EL, eds. *Complex and Revision Problems in Shoulder Surgery*, 2nd ed. Philadelphia: Lippincott Williams & Wilkins, 2005:222, with permission.)

(47,49,52,135), the capsule circumferentially or selectively around the glenoid, and the subscapularis (89,136), which is often lengthened and then securely repaired to maintain anterior stability. After each of these structures is addressed, the surgeon should assess the degree of regained motion and the necessity for further dissection and release.

Using a deltopectoral approach, the open procedure begins with the release of adhesions between the deltoid, acromion, coracoacromial ligament, coracoid, and coracoid muscles from the underlying rotator cuff. This can be accomplished sharply with a knife or bluntly using a soft-tissue elevator. Care is taken to stay lateral to the coracoid. This minimizes the risk of injuring neurovascular structures. The coracohumeral ligament and rotator interval are then released, dissecting the supraspinatus and subscapularis from the coracoid bluntly or sharply as needed.

Subscapularis tendon and underlying capsule are then incised. The method is usually determined by the degree of limitation of external rotation. This often includes (a) subscapularis tenotomy with capsular releases at the gle-

noid neck to increase excursion, (b) dissection of the subscapularis directly from its insertion at the lesser tuberosity with the option of a more medial reattachment to increase length and amount of external rotation, or (c) a true Z-plasty to achieve increased external rotation. At this point, the capsule is released selectively or circumferentially, depending on the degree and pattern of stiffness (Fig. 8-7). This is performed just lateral to the labrum and proceeds from anterosuperior to anteroinferior and then from posteroinferior to posterosuperior as needed. Care should be taken to protect the axillary nerve inferiorly. After the release of all of the contracted structures, if a significant internal rotation contracture is present, the subscapularis repair is performed based on the method of exposure. Each centimeter increase of subscapularis length increases external rotation by approximately 20 degrees.

Postoperative Treatment

Continuous passive motion machines have been used successfully after open release for frozen shoulder. Passive and active-assisted forward elevation and external rotation should begin immediately with the therapist. Because the subscapularis repair should be protected, external rotation should be limited based on intraoperative assessment after repair, and active internal rotation should be avoided for 4 to 6 weeks after surgery. There are few reported series with small numbers of patients and generally good results (135,137,138).

Management of Complications

In most cases, frozen shoulder runs a self-limited course. Most of the complications encountered with this disorder are iatrogenic. Potential complications of manipulation include fractures of the proximal humerus and shaft, dislocation of the shoulder, rotator cuff tears or tear extension, and injuries to the brachial plexus. The primary objective in the treatment of frozen shoulder is to increase the range of motion. This should be taken into account when deciding on a rational approach for the treatment of these complications. Iatrogenic fractures of the proximal humerus and shaft should be stabilized with internal fixation in such a way to permit early shoulder range of motion.

Rotator cuff tears or tear extension that occur after manipulation should be left alone, because repairing them immediately could lead to recurrent stiffness. After successful maintenance of motion, preferably active and passive, the patient should be reevaluated and a treatment program established. Generally, depending on the clinical situation, we try to avoid waiting longer than 6 months as this may compromise overall results. Prolonged overhead suspension of the arm after manipulation, which has been advocated by some surgeons (73), can cause neurologic injury. Traction injuries to the brachial plexus and peripheral nerves have been reported after closed manipulation of the shoulder (139). These injuries usually are neuropraxias that

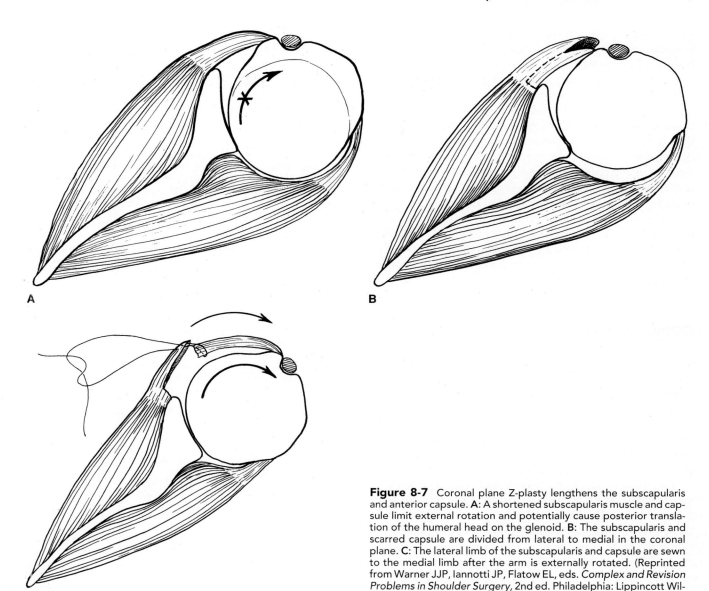

Figure 8-7 Coronal plane Z-plasty lengthens the subscapularis and anterior capsule. **A:** A shortened subscapularis muscle and capsule limit external rotation and potentially cause posterior translation of the humeral head on the glenoid. **B:** The subscapularis and scarred capsule are divided from lateral to medial in the coronal plane. **C:** The lateral limb of the subscapularis and capsule are sewn to the medial limb after the arm is externally rotated. (Reprinted from Warner JJP, Iannotti JP, Flatow EL, eds. *Complex and Revision Problems in Shoulder Surgery*, 2nd ed. Philadelphia: Lippincott Williams & Wilkins, 2005:245, with permission.)

recover spontaneously over time. It is critical to maintain passive range of motion while the nerves are recovering to avoid recurrent stiffness. Although a sling should be used to prevent excessive traction on the plexus while it is recovering, it should be removed for physical therapy and home exercise sessions. The patient and the physical therapist should be made aware of the problem so that extremes of range of motion, particularly forward elevation and abduction, are avoided to prevent further nerve injury. The diagnosis of middle and lower plexus injuries can be made almost immediately with somatosensory evoked potentials. Diminished sensory nerve action potentials at 5 days after the injury may also be helpful in diagnosing an early plexopathy. Definitive electrodiagnostic studies can be performed at 2 weeks after the injury to evaluate the extent of nerve damage and the potential for recovery.

AUTHOR'S PREFERRED TREATMENT APPROACH

Treatment for patients with frozen shoulder must be individualized based on patient, stage of disease, and response to treatment. It is important to classify the patient as having either primary or secondary frozen shoulder, as this will determine a specific treatment plan ultimately prognosis. Initial consultation with patients in stages 1 and 2 (painful, stiffening phases) of the disease process should include education about their condition. It is important to enlist patient participation, as physical therapy will play a major role in their recovery. The disease process needs to be explained and the natural history and treatments options reviewed. It must be emphasized that recovery can take a long time and that the best chance of regaining motion and function is through their own active participation. Patients are sent to physical therapy for exercise instruction but are told to perform the exercises four to five times per day at home. If patients are experiencing excessive pain with therapy and not responding to oral pain medication, a combined intra-articular/subacromial cortisone injection is given. We avoid surgical intervention in these phases as they can worsen the inflammatory phase. For stage 3 patients (stiff phase), nonoperative treatments should continue until the patient plateaus in ROM improvement or motion worsens. Usually, we continue nonoperative treatment for 6 months before any surgical intervention. However, this is not an absolute and we will base our decision on how the patient is progressing in therapy. It is important to note that most patients will not require surgical intervention. If surgical intervention is required, we proceed with arthroscopy and manipulation.

CONCLUSION

Frozen shoulder is one of the most poorly understood disorders of shoulder motion, posing significant diagnostic and therapeutic challenges for the clinician. This condition can be considered primary (idiopathic) or secondary in origin. Secondary frozen shoulder is associated with known intrinsic, extrinsic, or systemic abnormalities. This distinction is important in formulating an appropriate treatment plan and assessing treatment outcomes.

Treatment of frozen shoulder should begin with an exercise program aimed at maintaining and regaining range of motion. Manipulation under anesthesia is performed in those cases that do not respond to a structured rehabilitation program. Arthroscopic or open surgical lysis of adhesions is reserved for shoulders that remain stiff despite nonsurgical treatment or when manipulation is contraindicated.

ACKNOWLEDGMENTS

The authors would like to thank Dr. Charbel Y. Ishak for overall manuscript preparation and editing.

REFERENCES

1. Codman EA. Rupture of the supraspinatus tendon and other lesions in or about the subacromial bursa. In: Codman EA, ed. *The Shoulder*. Boston: Thomas Todd, 1934.
2. Kay NR. The clinical diagnosis and management of frozen shoulders. *Practitioner* 1981;225:164–167.
3. Lundberg BJ. The frozen shoulder. Clinical and radiographical observations. The effect of manipulation under general anesthesia. Structure and glycosaminoglycan content of the joint capsule. Local bone metabolism. *Acta Orthop Scand* 1969;119 (Suppl 1):1–59.
4. Neviaser RJ. *Arthrography of the Shoulder*. Springfield, IL: Charles Thomas, 1975:60–66.
5. Reeves B. Arthrography of the shoulder. *J Bone Joint Surg Br* 1966;48:424–435.
6. Withers RJW. The painful shoulder: review of one hundred personal cases with remarks on the pathology. *J Bone Joint Surg Am* 1949;31:414–417.
7. Jones R, Lovett RW. *Orthopedic Surgery*. New York: Williams & Wood, 1923:59.
8. Lundberg BJ. The frozen shoulder: clinical and radiographical observations. The effect of manipulation under general anesthesia: structure and glycosaminoglycan content of the joint capsule. *Acta Orthop Scand* 1969;119 (Suppl):1.
9. Zuckerman JD, Cuomo F. Frozen shoulder. In: Matsen FAI, Fu FU, Hawkins RI, eds. *The Shoulder: A Balance of Mobility and Stability*. Rosemont, IL: American Academy of Orthopaedic Surgeons, 1993:253.
10. Duplay ES. De la periarthrite scapulo-humerale. *Rev Frat Trav Med* 1896;53:226.
11. Putnam J. The treatment of a form of painful periarthritis of the shoulder. *Boston Med Surg* 1882;107:536–539.
12. Neviaser JS. Adhesive capsulitis of the shoulder. *J Bone Joint Surg Am* 1945;222.
13. Baslund B, Thomsen BS, Jensen EM. Frozen shoulder: current concepts. *Scand J Rheum* 1990;19:321–325.
14. DePalma AF. Loss of scapulohumeral motion (frozen shoulder). *Ann Surg* 1952;135:193–204.
15. Lippman RK. Frozen shoulder: periarthritis: bicipital tenosynovitis. *Arch Surg* 1943;47:283.
16. Binder A, Bulgen DY, Hazleman BL. Frozen shoulder: a long-term prospective study. *Ann Rheum Dis* 1984;43:361–364.
17. Bulgen DY, Binder AI, Hazleman BL, et al. Immunological studies in frozen shoulder. *J Rheum* 1982;9:893–898.
18. Reeves B. The natural history of the frozen shoulder syndrome. *J Rheumatol* 1975;4:193.
19. Bateman JE. *The Shoulder and Neck*, 2nd ed. Philadelphia: WB Saunders, 1978.
20. Rizk TE, Pinals RD. Frozen shoulder. *Semin Arthritis Rheum* 1982;11:440–452.
21. Hazleman BL. Frozen shoulder. In: Watson MS, ed. *Surgical Disorders of the Shoulder*. New York: Churchill-Livingstone, 1991:167–179.
22. Bulgen DY, Hazleman BL, Voak DL. HLA-B27 and frozen shoulder. *Lancet* 1976;1:1042–1044.
23. Bulgen D, Hazlen BL, Ward M, et al. Immunological studies in frozen shoulder. *Ann Rheum Dis* 1978;37:135–138.
24. Hazleman BL. The painful stiff shoulder. *Rheumatol Phys Med* 1972;11:413–421.
25. Kessel L, Bayley I, Young A. The upper limb: the frozen shoulder. *Br J Hosp Med* 1981;25:334–339.
26. Noy S, Dekel S, Orgad S, et al. HLA-B27 and frozen shoulder. *Tissue Antigens* 1981;17:251.
27. Rizk TE, Pinals RS. Histocompatibility type and racial incidence in frozen shoulder. *Arch Phys Med Rehabil* 1984;65:33–34.
28. Stodell MA, Sturrock RD. Frozen shoulder. *Lancet* 1981;2:527.
29. Lundberg BJ. Glycosaminoglycans of the normal and frozen shoulder joint capsule. *Clin Orthop Relat Res* 1970;69:279–284.
30. Kopell AP, Thompson WA. Pain and the frozen shoulder. *Surg Gyne Col Obstet* 1959;109:92–96.
31. Bridgman JF. Periarthritis of the shoulder and diabetes mellitus. *Ann Rheum Dis* 1972;31:69–71.
32. Lequesne M, Dang N, Bensasson M, et al. Increased association of diabetes mellitus with capsulitis of the shoulder and shoulder-hand I syndrome. *Scand J Rheumatol* 1977;6:53–56.
33. Bowman CA, Jeffcoate WJ, Pattrick M, et al. Bilateral adhesive capsulitis, oligoarthritis and proximal myopathy as presentation of hypothyroidism. *Br J Rheum* 1988;27:62.
34. Wohlgethan JR. Frozen shoulder in hyperthyroidism. *Arthritis Rheum* 1987;30:936.
35. Wiley AM: Arthroscopic appearance of frozen shoulder. *J Arthrosc Rel Surg* 1991;7:138.
36. Choy EH, Corhill M, Gibson T, et al. Isolated ACTH deficiency presenting with bilateral frozen shoulder. *Br J Rheum* 1991;30:226.

37. DePalma AF. Loss of scapulohumeral motion (frozen shoulder). *Ann Surg* 1952;135:193.

38. Quigley TB. Checkrein shoulder, a type of "frozen" shoulder: diagnosis and treatment by manipulation and ACTH or cortisone. *Clin Orthop* 1982;164:4.

39. Oesterreicher W, Van Dam G. Social and psychological researches into brachialgia and periarthritis. *Arthritis Rheum* 1964; 7:670.

40. Wright V, Haq AM. Periarthritis of the shoulder: I. Aetiological considerations with particular reference to personality factors. *Ann Rheum Dis* 1976;35:213.

41. Coventry MB. Problem of painful shoulder. *JAMA* 1953;151: 177.

42. Fleming A, Dodman S, Beer TC, et al. Personal in frozen shoulder. *Ann Rheum Dis* 1975;35:456.

43. Lorenz TH, Musser MJ. Life, stress, emotions, and the painful stiff shoulder. *Ann Arthritis Med* 1952;37:1232.

44. Macnab L. Rotator cuff tendonitis. *Ann Coll Surg Engl* 1973; 53.271.

45. Macnab L. Rotator cuff tendonitis. In: McKibbon G, ed. *Recent Advances in Orthopaedics*. Edinburgh: Churchill Livingstone, 1975.

46. Murnaghan JP. Frozen shoulder. In: Rockwood CA Jr, Matsen FA, eds. *The Shoulder*. Philadelphia: WB Saunders, 1990: 837.

47. Neer CS II. Frozen shoulder. In: Neer CS, ed. *Shoulder Reconstruction*. Philadelphia: WB Saunders, 1990: 422.

48. Neviaser JS. Adhesive capsulitis of the shoulder: study of pathological findings in periarthritis of the shoulder. *J Bone Joint Surg* 1945;27:211.

49. Ozaki J, Nakagawa Y, Sakurai G, et al. Recalcitrant chronic adhesive capsulitis of the shoulder: role of contracture of the coracohumeral ligament and rotator interval in pathogenesis and treatment. *J Bone Joint Surg Am* 1989;7:1511.

50. Rathbun JB, Macnab I. The microvascular pattern of the rotator cuff. *J Bone Joint Surg Br* 1970;52:540.

51. Simmonds FA. Shoulder pain, with particular reference to the "frozen shoulder." *J Bone Joint Surg Br* 1949;31:426.

52. Neer CS, Satterlee CC, Daisy R, et al. On the value of the coracohumeral ligament release. *Orthop Trans* 1985;34:199.

53. Smith SP, Devaraj VS, Bunker TD. The association between frozen shoulder and Dupuytren's disease. *J Shoulder Elbow Surg* 2001;10:149–151.

54. Bunket TD, Anthony PP. The pathology of frozen shoulder. A Dupuytren like disease. *J Bone Joint Surg Br* 1995;77:677–683.

55. McLaughlin HL. The "frozen shoulder." *Clin Orthop* 1961;20: 126–131.

56. Rodeo SA, Hannafin JA, Tom J, et al. Immunolocalization of cytokines and their receptors in adhesive capsulitis of the shoulder. *J Orthop Res* 1997;15:427–436.

57. Suzuki K, Attia ET, Hannafin JA, et al. The effect of cytokines on the migration of fibroblasts derived from different regions of the canine shoulder capsule. *J Shoulder Elbow Surg* 2001;10:62–67.

58. Hannafin JA, DiCarlo ED, Wickiewicz TL, et al. Adhesive capsulitis: capsular fibroplasia of the glenohumeral joint. *J Shoulder Elbow Surg* 1994;3:5.

59. Bunker TD, Reilly J, Baird KS, et al. Expression of growth factors, cytokines and mattix metalloproteinases in frozen shoulder. *J Bone Joint Surg Br* 2000;82:768–773.

60. Hutchinson JW, Tierney GM, Parsons SL, et al. Dupuytren's disease and frozen shoulder induced by treatment with a matrix metalloproteinase inhibitor. *J Bone Joint Surg Br* 1998;80: 907–908.

61. Hannafin JA, Chiaia TA. Adhesive capsulitis. *Clin Orthop* 2000; 372:95–109.

62. Mintner WT. The shoulder-hand syndrome in coronary disease. *J Med Assoc Ga* 1967;56:45.

63. Johnson JT. Frozen-shoulder syndrome in patents with pulmonary tuberculosis. *J Bone Joint Surg Am* 1959;41:877.

64. Saba NC. Painful shoulder in patients with chronic bronchitis and emphysema. *Am Rev Respir Dis* 1966;94:45.

65. Demaziere A, Wiley AM. Primary chest wall tumor appearing as frozen shoulder: review and case presentations. *J Rheumatol* 1991;18:911.

66. Kamieth H. Rontgenkefunde der Halswerbesaule und der Schulter bie der Periarthrits Humerscapularis und ihre einordnung in die pathogen. Iese dieser Erkrankung (Radiography of the cervical spine in shoulder periarthritis). *Z Orthop* 1965;100: 162.

67. Braun RM, West F, Mooney V, et al. Surgical treatment of the painful shoulder contracture in the stroke patient. *J Bone Joint Surg Am* 1971;53:1307.

68. Bruckner FE, Nye CJ. A prospective study of adhesive capsulitis of the shoulder (frozen shoulder) in a high risk population. *Q J Med* 1981;50:191.

69. Shaw DK, Deutsch DT, Bowling RI. Efficacy of shoulder range of motion exercise in hospitalized patents after coronary artery bypass graft surgery. *Heart Lung* 1989;18:364.

70. Smith CR, Binder AI, Paice EW. Lesions of the midshaft of the humerus presenting as shoulder capsulitis. *Br J Rheumatol* 1990; 29:386.

71. Riley D, Lang AE, Blair RD, et al. Frozen shoulder and other shoulder disturbances in Parkinson's disease. *J Neurol Psychiatry* 1989;52:63.

72. Binder AI, Bulgen DY, Hazleman BL, et al. Frozen shoulder: an arthrographic and radionuclear scan assessment. *Ann Rheum Dis* 1984;43:365.

73. Neviaser JS. Adhesive capsulitis and the stiff and painful shoulder. *Orthop Clin North Am* 1980;11:327.

74. Fareed DO, Gallivan WRJ. Office management of frozen shoulder syndrome: treatment with hydraulic distension under local anesthesia. *Clin Orthop* 1989;242:177.

75. Gilula L, Schoenecker PL, Murphy WA. Shoulder arthrography as a treatment modality. *Am J Roentgenol* 1978;131:1047.

76. Hsu SY, Chan KM. Arthrographic distension in the management of frozen shoulder. *Int Orthop* 1991;15:79.

77. Loyd JA, Loyd HM. Adhesive capsulitis of the shoulder: arthrographic diagnosis and treatment. *South Med J* 1983;76:879.

78. Older MW, McIntyre JL, Lloyd GJ. Distention arthrography of the shoulder joint. *Can J Surg* 1976;19:203.

79. McLaughlin HL. On the "frozen shoulder." *Bull Hosp Joint Dis Orthop Inst* 1951;12:383.

80. Itoi E, Tabata S. Range of motion and arthrography in the frozen shoulder. *J Shoulder Elbow Surg* 1992;1:106.

81. Mengiardi B, Pfirrmann CW, Gerber C, et al. Frozen shoulder: MR arthrographic findings. *Radiology* 2004;233:486–492.

82. Grey RG. The natural history of "idiopathic" frozen shoulder. *J Bone Joint Surg Am* 1978;60:564.

83. Watson JR. Simple treatment of the stiff shoulder. *J Bone Joint Surg Br* 1963;45:207.

84. Clarke GR, Willis LA, Fish WW, et al. Preliminary studies in measuring range of motion in normal and painful stiff shoulders. *Rheum Rehabil* 1975;14:39.

85. Shaffer B, Tibone JE, Kerlan RK. Frozen shoulder: a long-term follow-up. *J Bone Joint Surg Am* 1993;74:738.

86. Duke O, Zeclear E, Grahame R. Anti-inflammatory drugs in periarthritis of the shoulder: a double blind, between-patient study of naproxen versus indomethacin. *Rheumatol Rehabil* 1981;20: 54.

87. Huskisson EC, Bryans R. Diclofenac sodium in treatment of the painful stiff shoulder. *Curr Med Res Opin* 1983;8:350.

88. Rhind V, Downie WW, Bird HA, et al. Naproxen and indomethacin in periarthritis of the shoulder. *Rheumatol Rehabil* 1982;21: 51.

89. Binder A, Hazleman BL, Parr G, et al. A controlled study of oral prednisolone in frozen shoulder. *Br J Rheumatol* 1986;25:288.

90. Bland JH, Merrit JA, Boushey DR. The painful shoulder. *Semin Arthritis Rheum* 1977;7:21.

91. Blockey NJ, Wright JK, Kellgren JH. Oral cortisone therapy in periarthritis of the shoulder: a controlled trial. *Br Med J* 1954;1: 1455.

92. Ehrlich M, Carp SP, Berkowitz SS, et al. ACTH and cortisone in periarthritis of the shoulder ("frozen shoulder"). *Ann Rheum Dis* 1951;10:485.

93. Neviaser JS. Adhesive capsulitis of the shoulder (the frozen shoulder). *Med Times* 1962;90:783.

94. Barry H, Fernandes I, Bloom B, et al. Clinical study comparing acupuncture, physiotherapy, injection, oral anti-inflammatory therapy in shoulder cuff lesions. *Curr Med Res Opin* 1980;7:121.

95. Bulgen DY, Binder A, Hazleman BL, et al. Frozen shoulder: prospective clinical study with an evaluation of three treatment regimens. *Ann Rheum Dis* 1984;43:353.

96. Dacre IE, Beeney N, Scott DL. Injections and physiotherapy for the painful stiff shoulder. *Ann Rheum Dis* 1989;48:322.

97. Lee M, Haq AM, Wright V, et al. Periarthritis of the shoulder: a controlled trial of physiotherapy. *Physiotherapy* 1973;59:312.

98. Quin CE. "Frozen shoulder": evaluation of treatment with hydrocortisone injections and exercises. *Ann Phys Med* 1965;8:22.

99. Richardson AT. Enest Fletcher lecture: the painful shoulder. *Proc R Soc Med* 1975;68:731.

100. Roy S, Oldham R. Management of painful shoulder. *Lancet* 1976; 1:1322.

101. Steinbrocker I, Argyros TG. Frozen shoulder: treatment by local injection of depot corticosteroids. *Arch Phys Med Rehabil* 1974; 55:209.

102. Werrheim HM, Rovenstine EA. Suprascapular nerve block. *Anesthesiology* 1941;2:541–545.

103. Carron H. Relieving pain with nerve blocks. *Geriatrics* 1978;33: 49–57.

104. Dangoisse MJ, Wilson DJ, Glynn CJ. MRI and clinical study of an easy and safe technique of suprascapular nerve blockade. *Acta Anaesthesiol Belg* 1994;45:49–54.

105. Jones OS, Chattopadhyay C. Suprascapular nerve block for the treatment of frozen shoulder in primary care: a randomized trial. *Br J Gen Pract* 1999;49:39–41.

106. Harryman DT II. Shoulders. frozen and stiff. *Instruct Course Lect* 1993;42:247.

107. Andren L, Lundberg BJ. Treatment of rigid shoulders by joint distension during arthrography. *Acta Orthop Scand* 1965;36:45.

108. Helbig B, Wagner P, Dohler R. Mobilization of frozen shoulder under general anesthesia. *Acta Orthop Belg* 1983;49:267.

109. Hill JJ Jr, Hogumill H. Manipulation in the treatment of frozen shoulder. *Orthopedics* 1988;11:1255.

110. Lloyd-Roberts GG, French PR. Periarthritis of the shoulder: a study of the disease and its treatment. *Br Med J* 1959;1:1596.

111. Neviaser RJ, Neviaser TJ. The frozen shoulder: diagnosis and management. *Clin Orthop* 1987;223:59.

112. Parker RD, Froimson AL, Winsburg DD, et al. Frozen shoulder. Part 1. Chronology, pathogenesis, clinical picture and treatment. *Orthopedics* 1989;12:869.

113. Parker RD, Froimson AI, Winsburg DD, et al. Frozen shoulder. Part II. Treatment by manipulation under anesthesia. *Orthopedics* 1989;12:989.

114. Thomas D, Williams RA, Smith DS. The frozen shoulder: a review of manipulative treatment. *Rheumatol Rehabil* 1980;19:173.

115. DePalma AF. Loss of scapulohumeral motion (frozen shoulder). *Ann Surg* 1952;135:193–204.

116. Haines JFF, Hargadon EJ. Manipulation as the primary treatment of the frozen shoulder. *R Coll Surg Edinb* 1982;27:271–275.

117. Charnley J. Periarthritis of the shoulder. *Posrgrad Med* 1959;35: 384–388.

118. Quigley TB. Indications for manipulation and corticosteroids in the treatment of stiff shoulders. *Surg Clin North Am* 1969;43: 1715–1720.

119. Matsen FA III, Kirby RM. Office evaluation and management of shoulder pain. *Ortho Clin North Am* 1982;13:453–475.

120. Matsen FA III, Lippitt SB, Sidles JA, et al. The Stiff shoulder. In: Matsen FA, Lippitt SB, Sidles JA, et al., *Practical Evaluation and Management of the Shoulder*. Philadelphia: WB Saunders, 1994: 19–109.

121. Neviaser RJ. Painful conditions affecting the shoulder. *Clin Orthop* 1983;173:63.

122. Andersen NH, Sojbjerg JO, Johannsen HV, et al. Frozen shoulder: arthroscopy and manipulation under general anesthesia and early passive motion. *J Shoulder Elbow Surg* 1998;7:218–222.

123. Dodenhoff RM, Levy O, Wilson A, et al. Manipulation under anesthesia for primary frozen shoulder: Effect on early recovery and return to activity. *J Shoulder Elbow Surg* 2000;9:23–26.

124. Reichmister JP, Friedman SL. Long-term functional results after manipulation of the frozen shoulder. *Maryland Med J* 1999;48: 7–11.

125. Janda DH, Hawkins RJ. Shoulder manipulation in patients with adhesive Capsulitis and diabetes mellitus: a clinical note. *J Shoulder Elbow Surg* 1999;2:36–38.

126. Massoud SN, Pearse EO, Levy O, et al. Operative management of the frozen shoulder in patients with diabetes. *J Shoulder Elbow Surg* 2002;11:609–613.

127. Conti V. Arthroscopy in rehabilitation. *Orrhop Clin North Am* 1979;10:709–711.

128. McGraw JM, Turba IE. Frozen shoulder: treatment by arthroscopy and manipulation. *Orthop Trans* 1989;13:661.

129. Warner JP, Allen AA, Marks P, et al. Arthroscopic release of refractory capsular contracture of the shoulder. Video presentation. Orlando, FL: American Academy of Orthopaedic Surgeons 62nd Annual Meeting, 1995.

130. Harryman D II, Lazarus M. The stiff shoulder. In: Rockwood CA, Matsen FA, eds. *The Shoulder*. Philadelphia, WB Saunders, 2004: 1121–1172.

131. Yamaguchi K, Sethi N, Bauer G. Postoperative pain control following arthroscopic release of adhesive capsulitis: a short-term retrospective review study of the use of an intra-articular pain catheter. *Arthroscopy* 2002;18:359–365.

132. Zanotti RM, Kuhn JE. Arthroscopic capsular release for the stiff shoulder. Description of technique and anatomic considerations. *Am J Sports Med* 1997;25:294–298.

133. Pearsall AW, Holovacs TF, Speer KP. The intra-articular component of the subscapularis tendon: anatomic and histological correlation in reference to surgical release in patients with frozen-shoulder syndrome. *Arthroscopy* 2000;3:236–242.

134. Ogilvie-Harris OJ, Myerthall S. The diabetic frozen shoulder: arthroscopic release. *Arthroscopy* 1997;13:1–8.

135. Kieras DM, Matsen FA III. Open release in the management of refractory frozen shoulder. *Orthop Trans* 1991;15:801.

136. Ogilvie-Harris DJ, Wiley AM. Arthroscopic surgery of the shoulder: a general appraisal. *J Bone Joint Surg Br* 1986;68:201.

137. Ozaki J, Nakagawa Y, Sakurai G, et al. Recalcitrant chronic adhesive capsulitis of the shoulder: role of contracture of the coracohumeral ligament and rotator interval in pathogenesis and treatment. *JBJS* 1989;71A:1511–1515.

138. Matsen FA III, Lippitt, S, Sidles, J, et al. *Practical Evaluation and Management of the Shoulder*. Philadelphia: WB Saunders, 1994.

139. Birch R, Jessop J, Scott G. Brachial plexus palsy after manipulation of the shoulder. *J Bone Joint Surg Br* 1991;73:I72.

Complications of Glenohumeral Arthrodesis

9

Gregory J. Gilot   *David J. Clare*
Bertrand Coulet   *Charles A. Rockwood, Jr.*

INTRODUCTION

Humeroscapular arthrodesis is a well-established operative procedure that involves fusion of the humeral head to the glenoid. In some procedures, the fusion also includes an acromiohumeral arthrodesis. Humeroscapular arthrodesis is commonly called *shoulder arthrodesis*. Indications for this procedure early in the 20th century included the treatment of residual glenohumeral destruction resulting from tuberculosis and the treatment of upper extremity paralysis resulting from poliomyelitis. Additional historical indications included osteoarthritis, rheumatoid arthritis, irreparable injury of the rotator cuff, and severely comminuted fracture of the proximal aspect of the humerus. However, the advent of shoulder arthroplasty has resulted in a marked reduction in the number of shoulder arthrodesis performed, although there are instances when arthrodesis is favored over joint replacement arthroplasty. Current indications for shoulder arthrodesis include posttraumatic brachial plexus injury, paralytic disorders in infancy, insufficiency of the deltoid muscle and rotator cuff, chronic infection, failed revision arthroplasty, severe refractory instability, and bone deficiency following resection of tumor in the proximal aspect of the humerus (1).

Shoulder arthrodesis is an extensive procedure. The techniques for shoulder arthrodesis include internal fixation and external fixation. Rigid internal fixation with either single- or double-plating is probably the most commonly used technique for obtaining a solid fusion. Several factors have contributed to a high rate of successful fusion. These include the combination of rigid internal fixation as well as incorporation of both intra-articular (glenohumeral) and extra-articular (acromiohumeral) surfaces (1).

COMPLICATIONS

Complications with shoulder arthrodesis can occur and can be potentially devastating. This chapter will cover the most common complications associated with shoulder arthrodesis. The complications include wound healing problems, wound infection, fractures below the level of the fusion, nonunion of the arthrodesis, and malposition of the arthrodesis (1,2). Surgical corrections for a malpositioned arthrodesis will also be addressed. Less common complications include acromioclavicular dislocation, acromioclavicular arthrosis, and suprascapular traction neuritis, which is primarily caused by excessive abduction and forward flexion of the fusion resulting in increased tension on the scapular muscles, acromioclavicular joint and suprascapular nerve (3–6).

Many authors have stressed the value of internal fixation for maintenance of the position of the humeral and scapular surfaces, especially when the arthrodesis combines both intra-articular (glenohumeral) and extra-articular (acromiohumeral) techniques. This combination has resulted in a high rate of successful fusion, although complications continue to be reported (1).

INFECTION

Difficulties that may arise with shoulder arthrodesis are not unique to this long and difficult operative procedure. Wound infection at the operative site is managed with standard techniques, which include irrigation and drainage along with culture of specimens from the wound. Appropriate antibiotics (an intravenous course followed by an oral course) have been successful in the treatment of this wound problem. In the early postoperative period, hardware retention should be attempted at all costs. Infection with a more virulent gram-positive organism may make this difficult. Infections that are recalcitrant to conservative measures may require hardware removal to help eradicate the infection. In an unstable patient or an elderly patient with low functional demands, conversion to a resectional arthroplasty should be considered. In other patients and those infected with more common gram-positive organisms, a delayed revision arthrodesis should be considered once successful union has been achieved. In the late postoperative period with clinical and radiographic evidence of healing, hardware removal should be considered to help eradicate the infection. In short, hardware contributing to harboring of organisms leading to tissue destruction warrants removal.

Wick et al. (7) reported the long-term results of arthrodesis of the shoulder after septic arthritis in 15 patients. They were able to show an increased rate of complications in patients with active sepsis. Younger patients (<50 years) and those with fewer previous operations (<4 operations) had better outcomes. The main complication was persistent infection with failure of bony fusion. Considering the rate of complications, they recommended early surgery in these patients. Similarly, a wound hematoma may develop, particularly in association with harvest of iliac-crest bone graft. Evacuation of the hematoma is often indicated. Also related to the harvest of iliac-crest bone graft are the risk of injury to the lateral femoral cutaneous nerve and the potential development of meralgia paresthetica (1).

FRACTURES

Fracture about the shoulder may occur in a patient treated with a shoulder arthrodesis. The fracture may occur in association with the fixation device or distal to the site of the arthrodesis. Distal fractures have responded to nonoperative treatment with simple use of a coaptation splint. Union has been observed to occur without substantial change in the position of the shoulder. Fractures that occur more proximally in association with internal fixation devices have been successfully treated with removal of the devices

and repeat plate application and bone-grafting (1). It is important to span the fusion site as well as the fracture site with an appropriately sized 4.5-mm pelvic reconstruction or a 4.5-mm dynamic compression plate. The use of synthetic auto- or allograft should be considered at the surgeon's discretion.

NONUNION

Failure of union may occur after either primary or revision shoulder arthrodesis, but this is rare when current fixation techniques are used, consisting of internal fixation with one or two plates. Nonunions due to poor fixation techniques should be treated with hardware removal and revision arthrodesis. The use of bone graft is not necessary when bone coaptation can be achieved. In the setting of significant bone loss, the use of autogenous corticocancellous bone graft should be considered. Nonunions following an arthrodesis using adequate fixation techniques should be treated with revision arthrodesis. We recommend hardware removal, debridement of the nonunion site, and repeat plate application. The site of arthrodesis is stabilized with a 4.5-mm pelvic reconstruction plate. A 4.5-mm dynamic compression plate is preferred for patients who weigh more than 100 kg. Bone grafting with autogenous bone recovered from the pelvis is used to supplement and fill in deficient areas.

There seems to be a trend toward improved union rates with an increase in the utilization of internal fixation techniques. Miller et al. (8) used a cadaveric model to perform a biomechanical analysis of five fixation techniques used in glenohumeral arthrodesis. They were able to demonstrate that bending and torsional stiffness was greatest in double-plate fixation. The authors suggested that applying these biomechanical principles to surgical decision-making could minimize the risk of nonunion and malposition. To further minimize chances of failure, patients should be counseled preoperatively to abstain from tobacco use because of the association of smoking with an increased risk for nonunion in general. Optimal operative technique includes careful attention to elimination of all cartilage, maximum bone coaptation, and solid positioning of all implants (1).

The need for supplemental support with the use of external fixation is unnecessary provided that optimal operative techniques are utilized. In addition, the use of an external fixator is poorly tolerated. Although of no proven benefit for shoulder arthrodesis, a bone stimulator may be considered at the surgeon's discretion.

MALPOSITION

By far the most critical complication that may follow shoulder arthrodesis is malpositioning of the extremity, which is primarily the result of excessive abduction and flexion. When fusion occurs in malposition, the extremity does not hang comfortably at the patient's side. In Groh et al.'s series of fourteen patients treated for complications related to shoulder arthrodesis (2), malposition was primarily the result of either flexion or abduction or both, coupled with improper internal rotation, which was defined as rotation less than 40 degrees or more than 60 degrees. Excessive abduction and flexion produce malrotation or winging of the scapula, which results in a dull painful ache in the shoulder. In addition, excessive abduction can cause a traction neuritis on the brachial plexus and, specifically, on the suprascapular nerve (1,2). Once the diagnoses of nonunion and pseuodarthrosis have been excluded, symptomatic malposition should be corrected.

Nagy et al. (9) reported that correct positioning of the humerus on the scapula was the main determinant for the outcome of shoulder arthrodesis. To facilitate positioning of shoulder arthrodesis, the authors recommended clinically estimating the position by assessing both scapulae in a symmetrical position relative to the healthy arm. In 1974, Rowe and Leffert (10) recommended a fusion position of abduction and flexion of approximately 20 to 25 degrees each, and internal rotation to approximately 40 degrees. Rowe recommended positioning the extremity to provide enough abduction to clear the axilla, enough forward flexion to reach the face, and sufficient internal rotation to reach the midline of the body (11). Groh et al. (2) recommend a position of 10 to 15 degrees of abduction, 10 to 15 degrees of flexion, and 45 degrees of internal rotation.

PEARLS

In planning a corrective osteotomy for malposition, the arm is stabilized in a position of sufficient abduction and flexion to alleviate the pain in the shoulder resulting from strain on the scapulothoracic muscles. An osteotomy that will correct the malposition is then planned based on the difference between the malposition and the normal resting position in relation to the thorax. The operative technique for correcting a malpositioned arthrodesis has been described by Groh et al. (2).

Provided that there is a solid union, we recommend a correctional humeral osteotomy. After the arthrodesis is exposed, any hardware (if present) is removed. We prefer to leave the arthrodesis site intact and perform an osteotomy inferior to the arthrodesis, making sure that the site of the osteotomy exits inferior and lateral to the inferior rim of the original glenoid. A medial closing wedge osteotomy is performed corresponding to the amount of correction needed to obtain the desired abduction. An anterior closing wedge osteotomy is performed corresponding to the amount of correction needed to obtain the desired flexion. A mathematical formula is used to convert the desired degree of correction of flexion or abduction into the millimeters of thickness of bone that must be removed with a closing-wedge osteotomy to restore the proper angle of the arm, or a scale drawing can be used to determine the width of the wedge (Fig. 9-1). The amount of angular correction (in degrees) needed to obtain the desired position can be calculated from radiographs. An anteroposterior and lateral radiograph is used to calculate the amount of abduction and flexion, respectively. The width (in millimeters) of the proximal part of the humerus, inferior to the glenoid, is determined from the radiographs, after correction for magnification. These values are used to construct a right triangle. The base of the triangle (AB; Fig. 9-1) is the width of the proximal part of the humerus inferior to the glenoid. Angle A is the total amount of angular correction needed to obtain the desired position. From this, the width of the wedge (BC) either is determined from the mathematical formula $BC = \tan A \cdot AB$ or is measured directly from a scale drawing. The amount of internal rotation that is needed depends on the configuration of the torso. For thin patients, more internal rotation will be necessary; for obese patients less internal rotation is necessary.

The operative technique for correction is similar to the technique for primary arthrodesis (1). The transverse cut is made first, and rotation is corrected if necessary. The closing wedge osteotomy is then performed with the arm held in correct rotational alignment (Fig. 9-2). After the

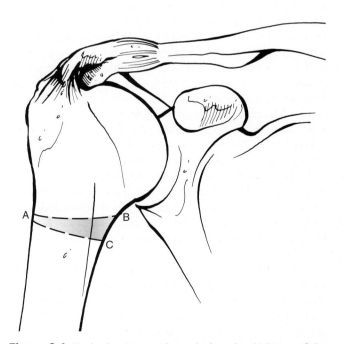

Figure 9-1 Scale drawing used to calculate the thickness of the closing-wedge osteotomy needed to correct malposition after arthrodesis. (Reprinted from Groh GI, Williams GR, Jarman RN, Rockwood CA. Treatment of complications of shoulder arthrodesis. *J Bone Joint Surg Am* 1997;79:881–887, with permission.)

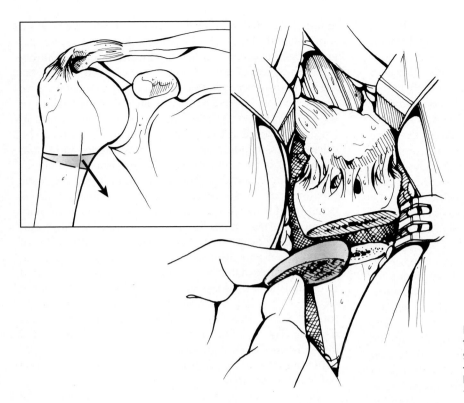

Figure 9-2 An inferior osteotomy is performed just inferior and lateral to the original glenoid. (Reprinted from Groh GI, Williams GR, Jarman RN, Rockwood CA. Treatment of complications of shoulder arthrodesis. *J Bone Joint Surg Am* 1997;79:881–887, with permission.)

wedge of bone has been removed, the osteotomy site is reduced and held provisionally. This position is then checked by moving the hand of the involved limb to the mouth, the abdomen, and the perineal area. The site of arthrodesis is stabilized with a 4.5-mm pelvic reconstruction plate. A 4.5-mm dynamic compression plate is preferred for patients who weigh more than 100 kg. The length of the plate is determined by the need to have three screws proximal to the acromion and three screws distal to the level of the osteotomy (Fig. 9-3). Bone grafting should be done when complete coaptation of the osteotomy site has not been achieved either from the autogenous bone recovered from the osteotomy; if not, sufficient additional bone should be taken from the pelvis.

In the Groh et al. series of 14 patients treated for complications related to shoulder arthrodesis (2), the complications were the result of a malpositioned arthrodesis in 9 cases. These patients underwent a reconstructive osteotomy of the fusion mass for correction of the malpositioned extremity, and their cases were reviewed at a mean of 6 years following the surgery. Preoperatively, the mean position of fusion was 47 degrees of forward flexion, 37 degrees of abduction, and 37 degrees of internal rotation. All patients had chronic, long-standing pain and difficulty with daily activities. Postoperatively, the mean position of the shoulder was 13 degrees of forward flexion, 16 degrees of abduction, and 48 degrees of internal rotation. All patients had substantial relief of pain and were able to perform their daily activities much more effectively.

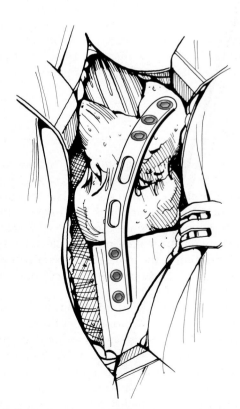

Figure 9-3 Final appearance, before closure and after application of a contoured plate. (Reprinted from Groh GI, Williams GR, Jarman RN, Rockwood CA. Treatment of complications of shoulder arthrodesis. *J Bone Joint Surg Am* 1997;79:881–887, with permission.)

REFERENCES

1. Clare DJ, Wirth MA, Groh GI, et al. Current concepts review: shoulder arthrodesis. *J Bone Joint Surg* 2001;83:593–600.
2. Groh GI, Williams GR, Jarman RN, et al. Treatment of complications of shoulder arthrodesis. *J Bone Joint Surg* 1997;79:881–887.
3. Gonzalez-Diaz R, Rodriguez-Merchan EC, Gilbert MS. The role of shoulder fusion in the era of arthroplasty. *Int Orthop* 1997;21: 204–209.
4. Diaz JA, Cohen SB, Warren RF, et al. Arthrodesis as a salvage procedure for recurrent instability of the shoulder. *J Shoulder Elbow Surg* 2003;12:237–241.
5. Carnesale PG, Stewart MJ. Complications of arthrodesis surgery. In: Epps CH Jr, ed. *Complications in Orthopaedic Surgery*, 3rd ed, Vol 2. Philadelphia: JB Lippincott, 1994: 1201–1218.
6. Wilde AH, Brems JJ, Boumphrey FR. Arthrodesis of the shoulder. Current indications and operative technique. *Orthop Clin North Am* 1987;18:463–472.
7. Wick M, Muller EJ, Ambacher T, et al. Arthrodesis of the shoulder after septic arthritis. Long-term results. *J Bone Joint Surg Br* 2003; 85:666–670.
8. Miller BS, Harper WP, Gillies RM, et al. Biomechanical analysis of five fixation techniques used in glenohumeral arthrodesis. *ANZ J Surg* 2003;73:1015–1017.
9. Nagy L, Koch PP, Gerber C. Functional analysis of shoulder arthrodesis. *J Shoulder Elbow Surg* 2004;13:386–395.
10. Rowe CR. Re-evaluation of the position of the arm in arthrodesis of the shoulder in the adult. *J Bone Joint Surg Am* 1974;56: 913–922.
11. Rowe CR, Leffert RD. *Advances in Arthrodesis of the Shoulder.* New York: Mosby, 1988:507–519.

Complications of Scapulothoracic Arthrodesis

10

Sumant G. Krishnan   Richard J. Hawkins   Wayne Z. Burkhead

INTRODUCTION

Refractory disorders of the scapulothoracic articulation have been reported to result in debilitating pain and dysfunction that may require surgical management (1–22). The most common clinical presentation, scapular winging (23), was first reported in the published literature in 1723, and several etiologies for scapular winging have been subsequently documented. Soft tissue operations (such as pectoralis major tendon transfer) have had reported success in stabilizing the dyskinetic scapula in the appropriate patient population (24–30).

However, despite these successful clinical outcomes, there exists a population of patients who experience recurrent symptomatic scapular winging even after pectoralis major transfer (23,25). Several authors (7,23,25,31) report that arthrodesis is the treatment of choice for these failed muscle transfers. For failed pectoralis transfer or significant (irreducible) fixed winging, scapulothoracic arthrodesis can be a successful salvage operation for these patients (12).

Unfortunately, the incidence of postoperative complications after scapulothoracic arthrodesis is significant, occurring in 33% to 48% of patients (12). The vast majority of complications can be grouped into four major categories:

1. Pulmonary complications
2. Hardware complications and/or nonunion
3. Neurologic complications
4. Wound complications

AUTHORS' PREFERRED SURGICAL TECHNIQUE FOR SCAPULOTHORACIC ARTHRODESIS

Although a detailed description of the technique for scapulothoracic arthrodesis can be found elsewhere (12), a brief review assists in the understanding of potential complications.

The patient is intubated with a double-lumen endotracheal tube (to allow for selective deflation of the ipsilateral lung during wire placement) and positioned prone. The entire involved arm, scapula, and ipsilateral posterior iliac crest are prepped and draped to the midline of the spine. The incision is placed along the medial border of the scapula from just superior to the scapular spine to the inferior angle. The superficial fascia is incised and the trapezius muscle is identified and retracted medially. The rhomboid muscles are incised off the medial edge of the scapula to allow for reattachment prior to closure.

Approximately one-third of the musculature of the serratus anterior and the subscapularis are resected from medial to lateral off the anterior surface of the scapula to allow for a wide fusion surface. The anterior surface of the scapula is now slightly roughened with a burr. Next, the scapula is reduced to the rib cage in approximately 20 to 25 degrees of external rotation from the midline. The ribs corresponding to the decorticated anterior surface of the scapula are identified and the scapula is again retracted to allow for rib preparation. Depending on the size and configuration of the scapula, typically three or four ribs will be utilized in the fusion (usually the third to sixth ribs). The periosteum is carefully incised in a longitudinal direction and stripped off each rib. The ribs are minimally roughened with a burr down to bleeding bone.

At this time, the involved lung is deflated prior to passage of cerclage wires around the ribs. Using rib and periosteal dissectors, 1.5-mm cerclage wire is carefully passed around each of the exposed ribs at the level where the medial border of the scapula will be placed on the rib cage (Fig. 10-1). After passage of the cerclage wires, a one-third semitubular large fragment plate (typically with five or six holes depending on the size of the scapula) is lined up on the posterior aspect of the medial border of the scapula (the thickest part of the scapula). A 3-mm burr is used to make holes through the scapula corresponding to the holes in the semitubular plate.

Cancellous bone is now harvested from the posterior iliac crest in routine fashion. The wires are now passed through the scapula and semitubular plate, and the bone graft is placed between the scapula and ribs. The wires are now sequentially tightened with the scapula held in 20 to 25 degrees of external rotation from the midline. The semitubular plate allows uniform stress distribution once the wires are tightened (Fig. 10-2).

The lung is reinflated and irrigation is used to assess for a pneumothorax. The rhomboids are then reattached to the medial aspect of the scapula, and the subcutaneous tissue and skin are closed in the usual fashion. A postoperative chest x-ray is then obtained prior to leaving the operating room.

Immobilization is used for 12 weeks in a "gunslinger" brace (Fig. 10-3). Rehabilitation is commenced at 12 weeks with a gentle passive range-of-motion program that emphasizes forward elevation and external rotation. Three weeks

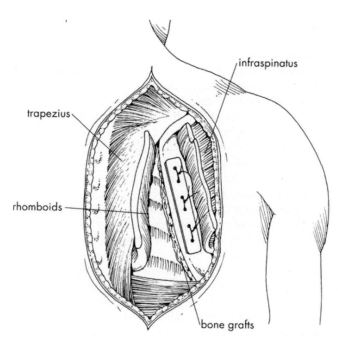

Figure 10-2 Final construct with plate on medial border of scapula.

later, the patient is progressed to an active range-of-motion program. A strengthening program involving resisted exercises is subsequently begun 6 weeks after the gunslinger was removed.

PULMONARY COMPLICATIONS

Pulmonary complications have been reported in up to 48% of patients undergoing scapulothoracic arthrodeses

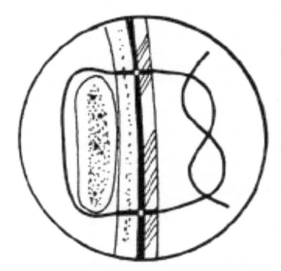

Figure 10-1 Sagittal plane view of cerclage wire through plate, through scapula, and around rib.

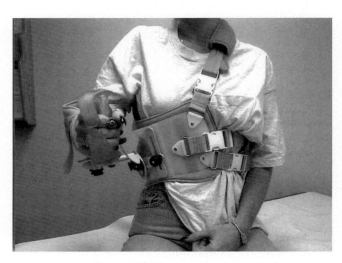

Figure 10-3 Gunslinger brace.

(12,24–27,31,32). Intraoperative or postoperative pneumothorax remains the most common problem. Some patients have also demonstrated "reactive" bilateral pleural effusions within 48 hours of the index procedure (10,12,25). Despite meticulous attention to surgical technique, pulmonary complications remain a very present problem with scapulothoracic fusions and must be considered in the preoperative discussions with patients. Any patient with previous pulmonary compromise or pulmonary disease must undergo a formal pulmonary evaluation with pulmonary function tests to assess ability to withstand the morbidity of this operation.

The most likely cause of any pneumothorax or hemothorax is undoubtedly penetration of the pleural cavity during passage of cerclage wires around the thoracic ribs (12). The first step in prevention involves the use of a double-lumen endotracheal tube by the anesthesiologist for intubation and anesthesia. When the ribs are being prepared, the ipsilateral lung should be deflated to keep the pleural surface as far from the ribs as possible. Meticulous surgical technique for subperiosteal exposure of the ribs must be respected. Passage of the cerclage wire places the pleura at most risk, and a right-angle clamp or modified Satinsky vascular clamp is extremely useful in maintaining complete contact with the rib during passage near the pleura.

Immediately after passage of all wires, irrigation fluid should be placed in the wound and the ipsilateral lung should be inflated multiple with large tidal volumes in an attempt to identify any air bubbles indicative of an air leak (or pneumothorax) (25). If a pneumothorax is present, a thoracostomy tube must be inserted at the completion of the surgical procedure (usually by a thoracic surgeon who has been placed on standby during the procedure).

If a reactive pleural effusion develops in the immediate perioperative period, a therapeutic thoracentesis must be considered based on patient symptoms and shortness of breath. The reason for this complication still remains unknown but must be related to intraoperatively induced changes in intrapleural pressure forcing third-spacing of fluid into the extrapleural cavity (1,12,25). If a thoracentesis cannot relieve the fluid buildup, a thoracostomy tube must again be considered to alleviate patient symptoms.

Pearls

- Use double-lumen tube and deflate lung
- Meticulous subperiosteal passage of rib cerclage wires
- Thoracostomy tube when necessary

HARDWARE COMPLICATIONS AND NONUNIONS

Hardware-related complications are second to pulmonary complications in incidence and have been reported in as many as 33% of patients after scapulothoracic arthrodesis (12,25). Such problems usually involve either breakage of the cerclage wires and/or nonunion of the fusion construct.

To minimize the occurrence of wire breakage, the recommended size of the wire is no smaller than 1.50 mm (12). This will provide not only strong compression at the plate/bone interface, but also will allow for enough static strength to withstand muscular contraction until a solid arthrodesis has developed.

Assuming that the strength of the wire/plate construct is as mentioned above, failure of fusion or pseudarthrosis at the scapulothoracic junction appears to be related to inadequate osteoinductive graft and/or inadequate mobilization prior to radiographic arthrodesis (5,12,25). The systematic use of iliac crest autograft (with or without allograft cancellous chips) should not be overlooked; this can be harvested easily from a posterior approach to the iliac crest as is performed in spinal fusion surgery. Use of cancellous autograft has been documented to increase the incidence of clinically and radiographically stable fusions.

Postoperative immobilization must be rigid enough to withstand both involuntary muscular contraction and also potential active motion. The use of a simple sling is contraindicated secondary to the high rate of nonunions associated with simple sling immobilization (12,33). Hence, a rigid orthosis (such as a "gunslinger" brace) that maintains both an appropriate neutral position of the arm and also prevents active motion should be employed.

Pearls

- Use minimum 1.50 mm size wire
- Use cancellous autograft
- Immobilize in gunslinger or similar brace

NEUROLOGIC COMPLICATIONS

Postoperative neuralgia has been documented in approximately 20% of patients following this operation (12). This pain and numbness most often follows an intercostal nerve dermatomal distribution and can be very troublesome to manage. Intercostal nerve blocks may provide some relief, but some patients even require eventual cerclage wire and hardware removal secondary to refractory intercostals neuralgia. Consequently, attempts to minimize damage or irritation to the intercostals nerves via meticulous surgical technique and true subperiosteal passage of the cerclage wires are paramount.

Pearls

- Prevention of intercostal neuralgia by minimizing trauma to intercostal nerves is the best method to reduce neurologic complications.

WOUND COMPLICATIONS

Despite the apparently morbid surgical approach and extensive tissue dissection necessary for successful scapulothoracic arthrodesis, the incidence of wound complications is actually quite low. Most series report few deep infections (<10%) and very few even superficial wound infections (5,12,25). This may be due to the highly vascular muscular bed that is elevated during this operation. Still, any wound problem should be treated aggressively and surgeons must maintain vigilance due to the potentially catastrophic nature of an unrecognized deep infection after attempted scapulothoracic arthrodesis.

Pearls

- Infection rare but surgeons must maintain vigilance.

CONCLUSION

Despite the significant complication rate (up to nearly 50%) that accompanies scapulothoracic arthrodesis, this operation has been documented to provide both improvements in pain and functional disability. High patient satisfaction after appropriate surgical indications and technique can make this operation rewarding for both patient and surgeon. Avoidance of complications via precise surgical technique appears to be the best method for prophylactically "treating" the complications associated with scapulothoracic fusions. Aggressive identification and management of any complications that arise will still allow for potentially successful outcomes.

REFERENCES

1. Atasoy EJ, Majd M. Scapulothoracic stabilization for winging of the scapula using strips of autogenous fascia lata. *J Bone Joint Surg Br* 2000;82:813–817.
2. Bunch WH, Siegel IM. Scapulothoracic arthrodesis in facioscapulohumeral muscular dystrophy. *J Bone Joint Surg Am* 1993;75:372–376.
3. Connor PM, Yamaguchi K, Manifold SG, et al. Split pectoralis major for serratus anterior palsy. *Clin Orthop* 1997;341:134–142.
4. Cooley LH, Torg JS. "Pseudowinging" of the scapula secondary to subscapular osteochondroma. *Clin Orthop* 1982;162:119–124.
5. Copeland SA, Howard RC. Thorascapular fusion for facioscapulohumeral dystrophy. *J Bone Joint Surg Br* 1978;60:547–551.
6. Fery A. Results of treatment of anterior serratus paralysis. In: Post M, Morrey BF, Hawkins RJ, eds. *Surgery of the Shoulder.* Philadelphia: Mosby, 1990:325–329.
7. Foo CL, Swann M. Isolated paralysis of the serratus anterior. A report of 20 cases. *J Bone Joint Surg Br* 1983;65:552–556.
8. Harper GD, McIlroy S, Bayley JIL, et al. Arthroscopic partial resection of the scapula for snapping scapula: a new technique. *J Shoulder Elbow Surg* 1999;8:53–57.
9. Iceton J, Harris WR. Treatment of winged scapula by pectoralis major transfer. *J Bone Joint Surg Br* 1987;69:108–110.
10. Ketenjian AY. Scapulocostal stabilization for scapular winging in facioscapulohumeral muscular dystrophy. *J Bone Joint Surg Am* 1978;60:476–480.
11. Kuhn JE, Plancher KD, Hawkins RJ. Symptomatic scapulothoracic crepitus and bursitis. *J Am Acad Orthop Surg* 1998;6:267–273.
12. Krishnan SG, Hawkins RJ, Michelotti JD, et al. Scapulothoracic arthrodesis: indications, technique, and results. *Clin Orthop* 2005;435:126–133.
13. Letournel E, Fardeau M, Lytle JO, et al. Scapulothoracic arthrodesis for patients who have facioscapulohumeral muscular dystrophy. *J Bone Joint Surg Am* 1990;72:78–84.
14. Marmor L, Bechtol CO. Paralysis of the serratus anterior due to electric shock relieved by transplantation of the pectoralis major muscle: a case report. *J Bone Joint Surg Am* 1963;45:156–160.
15. Milch H. Partial scapulectomy for snapping of the scapula. *J Bone Joint Surg Am* 1950;32:561–566.
16. Milch H. Snapping scapula. *Clin Orthop* 1961;20:139–150.
17. Perlmutter GS, Leffert RD. Results of transfer of the pectoralis major tendon to treat paralysis of the serratus anterior muscle. *J Bone Joint Surg* 1999;81:377–384.
18. Post MP. Pectoralis major transfer for winging of the scapula. *J Shoulder Elbow Surg* 1995;4:1–9.
19. Richards RR, An K-N, Bigliani LU, et al. A standardized method for assessment of shoulder function. *J Shoulder Elbow Surg* 1994;3:347–352.
20. Richards RR, McKee MD. Treatment of painful scapulothoracic crepitus by resection of the superomedial angle of the scapula. *Clin Orthop* 1989;247: 111–116.
21. Strizak AM, Cowen MH. The snapping scapula syndrome. *J Bone Joint Surg Am* 1982;64:941–942.
22. Wiater JM, Flatow EL. Long thoracic nerve injury. *Clin Orthop* 1999;368:17–27.
23. Kuhn JE, Plancher KD, Hawkins RJ. Scapular winging. *J Am Acad Orthop Surg* 1995;3:319–325.
24. Freedman L, Munro RR. Abduction of the arm in the scapular plane: scapular and glenohumeral movements. *J Bone Joint Surg Am* 1966;48:1503–1510.
25. Hawkins RJ, Willis RB, Litchfield RB. Scapulothoracic arthrodesis for scapular winging. In: Post M, Morrey BF, Hawkins RJ, eds. *Surgery of the Shoulder.* Philadelphia: Mosby, 1990:340–349.
26. Hays JM, Zehr DJ. Traumatic muscle avulsion causing winging of the scapula. *J Bone Joint Surg Am* 1981;63:495–497.
27. Johnson JT, Kendall HO. Isolated paralysis of the serratus anterior muscle. *J Bone Joint Surg Am* 1955;37:567–574.
28. Povacz P, Resch H. Dynamic stabilization of winging scapula by direct split pectoralis major transfer: a technical note. *J Shoulder Elbow Surg* 2000;9:76–78.
29. Warner JJP, Navarro RA. Serratus anterior dysfunction. *Clin Orthop* 1998;349:139–148.
30. Zeier FG. The treatment of winged scapula. *Clin Orthop* 1973;91:128–133.
31. Gozna ER, Harris WR. Traumatic winging of the scapula. *J Bone Joint Surg Am* 1979;61:1230–1233.
32. Gregg JR, LaBosky D, Harty M, et al. Serratus anterior paralysis in the young athlete. *J Bone Joint Surg Am* 1979;61:825–832.
33. Harryman DT, Walker ED, Harris SL, et al. Residual motion and function after glenohumeral or scapulothoracic arthrodesis. *J Shoulder Elbow Surg* 1993;2:275–285.

Arthroscopy

General Complications of Arthroscopic Shoulder Surgery

Sumant G. Krishnan **Scott D. Pennington**
Daniel E. Cooper **Wayne Z. Burkhead**

INTRODUCTION

The evolution of both arthroscopic surgical techniques and equipment over the past 75 years has revolutionized shoulder surgery. Arthroscopy has evolved from a simple diagnostic tool to an invaluable instrument for minimally invasive shoulder reconstructions. The potentially devastating complications of open shoulder surgery, such as subscapularis repair failures and deltoid dehiscence, are minimized with arthroscopy but are not eliminated if attention to detail is lost (1). In truth, the overall complication rate of arthroscopic shoulder surgery is low but not insignificant.

A 1998 study from Madrid reported one surgeon's arthroscopic complication rate of 10.63% (2). In 2002, Weber et al. (3) reported an overall complication rate in the published literature ranging from 5.8% to 9.5%. An exact rate is difficult to determine secondary to inaccuracies in reporting complications and disagreement over what constitutes a complication. For instance, some studies include postoperative shoulder stiffness as a complication, whereas others do not (2).

As Muller and Landsiedl stated, arthroscopy is not "band-aid surgery" (4). Specifically, problems can be encountered with patient positioning, surgical draping, and even arthroscopic portal placement. Patient selection, correct clinical diagnoses, and appropriate surgical indications remain critical to the success of any arthroscopic procedure,

as some shoulder pathologies are not correctable by arthroscopic techniques alone. Anatomic structures are at risk and anatomic variants can cause confusion. Poor implant selection or placement may lead to intraoperative difficulty and possibly iatrogenic chondral damage. However, most complications of shoulder arthroscopy can be avoided by meticulous attention to detail.

PATIENT SELECTION

The appropriate patient selection for shoulder surgical procedures is covered comprehensively throughout this text, but several points with respect to shoulder arthroscopy bear mentioning. Although surgeons are attracted to the comprehensive visualization, scar cosmesis, and brisk return to function provided by shoulder arthroscopy, not all shoulder pathologies are amenable to arthroscopic procedures. Instability secondary to significant glenoid bony deficiency or large engaging Hill-Sachs lesions may require an open stabilization with an osseous transfer (iliac crest or Latarjet-Bristow procedure) (5). Massive and irreparable rotator cuff tears can be debrided or partially repaired arthroscopically, but large retracted and irreparable tears with significant fatty infiltration may require a tendon transfer. Failure to appreciate these clinical situations preoperatively will undoubtedly lead to surgical frustration and potentially sub-optimal patient outcomes.

ANESTHESIA CONCERNS

There have been several reports in the recent orthopaedic and anesthesia literature of anesthetic complications encountered during arthroscopic shoulder surgery (4). These include tracheal compression caused by periarticular fluid accumulation, visual loss and opthalmoplegia, pneumomediastinum from subcutaneous emphysema, spontaneous pneumothorax, and negative pressure pulmonary edema (6–10). These complications are exceedingly rare and hence difficult to screen for or prevent. The keys to managing (and possibly even preventing) these catastrophic situations are constant communication between the surgeon and anesthesiologist during the surgical procedure and a thorough knowledge of advance cardiac life support (ACLS) should the need arise for emergent perioperative resuscitation.

The main decision for patients and surgeons remains choice of anesthesia: general anesthesia versus regional anesthesia. Although the complications of general anesthesia are beyond the scope of this text, the most common complications of the interscalene brachial plexus block must be reviewed because this is the most widely used regional technique for arthroscopic shoulder surgery (3). Such complications most often involve palsy of the phrenic nerve (shortness of breath with hemidiaphragmatic paralysis), Horner's syndrome (ipsilateral sympathetic blockade), and/or recurrent laryngeal nerve palsy (hoarseness and ipsilateral vocal cord paralysis). Although these complications are most often transient, they should be promptly evaluated when present by both the operating surgeon and the involved anesthesiologist.

Authors' Preferred Anesthesia

We prefer to use general anesthesia for nearly every shoulder arthroscopy case. Although regional anesthesia is attractive, in our experience this technique is clearly dependent on the skill of the treating anesthesiologist and the incidence of transient vocal cord/laryngeal paralysis and/or hemidiaphragmatic paralysis is not negligible. At times, for postoperative pain control, we will combine a regional interscalene block with general anesthesia, although this may incur the risks inherent to both techniques.

PATIENT POSITIONING

Inappropriate patient positioning is perhaps the leading cause of complications both during and after arthroscopic

shoulder surgery (11). Malpositioning can lead to significant upper and lower extremity neuropraxias as well as soft tissue injury away from the surgical site. The operating surgeon must be intimately involved during the installation of patients prior to shoulder arthroscopy, whether in the lateral decubitus position or the beach chair position. Surgeon participation at this level insures both the proper orientation of the patient for arthroscopic visualization as well as the optimal padding of bony prominences and susceptible neurovascular structures. Furthermore, preoperative planning by the operating surgeon may also dictate the type of positioning that may not be readily apparent to other physician or surgical assistants in the operating room. Arthroscopic posterior instability surgery may be more easily done in the lateral position, whereas the beach chair position may be preferred if the conversion to an open procedure is likely (3).

When placing the patient in the beach chair position, make certain the head is well-seated and secured in a fixed head holder with neutral position of the cervical spine (Fig. 11-1). Excessive pressure around the head can cause a neuropraxia of the posterior auricular nerve. The eyes should be free of any compression and the endotrachial tube should be directed away from the operative field. Flex the hips and knees comfortably such that the patient does not slide inferiorly during the procedure (Fig. 11-2). This also decreases both lumbosacral pressure and also the tension of the sciatic nerve. The neck must remain in a neutral position throughout the procedure to avoid any neuropraxias, and the anesthesiologist should be encouraged to frequently check the position of the head and neck during surgery (Fig. 11-3). Excessive flexion, extension, rotation,

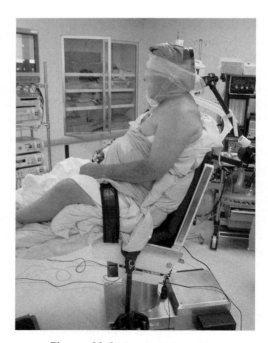

Figure 11-1 Beach chair position.

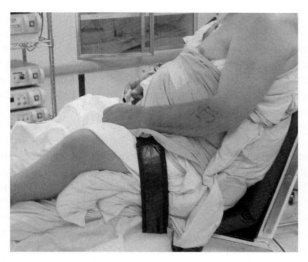

Figure 11-2 Appropriate flexion of hips and knees to relieve lumbosacral pressure and prevent traction on the long-tract nerves of the lower extremities.

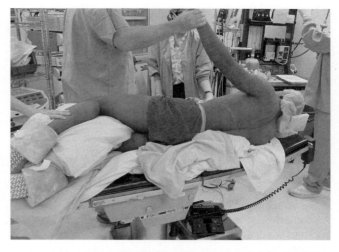

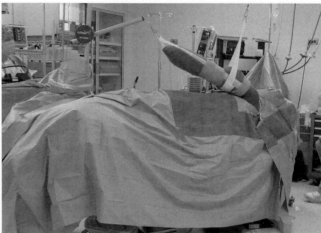

Figure 11-4 Lateral decubitus position.

or lateral bending of the cervical spine can lead to a brachial plexus injury (12,13).

When installing the patient in the lateral decubitus position, the same parameters for the head and neck should be respected: neutral cervical spine position, avoidance of excessive pressure on the cranium or eyes, and flexion of both hips and knees (Fig. 11-4). Because in the lateral position the patient will be applying direct pressure to the contralateral half of the body, several other measures must be undertaken (3). An axillary roll should be placed under the contralateral upper ribs to prevent direct pressure through the axilla on the brachial plexus (though pressure-induced plexus palsy in the lateral position may still occur, even with appropriate axillary padding, if the patient has a cervical rib) (12,13). The contralateral peroneal nerve must be padded at the fibular head, as this is the nerve anatomically

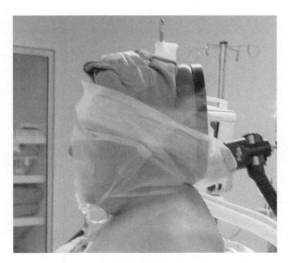

Figure 11-3 Neutral position of the cervical spine.

located in the most subcutaneous position that may be affected by prolonged direct pressure (14). The operative arm is often held in an abducted position by a longitudinal and perpendicular traction device. The appropriate amount of arm abduction to provide necessary visualization in the lateral position remains controversial and ranges from 0 to 90 degrees when combined with varying amounts of flexion. Published work has documented a reduced incidence of brachial plexus strain with increasing amounts of arm flexion (up to 90 degrees) and decreasing amounts of arm abduction (up to 0 degrees). We prefer to keep the arm in approximately 25 to 30 degrees of abduction in the scapular plane (approximately 30 degrees of forward flexion). Care must be taken to avoid excessive traction in either position (longitudinally or perpendicular to the glenohumeral joint). Neuropraxias have been documented by simple traction along the length of the operative arm. In addition, both abduction and traction changes the position of neurovascular structures at risk relative to the glenohumeral joint, and the potential for iatrogenic injury may increase if care is not taken when operating in the lateral position (14–20).

The brachial plexus is fixed at two positions: at the transverse processes by the prevertebral fascia and at the axillary fascia (21). Neck extension and lateral bending to the contralateral side puts traction on the plexus, as does excessive arm external rotation and abduction (11). Use of as little as 2 to 4 kg of longitudinal and perpendicular distraction while in the lateral position may be more than sufficient to distract the glenohumeral joint without producing a traction neuropraxia.

Pearls

■ Neutral cervical spine position
■ Pad all bony prominences and subcutaneous nerves
■ Flexion of hips and knees

DRAPING

Surgical draping is an important and often overlooked detail of arthroscopic shoulder surgery that may prevent unnecessary complications. Improper draping can contaminate the operative field, tempt the surgeon to create suboptimal portals secondary to insufficient medial shoulder exposure, and make seamless conversion to an open procedure impossible. Consequently, the surgeon must educate the entire surgical team in a consistent method of draping the operative field that provides for reproducible exposure of the shoulder for any arthroscopic or open procedure (14).

Pearls

■ Reproducible draping technique for reproducible exposure

ANATOMIC STRUCTURES AT RISK DURING ARTHROSCOPY

"Doctors without anatomy are like moles. They work in the dark and the work of their hands are mounds."
                                        Tiedemann (1781–1861)

"Anatomy is power . . . but the only constant in anatomy is variation."

                                        Henry (1957)

A fundamental and detailed knowledge of shoulder anatomy is critical to avoid iatrogenic neurovascular injury and to prevent catastrophic, irreparable complications.

Axillary Nerve

The axillary nerve arises from the posterior cord of the brachial plexus with contributions from C5 and C6. It courses

directly posterior to the coracoid and along the anteroinferior subscapularis muscle before traveling posteriorly just inferior and lateral to the glenoid with direct capsular contact while exiting the quadrilateral space. It then divides into the anterior branch (which innervates the anterior and middle deltoid from the subdeltoid surface and within the muscle of the deltoid) and the posterior branch (which innervates the teres minor and posterior deltoid) and terminates with the cutaneous innervation of the lateral shoulder. The nerve is held to the glenohumeral capsule with loose areolar tissue between the 5 and 7 o'clock positions of the glenoid face and is closer to the humeral attachment of the capsule than the glenoid attachment (18,20).

The nerve is potentially at risk with creation of the standard arthroscopic posterior viewing portal. The traditional location of this portal in the "soft spot" is 2 cm inferior and 2 cm medial to the posteriolateral corner of the acromion, thereby entering the joint through the infraspinatus or between the infraspinatus and the teres minor. This is safely superior to the quadrilateral space but the axillary nerve can still run 0.5 to 2.5 cm inferior to this portal (12). Hence, some surgeons advocate the use of a "high" lateral portal located approximately 1 cm inferior and 1 cm medial to the posterolateral acromion. (Fig. 11-5) (22). Any lateral working portal can also place the axillary nerve in jeopardy if it is created more than 3 cm distal to the edge of the acromion (13). A safe 7 o'clock accessory posterior portal has recently been described with mean distance from the axillary nerve of 39 mm (23).

Specific surgical procedures within the glenohumeral joint capsule also place the axillary nerve at risk. Glenohumeral capsular releases through the anteroinferior and posteroinferior axillary pouch and recesses place the nerve in jeopardy as indicated by its anatomical course. However, adhesive capsulitis makes the joint capsule taut and the distance between the glenoid and the axillary nerve may

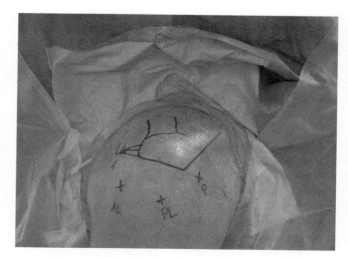

Figure 11-5 High posterior portal 1 cm inferior to and 1 cm medial to the posterolateral acromion.

actually be increased when the arm is in more abduction and external rotation (18).

Capsulolabral sutures for arthroscopic glenohumeral instability reconstructions have been implicated in potential axillary nerve damage, especially when arthroscopically performing a capsular shift of the anteroinferior band of the inferior glenohumeral ligament (3). However, recent anatomical work has demonstrated that when sutures are placed in the glenohumeral capsule no further lateral than 1 cm from the glenoid rim, the axillary nerve still maintains a minimum distance of 7 mm (17).

Suprascapular Nerve

The suprascapular nerve originates from the C5 and C6 nerve roots at the junction of the upper trunk of the brachial plexus and its divisions. After following the omohyoid muscle posteriorly, the nerve runs inferiorly through the suprascapular notch under the superior transverse scapular ligament where it is relatively fixed in position. After exiting the notch, the nerve provides innervation to the supraspinatus and then continues medial to the superior edge of the glenoid and enters the spinoglenoid notch at the lateral scapular border while traveling posteriorly to innervate the infraspinatus via two to four branches. At its closest point, the nerve may be less than 2 cm from the glenoid rim as it travels posteriorly (19).

Although the use of suture anchors has all but eliminated injury to the suprascapular nerve previously caused by "blind" transglenoid drilling during instability surgeries, injury to the nerve still remains a concern with both glenohumeral and subacromial surgeries. The safe zone for the nerve remains approximately 1 to 2 cm from the glenoid rim for any superior or posterosuperior procedure, so the often-used Neviaser "superior" portal (just medial to the acromioclavicular joint) maintains this safe zone (3). However, excessive medial placement of this superior portal or medially-directed instruments could still damage the nerve at it traverses the supraspinatus fossa.

Though not unique to arthroscopic shoulder surgery, injury to the suprascapular nerve has been documented with overly aggressive lateral mobilization of a retracted rotator cuff tear (24). Hence, the safe zone of no more than 2 cm of mobilization medial to the superior glenoid rim must be respected during juxtaglenoid capsulotomy and mobilization during arthroscopic rotator cuff repair.

Musclocutaneous Nerve

The main trunk of the musclocutaneous nerve enters the coracobrachialis 3.1 to 8.2 cm inferior to the tip of the coracoid, with smaller branches entering as close as 1.7 cm distal to the coracoid tip (25). Standard anterior arthroscopic working portal placement is usually midway between the coracoid and anterolateral corner of the acromion (Fig. 11-6). Either inferior or medial placement of

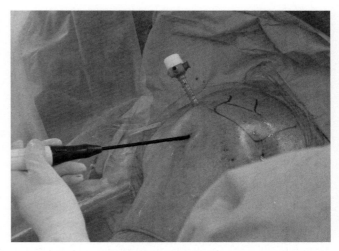

Figure 11-6 Anterior arthroscopic working portal midway between the coracoid and anterolateral acromion.

this anterior portal can place the musculocutaneous nerve at risk. Use of a spinal needle through the rotator interval under direct visualization or creation of an inside-out portal can diminish this risk.

Anatomical Variants and Miscellaneous Concerns

"Primum non nocerum (First, do no harm).*"*

Familiarity with normal anatomic variants can prevent both intraoperative confusion and unnecessary procedures. Although the discussion of these variants is provided elsewhere, surgeons should seek to understand intimately the normal anatomy because the only constant in anatomy is truly variation. Just as the "peel-back" maneuver can distinguish a meniscoid labrum or sublabral foramen from a superior labral anterior posterior (SLAP) tear (26), so too can the recognition of the sublabral foramen associated with a cordlike middle glenohumeral ligament (Buford) complex prevent an unwarranted anterosuperior labral "repair."

Iatrogenic chondral damage from shoulder arthoscopy can be catastrophic and may even result in humeral head collapse requiring prosthetic replacement (3). Consequently, surgeons strive to minimize any potential for chondral damage by surgical instruments. For example, even in patients with a contracted capsule from adhesive capsulitis, damage to the articular surface of the humerus can be avoided if the joint is entered at the superior aspect of the glenohumeral articulation rather than at the midline of the glenoid.

Vascular injuries during or after shoulder arthroscopy are exceedingly rare. The cephalic vein is anterior and lateral to the anterolateral acromion and sequela from its injury are both infrequent and often overlooked. No other reports of major vascular injuries after routine shoulder arthroscopy have been documented.

Pearls

- Understand and review anatomy
- Respect neurovascular structures

COMPLICATIONS FROM SURGICAL IMPLANTS AND DEVICES

Implant-related complications can be divided into four types: improper placement, migration after placement, loosening, and breakage (27–31). Synovitis associated with absorbable devices can also occur (30). With the advent of stronger sutures and improved anchor eyelets, breakage of suture is less common. Rather, some sutures are stouter than the tissue they are securing and can actually tear through poor tissue.

Implant choice is also critical to preventing complication and thereby optimizing patient outcome. Documented loosening of metallic anchors placed within the glenohumeral joint has been shown to lead to extreme third-body wear and severe glenohumeral arthrosis. Consequently, bioabsorbable implants have been advocated in an attempt to reduce that incidence should the implant either fail or "pull out." Unfortunately, the exact degradation of bioabsorbable and bioresorbable products in vivo still remains unknown, and the relative makeup of the absorbable implant can be responsible for both faster breakdown and also for inciting an inflammatory reaction. Predominantly polyglycolic (PLGA) acid implants have demonstrated a larger inflammatory response when compared to polylactic (PLLA) acid implants, though PLLA implants degrade at a faster rate than PLGA implants. Hence, although failure of an implant is occasionally out of the control of the surgeon, appropriate implant selection, skillful surgical technique, and attention to detail can diminish untoward outcomes.

Pearls

- Know the surgical implants intimately prior to surgery

EXTRAVASATION

Excessive intra-articular bleeding, extravasation of irrigant, and choice of irrigant can complicate shoulder arthroscopy. Maintaining the patient's systolic blood pressure between 90 to 100 mm Hg and use of pump-controlled irrigation can provide outstanding visualization without significant bleeding. Commercially available arthroscopic pumps can either control pressure alone or separately control both pressure and flow. Recent work has demonstrated that, although the total amount of fluid used does not seem to vary between pump types, the use of a pump that separately

controls both pressure and flow appears to result in less soft tissue extravasation, better visualization, and shorter operative time. We currently utilize both types of pumps and maintain the pump pressure between 35 and 40 mm Hg regardless of pump used.

The solution used for irrigation has been documented to create difficulties. Although a randomized, double-blinded, placebo-controlled study of dilute epinephrine in saline has been shown to improve visualization during arthroscopy with no cardiovascular adverse reactions (32), a published case report has described an "epinephrine-induced potentially lethal arrhythmia" that was attributed to "intraosseous infusion" of irrigation (33). Others have also reported an episode of transient blindness associated with glycine in the irrigation (34). Nevertheless, because the benefits for visualization and hemostasis appear to outweigh these miniscule risks, we currently utilize dilute epinephrine (1 cc epinephrine per 3000 cc fluid) in all of our arthroscopic irrigation fluid and have never experienced complications related to the epinephrine.

Extravasation of fluid is associated with prolonged operative times and elevated irrigation pump pressures. Although fluid extravasation has been felt by many to increase the potential for postoperative pain, some authors have found no clinical or electromyographical evidence of muscle damage with soft-tissue extravasation and noted that intramuscular pressure returned to baseline within minutes after the arthroscopic procedure was completed (35).

Pearls

- Minimize pump pressure to prevent extravasation (35 to 40 mm Hg)
- Meticulous hemostasis is paramount
- Use diluted epinephrine in the irrigation bags

INFECTION

Deep infection is a rare complication of arthroscopic shoulder surgery with an incidence of far less than 1% (3). Careful attention to the surgical preparation and draping, meticulous surgical technique, avoidance of tissue necrosis, and preoperative antibiotics are important factors in keeping the incidence of infection so exceedingly rare.

POSTOPERATIVE PAIN

Although open shoulder surgeries are traditionally considered significantly painful procedures, shoulder arthroscopy has developed a reputation for markedly reduced postoperative pain (16,36). Some even view postoperative pain from shoulder arthroscopy as a potentially preventable complication (22). As mentioned previously, appropriate attention to surgical technique, minimization of fluid extravasation, and the use of periportal anesthetic injections can all reduce patient discomfort following shoulder surgery.

CONCLUSION

Although not all complications are preventable, it does appear that the majority of complications associated with shoulder arthroscopic surgery can be avoided with meticulous attention to detail. Surgeons should seek to implement a reproducible system of patient anesthesia and installation/positioning to minimize variables out of the surgeon's control. Surgical anatomy and surgical techniques should be frequently reviewed so that precise portal placement and execution of the predetermined operative plan can lead to efficient surgical performance and minimized intraoperative and postoperative morbidity to the patient.

REFERENCES

1. Bonsell S. Detached deltoid during arthroscopic subacromial decompression. *Arthroscopy* 2000;16:745–748.
2. Berjano P, Gonzalez BG, Olmedo JF, et al. Complications on arthroscopic shoulder surgery. *Arthroscopy* 1998;14:785–788.
3. Weber SC, Abrams JS, Nottage WM. Complications associated with arthroscopic shoulder surgery. *Arthroscopy* 2002;18:88–95.
4. Muller D, Landsiedl F. Arthroscopy of the shoulder joint: a minimal invasive procedure and harmless procedure? *Arthroscopy* 2000;16(4):425.
5. Burkhart SS, DeBeer JF. Traumatic glenohumeral bone defects and their relationship to failure of arthroscopic Bankhart reapirs: significance of the inverted-pear glenoid and the humeral engaging Hill-Sachs lesion. *Arthroscopy* 2000;16:677–694.
6. Bhatti MT, Enneking FK. Visual loss and opthalmoplegia after shoulder surgery. *Anesth Analg* 2003;96:899–902.
7. Borgeat A, Bird P, Ekatodramis G, et al. Tracheal compression caused by periarticular fluid accumulation: a rare complication of shoulder surgery. *J Shoulder Elbow Surg* 2000;9:443–445.
8. Dietzel DP, Ciullo JV. Spontaneous pneumothorax after shoulder arthroscopy: a report of four cases. *Arthroscopy* 1996;12:99–102.
9. Langan P, Michaels R. Negative-pressure pulmonary edema: a complication of shoulder arthroscopy. *Am J Orthoped* 1999;28:56–58.
10. Lau KY. Pneumomediastinum caused by subcutaneous emphysema in the shoulder. A rare complication of arthroscopy. *Chest* 1993;103:1606–1607.
11. Cooper DE, Jenkins RS, Bready L, et al. The prevention of injuries of the brachial plexus secondary to malposition of the patient during surgery. *Clin Orthopaed Relat Res* 1988;228:33–41.
12. Pavlik A, Ang KC, Bell SN. Contralateral brachila plexus neuropathy after arthroscopic shoulder surgery. *Arthroscopy* 2002;18:658–659.
13. Perlmutter GS. Axillary nerve injury. *Clin Orthoped Relat Res* 1999;368:28–36.
14. Stanish WD, Peterson DC. Shoulder arthroscopy and nerve injury: pitfalls and prevention. *Arthroscopy* 1995;11:458–466.
15. Bigliani LU, Dalsey RM, McCann PD, et al. An anatomical study of the suprascapular nerve. *Arthroscopy* 1990;6:301–305.
16. Bigliani LU, Flatow EL, Deliz ED. Complications of shoulder arthroscopy. *Orthopedic Rev* 1991;20:743–751.
17. Eakin CL, Dvirnak P, Miller CM, et al. The relationship of the axillary nerve to arthroscopically placed capsulolabral sutures. *Am J Sports Med* 1998;26:505–509.
18. Jerosch J, Filler TJ, Peuker ET. Which joint position puts the axillary nerve at lowest risk when performing arthroscopic capsular release in patients with adhesive capsulitis of the shoulder. *Knee Surg Sport Tr A* 2002, 10:126–129.
19. Shishido H, Kikuchi S. Injury of the suprascapular nerve in shoulder surgery: an anatomic study. *J Shoulder Elbow Surg* 2001;10:372–376.
20. Uno A, Bain GI, Mehta JA. Athroscopic relationship of the axillary nerve to the shoulder joint capsule: an anatomic study. *J Shoulder Elbow Surg* 1999;8:226–230.
21. Clausen EG. Postoperative ("anesthetic") paralysis of the brachial plexus. *Surgery* 1942;12:933–942.
22. Krishnan SG, Burkhead WZ. *Arthroscopic rotator cuff repair in patients under the age of 40.* Orlando, FL: Arthoscopy Association of North America meeting, 2004.
23. Davidson PA, Rivenburgh DW. The 7 o'clock posteroinferior portal for shoulder arthroscopy. *Am J Sports Med* 2002;30:693–696.
24. Warner JP, Krushell RJ, Masquelet A, et al. Anatomy and relationships of the suprascapular nerve: anatomical constraints to mobilization of the supraspinatus and infraspinatus muscles in the management of massive rotator-cuff tears. *J Bone Joint Surg Am* 1992;74:36–45.
25. Flatow EL, Bigliani LU, April EW. An anatomic study of the musclocutaneous nerve and its relationship to the coracoid. *Clin Orthoped Relat Res* 1989;244:166–171.
26. Burkhart SS, Morgan CD. The peel-back mechanism: its role in producing and extending posterior type II SLAP lesions and its effect on SLAP repair rehabilitation. *Arthroscopy* 1998;14:637–640.
27. Antonogiannakis E, Yinnakopoulos CK, Karliaftis K, et al. Late disengagement of a knotless anchor. *Arthroscopy* 2002;18:E40.
28. Freehill MQ, Harms DJ, Huber SM, et al. Ploy-L-lactic acid tack synovitis after arthroscopic stabilization of the shoulder. *Am J Sports Med* 2003;31:643–647.
29. Mallik K, Barr MS, Anderson MW, et al. Intra-articular migration of sutureless arthroscopic rotator cuff fixation device. *Arthroscopy* 2003;19:E5–8.
30. Silver MD, Diagneault JP. Symptomatic intrasrticular migration of glenoid suture anchors. *Arthroscopy* 2000;16:102–105.
31. Wilkerson JP, Zvijac JE, Uribe JW, et al. Failure of polymerized lactic acid tacks in shoulder surgery. *J Shoulder Elbow Surg* 2003;12:117–121.
32. Jensen KH, Werther K, Stryger V, et al. Arthroscopic shoulder surgery with epinephrine saline irrigation. *Arthroscopy* 2001;17:578–581.
33. Karns JL. Epinephrine-induced potentially lethal arrhythmia during arthroscopic shoulder surgery: a case report. *AANA J* 1999;67:419–421.
34. Burkhart SS, Arnett CR, Synder SJ. Transient postoperative blindness as a possible effect of glycine toxicity. *Arthroscopy* 1990;6:112–114.
35. Ogilvie-Harris DJ, Boynton E. Arthroscopic acromioplasty: extravasation of fluid into the deltoid muscle. *Arthroscopy* 1990;6:52–54.
36. Scarlat MM, Harryman DT II. Management of the diabetic stiff shoulder. *Instruct Course Lect* 2000;49:283–294.

Arthroscopy: Complications of Surgery for Instability

Carlos A. Guanche   Stephen J. Snyder

INTRODUCTION

In the last decade, arthroscopic management of a multitude of orthopaedic problems has become commonplace. One of the most frequent scenarios addressed is glenohumeral instability, a diagnosis fraught with pitfalls. The challenge begins with making the appropriate diagnosis and ends with a likely complex surgical procedure that requires individualized rehabilitation. The incidence of complications arising from the arthroscopic management of instability, however, has not been clearly elucidated in the literature. There are many case reports of various untoward scenarios, yet there is no organized compilation of all the wisdom acquired through these cases.

In one of the earliest attempts to stratify the risks associated with arthroscopic surgery in general, Small (1) documented an overall complication rate of 1% with shoulder arthroscopy. According to his report, the highest rate of complications (5.3%) was from arthroscopic staple capsulorrhaphy. More recently, Curtis et al. (2) have shown an overall rate of complications of 6% for shoulder arthroscopy with some gradation of the procedures from minor to major. In procedures where arthroscopy alone was performed, there was an overall complication rate of 4.5%, with most of those being postoperative stiffness. With procedures that added an open component, the complication rate increased to 6%. More recently, Weber et al. (3) have estimated that there is a 5.8% to 9.5% incidence of complications with shoulder arthroscopy in general. They also al-

lude to the probable increased incidence with more complex procedures.

RECURRENT INSTABILITY

Despite the advances in arthroscopic stabilization, recurrence of instability continues to be the most common complication. The rates of recurrence have varied widely depending on the type of procedure performed. The rates have been documented as 16% to 33% with the use of staple capsulorrhaphy, 0% to 60% with transglenoid suturing, and 0% to 30% with suture anchor repair (4–6). In some situations, however, no amount of anchoring will maintain stability (Fig. 12-1).

There are many reasons for failure in the reconstruction of the unstable shoulder and these are not necessarily unique to arthroscopic stabilization. They can be divided into a variety of errors attributable to incorrect diagnosis (direction), surgical error, or rehabilitation error. In addition, the episode leading to recurrence is likely to offer some clues as to the etiology. An atraumatic event leading to recurrence in a patient following stabilization may indicate failure to address some component of the instability, whereas a more significant trauma may indicate simple recurrence from a macrotraumatic event. The patient should be questioned with regards to their postoperative satisfaction with the procedure. If the patient indicates that func-

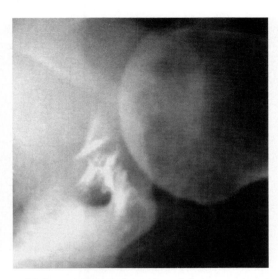

Figure 12-1 Multiple suture anchors following two attempted arthroscopic procedures in a patient with multidirectional instability.

tional return had not occurred prior to the recurrence event, then they are likely to have undergone inadequate rehabilitation or, in worse cases, sustained a surgical failure.

The most common error made by the surgeon is incomplete diagnosis or, more specifically, failure to address the primary component and/or often the secondary component of instability. This is especially true in cases of multidirectional instability. The reason for this problem is the vagueness of symptoms in most patients. Examination under anesthesia prior to beginning the arthroscopic procedure is critical in that regard. This portion of the procedure is either neglected or not performed at all in many cases. This step should be the final determining factor with respect to any surgical intervention that is undertaken.

Beyond misdiagnosis of the type of instability, failures can be attributable to a lack of understanding of surgical principles. In some situations, a labral detachment is properly addressed but the remaining capsular redundancy is not. This important element of instability correction has historically been described for open procedures, but certainly applies to arthroscopic stabilizations (7). Judicious use of the arthroscope and thorough examination under anesthesia go a long way toward preventing those unfortunate mistakes. A diagnostic arthroscopy should be entertained in any case where there is no significant obvious bony deficiency. Whether the procedure is actually performed arthroscopically or not must be determined by the pathology encountered as well as the arthroscopic skill of the surgeon.

The typical patient will spend 2 hours in the operating room but many days in the therapist's office. This fact is simply forgotten by many, not the least of whom is the surgeon. To that end, the most common rehabilitation

error is that of failure to complete the process (and in some cases, not to institute it at all). A thorough rehabilitation focus beginning with scapulothoracic stabilization and strengthening with a progression to proprioceptive neuromuscular facilitation is integral to returning the patient to his or her preoperative activity level.

A thorough evaluation of the soft tissues is the key to diagnosing the entire spectrum of injuries that is commonly seen with instability. One area that deserves special attention is the anterior labrum periosteal sleeve avulsion (ALPSA) lesion (8). In this situation, the glenoid labrum, along with the capsule, has been avulsed and then healed in a more medial position on the glenoid neck. This leads to mechanical incompetence of the labrum's stabilizing effect. This lesion is often missed because it may not be recognized on magnetic resonance imaging (MRI) or it may not be seen from the standard posterior portal.

Other variants in the spectrum of pathologies are the humeral avulsion of the glenohumeral ligament (HAGL) and reverse humeral avulsion of the glenohumeral ligaments (RHAGL) lesions. These rare anterior or posterior ligament detachments have been recognized for many years since first described by Nicola in 1942 (9). However, despite being known, they are often also difficult to identify on imaging studies or arthroscopic evaluation. HAGL or RHAGL lesions are commonly seen after failure of the original stabilization procedure, as has been noted by Savoie (10). Finally, the rotator interval capsule is a complex and poorly understood portion of the anatomy. Although insufficiency of this area contributes to instability in several directions (11), there is a paucity of guidelines for the treatment of rotator interval pathology.

Mologne et al. (12) have analyzed 20 patients that had failed arthroscopic stabilization procedures. In their study (in which the patients were revised with open surgery), they found that 40% of the patients had an unhealed Bankart lesion and 75% were found to have redundant anterior capsules (12). They concluded that capsular laxity is difficult to quantify arthroscopically and is present in a significant percentage of patients with chronic traumatic shoulder instability.

Bony deficiency is another area that warrants careful consideration (13). Historically, the focus on arthroscopic repairs has centered on the reattachment of soft tissue to bone, while ignoring the bony deficiencies. In situations where multiple episodes of instability have occurred, patients may develop a significant bony defect (Fig. 12-2). This is particularly important on the glenoid side, but can also be seen in the form of a large Hill-Sachs lesion of the humeral head. Burkhart and DeBeer (13) have documented that their arthroscopic stabilization patients are more likely to have instability recur when an insufficient glenoid surface was found intraoperatively. In their study of 21 patients having recurrent instability following arthroscopic suture anchor fixation, 14 had sizeable bone defects, with 3

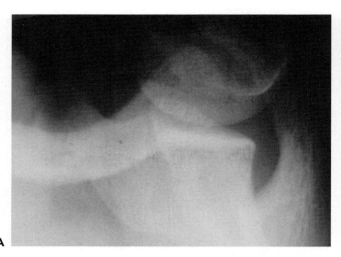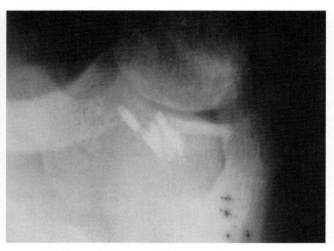

A   B

Figure 12-2 Axillary profile views (Bernageau) of the symptomatic and asymptomatic shoulders of a patient having undergone an open and an arthroscopic procedure for recurrent instability, now with continued dislocation episodes. **A:** Normal glenoid profile view. **B:** Abnormal profile with significant deficiency of the anterior portion as compared to the normal side. Note the multiple anchors within the deficient portion of the glenoid.

engaging Hill-Sachs lesions and 11 "inverted-pear" glenoid defects.

The diagnosis of a significant glenoid deficiency can be made radiographically with the use of the Bernageau or glenoid profile view (Fig. 12-2) (14). Confirmation of the deficiency can also be made arthroscopically by measuring the size of the glenoid from the central bare spot to the anterior and posterior edges of the labrum. A size difference of more than 2.5 mm between the two measurements is thought to be indicative of a relatively deficient glenoid (15). Most commonly, these cases are corrected with either a Laterjet-type coracoid transfer procedure (Fig. 12-3) (13),

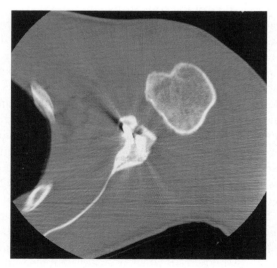

Figure 12-3 Postoperative computed tomography scan of a professional football player following Laterjet procedure. Note the interface between the original glenoid and the substantial bony fragment used to reconstruct the glenoid.

or reconstruction of the glenoid using iliac crest bone graft (16).

In some situations, a substantial avulsion fracture of the glenoid is either neglected or not addressed at the time of the initial surgical procedure (Fig. 12-4). In these cases, a solid labral repair may still fail as a result of the lack of surface for articulation of the humeral head and the glenoid. Although the etiology of the glenoid deficiency is an acute defect, the same treatment principles apply. The initial surgical approach should address the avulsion and an attempt should be made to reapproximate the bony fragment in as near an anatomical position as possible.

The engaging Hill-Sachs lesion should also be ruled out as a source of recurrent instability. The engaging lesion is defined as a large posterior-lateral humeral head compression fracture situated with its long axis parallel to the anterior glenoid with the shoulder in a functional position of abduction and external rotation. In this location, the Hill-Sachs defect engages the corner of the glenoid (13). If an engaging lesion is documented, the surgery should involve not only a labral repair, but also a restriction of external rotation by capsular plication (performed either open or arthroscopically). Alternatively, the humeral head defect can be extended by filling it with either autogenous or allograft bone (17). A rotational proximal humeral osteotomy can also be performed in severe cases (18). This operation, however, is limited to the most severe cases, often where other measures have failed.

Another area that has received little attention is the lack of healing ability. This is particularly true in older patients where an instability episode is followed by surgical reconstruction. Intraoperatively, the tissue available for repair may be friable or atrophic and minimal trauma may result in a recurrence of the instability, causing a retear of the

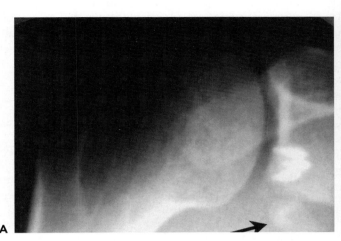
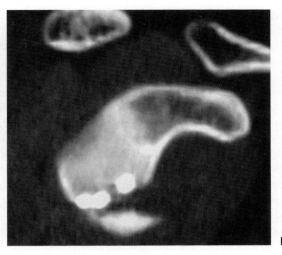

Figure 12-4 Patient with recurrent instability following arthroscopic reconstruction with minimal trauma. **A:** Radiograph depicting the bony fragment inferiorly. **B:** Computed tomography scan showing the position of the suture anchors within the fracture defect with significant displacement of the fragment.

labral repair (Fig. 12-5). This is a particularly troublesome situation that has no easy solution, although some attempts have been made to quantify the healing ability based on the appearance of the perilabral tissues (19). The referenced study analyzed the issue relating to the arthroscopic transglenoid technique, the principles of which apply to both arthroscopic reconstruction and open reconstruction. In these cases, open repairs may be more appropriate if the tissue mobilization that is necessary to obtain a solid repair cannot be performed arthroscopically. This concept has especially significant implications with respect to the surgeon's individual abilities in performing arthroscopic mobilization.

In summary, although the pathological areas to consider in revision surgery are many, a few principles can be applied to guide one through the process. In general, the arthroscope is a useful tool to delineate the extent of the pathology involved. In some cases, the arthroscopic visualization of the pathology is more readily visible than when assessed in an open fashion. An excellent example would be a HAGL lesion.

In cases where severe bony deficiency is suspected, plain films should serve as a guide for the need for further diagnostic studies, such as a computed tomography (CT) scan. Where the history and radiographs are questionable with regards to the remaining bone stock, a reasonable option is to perform a diagnostic arthroscopy and be prepared to perform an open reconstruction (such as a Laterjet) at the same sitting.

In situations where a severe bony deficiency is present, the arthroscope is not helpful in most cases. In these cases, a single open procedure is typically indicated without the need for a diagnostic arthroscopy. That being said, however, in cases where additional pathology is suspected (such as a rotator cuff deficiency), a diagnostic arthroscopy can help plan the appropriate procedure(s).

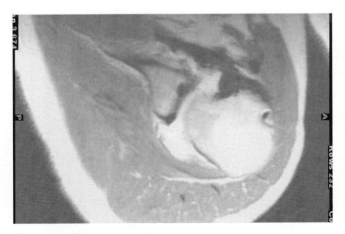

Figure 12-5 Recurrent Bankart lesion in a postoperative patient following minimal traumatic episode. Patient was 35 years of age at the time of the surgical procedure, with tissue being documented as frayed and relatively avascular.

LOSS OF MOTION WITHOUT ARTHROSIS

Although the major goal in the treatment of recurrent instability is the restoration of stability and the maintenance of pain-free motion, in some cases excessive tightening results in significant and often disabling painful limitation of motion. Excessive loss of motion, most often external rotation, has been implicated as a cause of degenerative arthrosis (20–22).

Historically, several open procedures sought to limit the incidence of dislocation and subluxation episodes by intentionally restricting motion. To date, this has not been a significant source of concern with respect to arthroscopic repairs. Arthroscopic repairs generally tend to recreate the normal anatomy, especially as it concerns a reattachment of the detached capsulolabral complex. It is technically more difficult to perform significant capsular shifts and imbrications as has been described and documented with open procedures. As a result, the more likely scenario following arthroscopic procedures has involved the recurrence of dislocation or subluxation episodes rather than excessive tightness. When stiffness does occur, it is often associated with hardware complications resulting from prominent suture anchors or degradative products of absorbable devices (23–27).

In summary, it is important to realize that the anatomical reconstruction of the joint is integral to a good outcome. Positioning of suture anchors appropriately on the articular margin is important, as is tightening the capsuloligamentous complex to its original configuration and tension. Advancing the tissue too far may cause an excessive restriction of motion and subsequent stiffness in the joint. When performing arthroscopic capsular closure procedures, it is important to avoid suturing and thus overtightening specific anatomic structures such as the middle or superior glenohumeral ligaments, unless the specific motion restrictions associated with their tightening is desired (11). This is especially dangerous in cases where a rotator interval closure is performed or when the cordlike middle ligament of a Buford complex is mistakenly fixed to the glenoid.

In a patient with restricted range of motion, one must rule out other pathologic entities such as reflex sympathetic dystrophy, rotator cuff tendinitis, inflammatory and crystalline arthropathy, avascular necrosis, secondary gain and psychological dysfunction. In addition, the patient's surgical procedure, postoperative immobilization, and rehabilitation regimen should all be critically analyzed. The causes of stiffness may be either capsular or extracapsular and a careful examination of the surrounding musculature is important in this respect (28).

ARTHROSIS

Although extremely rare in arthroscopic procedures, patients who have severe arthrosis following an arthroscopic reconstruction may require prosthetic replacement with careful attention to soft-tissue balancing. Long-standing contractures tend to force the humeral head posteriorly as a result of the anterior capsular restriction that tends to develop. This can result in a fixed posterior subluxation with significant posterior glenoid erosion (29).

There are two important considerations when treating a poststabilization arthritic shoulder with shoulder replacement: significant posterior capsular redundancy and posterior glenoid wear. Both problems can contribute to a difficult reconstructive procedure. Careful preoperative

planning must address the likelihood of the need to perform a posterior capsulorrhaphy. This may require either an anterior incision or a separate posterior surgical approach. In more severe cases, a glenoid bony reconstruction may be warranted (20).

HARDWARE/IMPLANT-RELATED

Implants placed arthroscopically have not been reported to cause life-threatening hardware migration as have implants placed in open procedures (30,31). It must be assumed that these implants will behave the same as when they are poorly placed in open surgery (Fig. 12-6).

In the early reports of transglenoid suturing techniques, fistula and cyst formation were documented (32) as well as intrathoracic penetration with a Beath pin (33). This type of procedure is no longer employed and the documentation of any of associated complications is largely historical.

The use of absorbable tack devices is relatively commonplace in arthroscopic labral repairs. The biological process of degradation of these devices has been elucidated in scientific literature and it is important to review the process to understand why failures occur. The polymers that are used to fabricate these devices include polydioxanone (PDS) and either combinations or racemic mixtures of polyglycolic acid (PGA) or polylactic acid (PLA).

Degradation of PLA and PGA occurs in a continuum of five stages (34). Initially, *hydrolysis* from local tissue fluids occurs. The hematoma from the surgery then leads to a fibrous capsule forming with granulation tissue and giant cells. The next stage is *depolymerization*, which begins with a loss of strength of the device. The kinetics of this mechanism depends on the material's physical qualities, surface area, and the environment to which it is exposed. The third

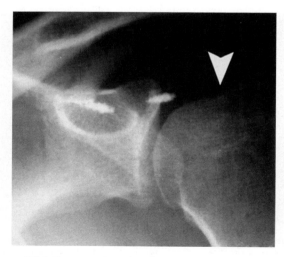

Figure 12-6 Suture anchor placed in a prominent position causing significant erosion (arrow) of the humeral head.

stage involves *loss of mass integrity* as the implant begins to fragment. At this point a mild inflammatory reaction may occur, although this varies with the actual material employed. The fourth stage, *absorption*, is where hydrolysis allows for phagocytosis and dissolution. Finally, *elimination* allows for the monomers to be broken down and excreted primarily as carbon dioxide and water from the lungs (PLA/PGA) or via the urinary system (PDS).

Tack capsulorrhaphy has been fraught with complications that are unique to the headed, absorbable devices. The synovitis that occurs as a result of the degradation products has been well documented (23,35,36). In many cases, a refractory capsulitis develops and leads to stiffness, which then leads to the need for further surgical intervention. Freehill et al. (23) have documented a 19% incidence of capsulitis and significant chondral injury in 52 patients who had undergone labral surgery with poly-L-lactic tacks. All of the patients underwent second look arthroscopy with extensive debridement and manipulation under anesthesia (23). Interestingly, despite the significant synovial reaction, the labral repairs were completely healed. In their histological analyses, they found extensive synovial hyperplasia and increased cellularity with an infiltration of giant cells and histiocytes with associated foreign bodies.

Besides the degradative inflammatory process described above, there are many reports of failing implants causing intra-articular symptoms similar to a loose body (Fig. 12-7). If the symptoms are mild, these situations can be observed until the material dissolves and the symptomatology abates. In many cases, however, not only are there symptoms associated with the loose material within the joint, but also there is a recurrence of the tear that was repaired (Fig. 12-8). The more significant danger with simply observing these patients is that often the degree of damage to the articular cartilage is difficult to assess and is fre-

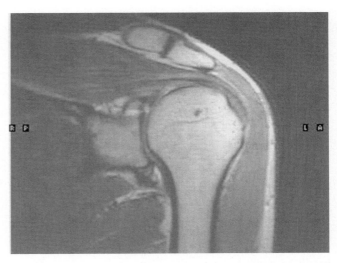

Figure 12-8 Recurrent SLAP lesion in a patient 6 weeks after tack repair of the labrum. Simple forward flexion of the arm caused significant pain and mechanical symptomatology prompting this magnetic resonance imaging.

quently underestimated (26). In an analysis of four patients undergoing repairs with bioabsorbable tacks (three for labral repair and one for rotator cuff repair), Wilkerson et al. (27) documented mechanical failure of the headed portion of the devices that occurred at the head-shaft junction (27). They theorized that the reason for the failure at this position was the variable microenvironments to which the head, neck, and shaft of the devices were exposed. It has been reported that degradation occurs more rapidly in soft tissue and or when the implant is exposed to mechanical stress (37). The intraosseous location of the polymer will have a different mechanism for debris clearance, neoangiogenesis, and the placement of implant within tissue versus the extraosseous location (38).

Extraosseous migration of the bioabsorbable implants has also been reported (39). This creates significant problem because the devices are radiolucent and thus may potentially cause permanent articular surface damage before the diagnosis is made.

In the analysis of patients following repairs with absorbable tacks, a high degree of suspicion must be had with regards to the occurrence of breakage and the subsequent synovitis that ensues. In general, patients that begin to increase their perceived pain level without increasing their activity level in rehabilitation are likely to have symptoms attributable to the side effects of degradation of the devices. In addition, a significant and relatively acute decrease in active or passive range of motion also indicates the possibility of synovitis. Radiographs are typically unrewarding and a magnetic resonance arthrogram (with gadolinium enhancement) should be performed in these questionable cases. A significant amount of synovitis is often seen in these cases and, not infrequently, large loose bodies.

The treatment once the diagnosis is made is highly indi-

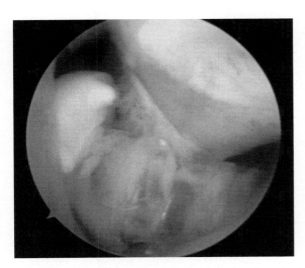

Figure 12-7 Bioabsorbable suture tack whose head portion has broken off postoperatively. The device was migrating about the joint, causing mechanical symptoms. Note the lack of degradation of the device.

vidualized. The use of corticosteroid injections in cases where there is a large inflammatory component without significant mechanical symptomatology is certainly acceptable. The most common problem that is seen in these patients is the significant capsular contracture that accompanies the inflammatory reaction. This is often the factor that delays their recovery most significantly.

In cases where there is a large mechanical component as well as pain that is refractory to corticosteroid injection, a reasonable course of action is to arthroscopically evaluate the joint and debride the synovium, along with removal of any loose debris. At this point, the treatment should not involve a new reconstruction of the joint, even in cases where the repair is clearly disrupted. The significant inflammatory component that accompanies these procedures warrants observation and later determination if instability is still an issue.

Bioabsorbable suture anchors have been implanted in the glenoid for repair of instability and superior labral anterior posterior (SLAP) lesions. Unlike the problems associated with the absorbable tacking devices, these anchors have met with success and no significant reports to date have been made of adverse reactions. In one multicenter study, the use of an L-lactic acid suture anchor with nonabsorbable sutures was found to be successful in 55 out of 57 patients with no adverse reactions to the biomaterial (40). Postoperative radiographs were analyzed at 2-year follow-up and no evidence of lytic or resorptive changes was found. Furthermore, there were no patients with inflammatory complications associated with the implants.

Arthroscopic staple capsulorrhaphy was the first attempt to use metal implants to stabilize the shoulder. Most of the early studies using staples documented high recurrence rates with significant complications caused by the migration of the device or breakage causing significant cartilage damage (1).

Suture anchor capsulorrhaphy is the current gold standard for arthroscopic stabilization. Early results in the literature vary from study to study, but current trends favor this technique as appropriate in most situations of instability. The recent results approximate the historical results of open surgery (13,41–43). Migration of metal anchors, however, has created problems in many situations, similar to those encountered with open procedures (Fig. 12-9) (44–46).

Historically, suture anchors were developed in tandem with arthroscopic procedures for the shoulder. Most reports have focused on the mechanical pullout resistance associated with the various anchors. Researchers agree the strength of the suture anchor construct is related mostly to the type of bone in which the anchor is placed and is ultimately dependent on the strength of suture material, the knots and quality of the tissues repaired.

There are few articles documenting the problems associated with metallic anchors. One study documented eight cases of complications associated with these anchors; however, only one case was performed arthroscopically (24).

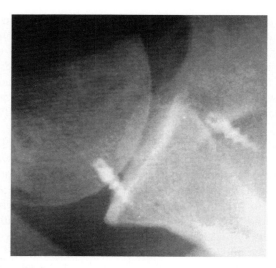

Figure 12-9 Axillary view of a metal suture anchor which has backed out following insertion, causing mechanical symptoms.

Another series documented glenohumeral arthropathy following arthroscopic anterior stabilization in five patients (25). In this retrospective review, all of the patients had anchors that were prominent. The heads of the anchors rubbed on the humeral head and caused severe arthritic changes. All of the patients were unsatisfied following a second surgical procedure for hardware removal.

The foremost causes of complications associated with metal anchors fall into two categories: technical problems associated with the mechanics of insertion, and incorrect location of anchor placement. The problems associated with the technical aspects of the devices vary from one manufacturer to another. One example of a common problem is the lack of control of insertion when using power-driven instruments (Fig. 12-10). In these cases, the anchor can be

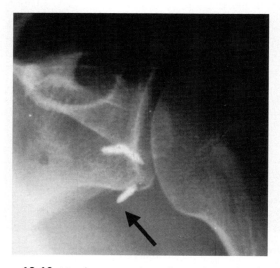

Figure 12-10 Metal suture anchor advanced past the glenoid as result of insertion with a motorized drill.

driven too deeply into the bone and penetrate the opposite side. The best solution is to avoid the mechanized or powered insertion of anchors. It is mandatory that the surgeon be thoroughly familiar with the mechanics of each individual device. Any questionable recommended insertion techniques should be evaluated and tested in the model lab prior to the implantation so as to avoid a major complication in surgery.

The position of insertion of the suture anchors is likewise crucial. It is important to be comfortable with the angle of approach to the various areas of the glenoid as well as the entire glenohumeral joint. There are two areas that are most difficult to access. The first is the area around superior labrum when repairing a SLAP lesion. Proper placement of the anchor requires a steep angle of insertion and potentially risks fracture of the cortex (Fig. 12-6). The second area that is commonly a problem is the lowest extent of Bankart lesions near the inferior pole of the glenoid. The areas below about 5 o'clock (on a right shoulder) can be difficult to access from a standard anterior portal as an anchor is inserted. The surgeon must assure that there is adequate circumferential bone around the anchor to ensure it remains in place. In addition, pulling on the anchor once it is inserted into the glenoid is important to assure that there is sufficient strength of fixation to sustain the postoperative physiologic load.

REVISION OF ARTHROSCOPIC REPAIRS

Addressing a failed instability procedure arthroscopically is certainly reasonable. There are many factors to consider in the preoperative plan including all those discussed above, in addition to the potential problems with any previously placed hardware.

If the factors of soft-tissue quality, adequate bone stock, and ability of the surgeon allow the management of the recurrence in an arthroscopic fashion, then it is appropriate. Surgical techniques are the same of those where there has been no previous surgery. As a frame of reference, Levine et al. (47) reviewed the results in 54 shoulders that had undergone a revision stabilization procedure after an operation for anterior instability had failed (47). At an average of 4.5 years, there were 40 excellent and 3 good results. All of the patients who had had a failed arthroscopic stabilization had an excellent result after an open revision operation.

Existing literature includes only one prospective study evaluating the results of arthroscopically revised instability surgery (48). Twenty-four consecutive patients who developed recurrent instability following a single surgical procedure were revised using arthroscopic techniques. All patients had a Bankart lesion visualized on preoperative MRI. At revision arthroscopy, three patients were noted to have anchor fixation that failed to address the anteroinferior capsular laxity, whereas five patients had failed as a result of

a nonanatomic repair, with the labral tissue fixed either proximal or medial to the glenoid margin. There were eight patients who had had suture anchors placed for labral repair. Eighteen anchors had been used in these patients with none having dislodged as a result of the dislocation episode. Failure of the suture occurred either by tear of the suture from the anchor in six patients or by avulsion of the suture from the capsulolabral tissue in seven. The authors recommended using an adequate number of suture anchors to increase the stress distribution and avoid failure of the repair with the disruption of any one suture.

The revision surgical procedure consisted of repairing the labrum using metal suture anchors and plicating the rotator interval with sutures in cases where there was residual laxity following knot tying. Five patients (22%) had failure of the arthroscopic revision procedure, three of the patients had recurrent instability, and two had positive anterior apprehension signs and relocation tests. With an increasing number of sutures, the stresses are distributed more widely and perhaps a recurrence can be avoided.

Finally, the study included only patients with failed Bankart repairs. Any patient having had additional procedures such as bony-block procedures or muscle-tightening procedures were excluded. Any patient with more than a 30% defect of the anterior glenoid was also excluded. Based on this prospective study, we can only make conclusions about patients having failed a straightforward labral repair.

NEUROVASCULAR INJURY

Aside from unresolved or recurrent laxity, nerve injury is the most common complication associated with shoulder arthroscopy. The incidence varies from 0% to 30%. The vast majority of these injuries are neuropraxias that resolve spontaneously with time. The most common sites are cutaneous nerve injuries that occur during portal placement (49). Neurological injuries associated with shoulder arthroscopy have been documented in two large series (1,2). Curtis et al. (2) have demonstrated a 0.8% rate of neurologic injury in their study of 711 patients undergoing arthroscopy of the shoulder in the lateral position. There were six cases of neuropraxia that appeared to result from three mechanisms. Two patients had an ulnar nerve paresthesia apparently secondary to a stretch injury, whereas three had symptoms in the distribution of the sensory branch of the radial nerve probably caused by compression at the wrist from the traction device used to support the arm. The final patient developed ulnar nerve paresthesias on the nonoperative side as a result of inadequate intraoperative padding. Similarly, Berjano et al. (50) showed that 2 of their 179 patients undergoing arthroscopy of the shoulder sustained transient ulnar nerve palsies secondary to application of the traction apparatus applied across the elbow.

Several authors have documented between a 10% to 30% incidence of neurologic injury following shoulder arthroscopy as diagnosed with somatosensory-evoked potentials and measurement of brachial plexus strain (51,52). Traction injury to the brachial plexus is the postulated etiology. Klein et al. (51) demonstrated this strain on the brachial plexus in cadaver studies with the arm in standard arthroscopic positions. Similarly, contralateral brachial plexus neuropathy has been documented following arthroscopic surgery in the lateral position in a patient with an unknown preexistent cervical rib (53).

The suprascapular nerve is also at risk with transglenoid repairs. Permanent injury has been reported (6,54–56). As mentioned earlier, this type of procedure is largely historical and these types of complications are infrequent in nature.

Schaffer and Tibone (6) have reviewed complications of thermal modification of capsular tissue. They have documented the occurrence of adhesive capsulitis, permanent changes to the capsule causing dissolution of the tissue, and, most importantly, a frequent incidence of axillary nerve injury, which in some cases has been permanent. This area is covered more extensively in a separate chapter of this text.

Arterial injury is rare but has been reported on few occasions. There is no specific association with stabilization procedures, but arthroscopy of the shoulder in general. A more common risk is the cephalic vein, particularly if using an inferior "5 o'clock" portal during anterior stabilization. This portal comes within 2 mm of the cephalic vein in cadaver (57), but injury to it has not been reported as a clinical problem (58).

PEARLS

Recurrent Instability

The most important consideration in these cases is to assess all of the variables discussed above with respect to the factors that contribute to recurrence. A thorough history, physical examination, careful review of any preoperative and postoperative imaging, and a review of the operative note with any available still images and/or video are important first steps.

Analysis of remaining bone stock on both the humerus and glenoid is the key to understanding a significant portion of recurrences. In addition, the original diagnosis must be either confirmed or discarded in those cases where a significant component of the instability has not been addressed.

The type of arthroscopic stabilization should also be carefully chosen. Although the results of suture anchor repair appear to be promising and are approaching the historical results of open repairs, other types of techniques do not appear to be as predictable. Specifically, the use of headed, bioabsorbable devices initially showed some promise in arthroscopic stabilization (59,60). The simplicity of inser-

tion and the lack of suture management made these devices tempting. However, with further analysis and follow-up, several studies have reported at least a 20% failure rate with the use of these headed devices in the treatment of anterior labral pathology (61,62). The current indications for these devices appear to be limited to those patients with robust labral detachments and no additional capsular laxity (62). Even in those situations, the results of suture anchor repairs appear to be superior and more predictable.

Loss of Motion Without Arthrosis

Treatment of the stiff postoperative shoulder should be individualized to a great extent depending on the patient's demands on the shoulder, the level of pain, and the desired activities. The first line of treatment, following a thorough evaluation and ruling out pathology other than intrinsic capsular or muscular contracture, should be aggressive physical therapy with periodic use of analgesics and nonsteroidal anti-inflammatory medications. This protocol has been documented to be effective in the management of even severe contractures in some studies (21). Operative release is indicated when pain or disability or both do not improve after an adequate course of nonoperative treatment. It may also be advisable in cases where early osteoarthrosis and reduced motion are evident because the progression of the arthrosis may be delayed (28). The guidelines for considering a surgical release include external rotation less than 0 degrees and to individualize the decision when external rotation is between 0 and 30 degrees (28). In addition, external rotation in abduction is important for the throwing athlete; certainly less than 90 degrees of external rotation with 90 degrees of abduction can significantly impair the throwing ability of most athletes, especially in those desirous of returning to throwing sports (28).

Arthrosis

As discussed earlier, arthrosis as a result of excessive tightness following arthroscopic stabilization is rare. One area that is commonly overlooked is the occurrence of mild to moderate pre-existing degenerative changes in a patient with instability. The preoperative realization of this problem is important since in some cases the pre-existing degenerative symptomatology may be exacerbated by the stabilization procedure. In such cases, the most important consideration goes back to the patient's initial complaint. When instability is the predominant factor, the patient will complain of either frank dislocation or perhaps subluxation episodes, but not of significant pain. Where the predominant problem is arthrosis, most patients will relate that pain and stiffness are their primary symptoms. There has been some effort to separate these patients by physical examination findings. In patients where there is significant arthrosis, loading the glenohumeral joint while internally and externally rotating the joint will exacerbate their pain, whereas those with instability will not be affected by the maneuver (63). The possibility of arthrosis should be entertained by the surgeon prior to performing the arthroscopic procedure.

Hardware/Implant-Related

When metal anchors are used for labral stabilization procedures, there are many pitfalls that can be avoided with meticulous surgical technique. The first is to assure proper portal placement, especially as it relates to the insertion of the lowest anchor in anterior stabilization procedures. The position can first be checked with the use of a spinal needle to assure that the appropriate angle of approach can be achieved with the intended portal site. The same applies in the stabilization of SLAP lesions.

Once the anchor insertion mechanics begin, it is critical to have an idea as to the thickness of the articular cartilage about the glenoid face. Prominence of the metal portion of the anchor in the cartilage can lead to articular surface damage on the humeral head. Insertion of the initial bone punch for marking of the subsequent anchor site should be 2 mm posterior to the anterior edge of the glenoid rim with about a 45-degree medial inclination. The subsequent drill hole should also follow this angle and position separated from the previous anchor by 6 or 7 mm.

Anchor insertion should be done manually with slow methodical advancement and assurance that the implant is fully seated prior to disengagement of the insertion device. It is recommended that the small pilot holes be tapped to cut a thread in the hard glenoid bone to avoid breaking the head of the miniature titanium screw-in anchors. Mechanized insertion of the devices using drills should be discouraged due to the lack of control upon insertion.

At the first postoperative visit, an x-ray should be taken to document the position of the anchors and assure that there is complete bony coverage of the device. These radiographs are also important as a baseline for further follow-up should the patient develop unusual symptoms consistent with prominent or migrating hardware (25).

Finally, if a patient complains of unusual symptoms such as a sharp pain and catching sensation, or an unexpected motion limitation during early rehabilitation following anchor implantation, the surgeon should consider the possibility of a malpositioned anchor (25). Radiographs or other imaging modalities (particularly in cases where bioabsorbable anchors were implanted) should be considered at this point to assure appropriate placement.

Revision of Arthroscopic Repairs

There are several factors that should be considered when repairing a failed arthroscopic surgical repair of instability. Making the proper diagnosis is certainly a critical factor that is often underestimated as has been discussed above.

Assuming the proper diagnosis was made, there are a number of intraoperative factors that are key to restoring stability to the shoulder. The soft-tissue anatomy is known to vary and certainly the surgeon should be familiar with normal and pathologic variations. As mentioned, two critical areas that are often overlooked are the ALPSA and HAGL lesions. Along with this, the quality of the soft tissues plays a key role (19).

There are many important technical steps in the arthroscopy that require meticulous attention, including mobilization and tensioning of the soft tissue and preparation of the bony bed (64,65). A mistake in the management of these steps can certainly explain a significant portion of failed repairs. Unfortunately, this chapter will not cover these steps in detail, but the reader is directed to review the appropriate references.

Finally, failed arthroscopic surgical knots can ruin the entire procedure. Failure to establish a secure initial loop of suture in which the soft tissues are snugly approximated against the glenoid may compromise security despite effective subsequent knots (66). To this end, the surgeon should be familiar with one sliding-locking knot (67–69) and a nonsliding multiple half-hitch knot with alternating posts. Proficiency with these techniques is an integral part of the repair, which should not be underestimated.

Neurovascular Injury

The most common situation is that of neuropraxia caused by improper positioning of patients during the arthroscopic procedure, particularly when using the lateral position. All prominent areas should be padded, including the lateral ankle and the peroneal nerve. The head and neck should be supported on a contoured pillow in a neutral position and an axillary roll should be placed under the dependent hemithorax to protect the dependent shoulder and its neurovascular structures.

Traction should be kept to a minimum, with 10 pounds being appropriate in most situations in the lateral position. Finally, padding of the area that is applied to the arm for traction should be carefully done in order to distribute the stresses throughout the extremity and avoid areas of excess pressure.

The usual considerations with respect to the known vascular and neural elements apply to stabilization procedures as well in shoulder arthroscopy. An improperly placed portal created near a neurovascular structure introduces the risk of a major complication for the patient. Attention to detail is paramount. If one is thoroughly familiar with the normal anatomy, the risk of these problems is significantly diminished.

CONCLUSION

Shoulder arthroscopy in general and stabilization surgery in particular appear to be safe and effective for the treatment of shoulder pathology. Despite the increasing complexity of the procedures, complication rates do not appear to have increased dramatically. Serious complications can and do occur and recognizing that this is not "band-aid" surgery remains important, not only for the patient but also the surgeon (3). The most important principle to keep in mind is that complications that can and do occasionally occur, and must be recognized and treated early in order to avoid long-term sequelae.

Arthroscopic stabilization is technically demanding and requires careful attention to detail in all aspects of the patient's care. This includes a thorough understanding of the underlying instability pattern as well as careful consideration of the technique chosen for repair, patient positioning, and physical therapy to optimize results. With adherence to these principles, the complication rates can be kept to a minimum and the results of arthroscopic stabilization may approach the historical rates of open stabilization procedures.

REFERENCES

1. Small NC. Complications in arthroscopic surgery performed by experienced arthroscopists. *Arthroscopy* 1988;4:215–221.
2. Curtis AS, Snyder SJ, Del Pizzo W, et al. Complications of shoulder arthroscopy. *Arthroscopy* 1992;8:395–401.
3. Weber SC, Abrams JS, Nottage WM. Complications associated with arthroscopic shoulder surgery. *Arthroscopy* 2002;18:88–95.
4. Geiger DF, Hurley JA, Tovey JA, et al. Results of arthroscopic versus open Bankart suture repair. *Clin Orthop* 1997;337:111–117.
5. Guanche CA, Quick DC, Sodergren K, et al. Arthroscopic versus open reconstruction of the shoulder in patients with isolated Bankart lesions. *Am J Sports Med* 1996;24:144–148.
6. Shaffer BS, Tibone JE. Arthroscopic shoulder instability surgery. Complications. *Clin Sports Med* 1999;18:737–767.
7. Neer CS II, Foster CR. Inferior capsular shift for involuntary inferior and multidirectional instability of the shoulder: a preliminary report. *J Bone Joint Surg Am* 1980;62:897–908.
8. Neviaser T. The anterior labroligamentous periosteal sleeve avulsion lesion: a cause of anterior instability of the shoulder. *Arthroscopy* 1993;9:17–21.
9. Nicola T. Anterior dislocation of the shoulder. The role of the articular capsule. *J Bone Joint Surg* 1942;24:614–616.
10. Savoie FH, Miller CD, Field LD. Arthroscopic reconstruction of traumatic anterior instability of the shoulder. The Caspari technique. *Arthroscopy* 1997;13:201–209.
11. Harryman DT, Sidles JA, Harris SL, et al. The role of the rotator interval capsule in passive motion and stability of the shoulder. *J Bone Joint Surg Am* 1992;74:53–66.
12. Mologne TS, McBride MT, Lapoint JM. Assessment of failed arthroscopic anterior labral repair. Findings at open surgery. *Am J Sports Med* 1997;25:813–817.
13. Burkhart SS, DeBeer JF. Traumatic glenohumeral bone defects and their relationship to failure of arthroscopic Bankart repairs: significance of the inverted-pear glenoid and the humeral engaging Hill-Sachs lesion. *Arthroscopy* 2000;16:677–694.
14. Bernageau J, Patte D, Debeyre J, et al. Value of the glenoid profile in recurrent luxations of the shoulder. *Rev Chir Orthop Reparatrice Appar Mot* 1975;61(Suppl 2):286–290.
15. Lo IK, Parten PM, Burkhart SS. The inverted pear glenoid: an indicator of significant glenoid bone loss. *Arthroscopy* 2004;20: 169–174.
16. Gill TJ, Millett PJ, O'Holleran J, et al. Glenoid reconstruction for recurrent traumatic anterior shoulder instability. San Francisco, CA: Annual Meeting of the American Academy of Orthopaedic Surgeons, March 11–14, 2004.
17. Yagishita K, Thomas BJ. Use of allograft for large Hill-Sachs lesion associated with anterior glenohumeral dislocation. A case report. *Injury* 2004;35:96.
18. Weber BG, Simpson LA, Hardegger F. Rotational humeral osteotomy for recurrent anterior dislocation of the shoulder associated with a large Hill-Sachs lesion. *J Bone Joint Surg Am* 1984;66: 1443–1446.
19. Hayashida K, Yoneda M, Nakagawa S, et al. Arthroscopic Bankart suture repair for traumatic anterior shoulder instability: analysis of the causes of a recurrence. *Arthroscopy* 1998;14:295–301.
20. Bigliani LU, Weinstein DM, Glasgow MT, et al. Glenohumeral arthroplasty for arthritis after instability surgery. *J Shoulder Elbow Surg* 1995;4:87–94.
21. Hawkins RJ, Angelo RL. Glenohumeral osteoarthrosis. A late complication of the Putti-Platt repair. *J Bone Joint Surg Am* 1990;72: 1193–1197.
22. MacDonald PB, Hawkins RJ, Fowler PJ, et al. Release of the subscapularis for internal rotation contracture and pain after anterior repair for recurrent anterior dislocation of the shoulder. *J Bone Joint Surg Am* 1992;74:734–377.
23. Freehill MQ, Harms DJ, Huber SM, et al. Poly-L-Lactic acid tack synovitis after arthroscopic stabilization of the shoulder. *Am J Sports Med* 2003;31:643–647.
24. Kaar TK, Schenck RC, Wirth MA, et al. Complications of metallic suture anchors in shoulder surgery: a report of 8 cases. *Arthroscopy* 2001;17:31–37.
25. Rhee YG, Lee DH, Chun IH, et al. Glenohumeral arthropathy after arthroscopic anterior shoulder stabilization. *Arthroscopy* 2004;4: 402–406.
26. Tetik O, Sumoda L. Nyland J, et al. Humeral head articular surface damage due to bioabsorbable tack placement: a case report. *J Shoulder Elbow Surg* 2004;13:463–466.
27. Wilkerson JP, Zvijac JE, Uribe JW, et al. Failure of polymerized lactic acid tacks in shoulder surgery. *J Shoulder Elbow Surg* 2003; 12:117–121.
28. Flatow EL, Miniaci A, Evans PJ, et al. Instability of the shoulder: complex problems and failed repairs. *J Bone Joint Surg Am* 1998; 80:284–298.
29. Bigliani LU, Flatow EL, Kelkar R, et al. The effect of anterior capsular tightening on shoulder kinematics and contact (abstract). *J Shoulder Elbow Surg* 1994;3(Suppl):S65.
30. Rosenberg BN, Richmond JC, Levine WN. Long-term follow-up of Bankart reconstruction. Incidence of late degenerative glenohumeral arthrosis. *Am J Sports Med* 1995;23:538–544.
31. Wirth MA, Rockwood CA. Migrations of a broken cerclage wire form the shoulder girdle into the heart: A case report. *J Shoulder Elbow Surg* 2000;9:543.
32. Moran MC, Warren RF. Development of a synovial cyst after arthroscopy of the shoulder. *J Bone Joint Surg Am* 1989;71:127–129.
33. Shea KP, Lovallo LJ. Scapulothoracic penetration of a Beath pin: an unusual complication of arthroscopic Bankart suture repair. *Arthroscopy* 1991;7:115–117.
34. Warme WJ, Arciero RA, Savoie FH, et al. Nonabsorbable versus absorbable suture anchors for open Bankart repair. *Am J Sports Med* 1999;27:747.
35. Edwards DJ, Hoy G, Saies AD, et al. Adverse reactions to an absorbable shoulder fixation device. *J Shoulder Elbow Surg* 1994;3: 230–233.
36. Burkart A, Imhoff AB, Roscher E. Foreign body reaction to the bioabsorbable Suretac device. *Arthroscopy* 2000;16:91–95.
37. Maitra RS, Brand JC, Caborn DN. Biodegradable implants. *Sports Med Athrosc Rev* 1998;6:103–117.
38. Bostman OM, Pihlajamaki HK. Late foreign-body reaction to an intraosseous bioabsorbable polylactic acid screw. *J Bone Joint Surg Am* 1998;80:1791–1794.
39. Berg EE, Oblesby JW. Loosening of a biodegradable shoulder staple. *J Shoulder Elbow Surg* 1996;5:76–78.
40. Barber FA, Snyder SJ, Abrams JS. Arthroscopic Bankart reconstruction with a bioabsorbable anchor. *J Shoulder and Elbow Surg* 2003; 12:535–538.
41. Bottoni CR, Wickens JH, DeBerardino TM, et al. A prospective, randomized evaluation of arthroscopic stabilization versus nonoperative treatment in patients with acute, traumatic, first-time shoulder dislocations. *Am J Sports Med* 2002;30:576–580.

42. Fabbriciani C, Milano G, Demontis A, et al. Arthroscopic versus open treatment of Bankart lesion of the shoulder: a prospective randomized study. *Arthroscopy* 2004;20:456–462.

43. Kim SH, Ha KI, Cho YB, et al. Arthroscopic anterior stabilization of the shoulder: two to six year follow-up. *J Bone Joint Surg Am* 2003;85:1511–1518.

44. Ekelund A. Case report: Cartilage injuries in the shoulder caused by migration of suture anchors or mini screw. *J Shoulder Elbow Surg* 1998;7:537–539.

45. Silver MD, Daigneault JP. Symptomatic interarticular migration of glenoid suture anchor. *Arthroscopy* 2000;16:102–105.

46. Zuckerman JD, Matsen FA III. Complications about the glenohumeral joint related to the use of screw and staples. *J Bone Joint Surg Am* 1984;66:175–180.

47. Levine WN, Connor PM, Arroyo JS, et al. Revision instability surgery for failed glenohumeral stabilization procedures. San Francisco, CA: American Orthopaedic Society for Sports Medicine, February 16, 1997.

48. Kim SH, Ha KI, Kim YM. Arthroscopic revision Bankart repair: a prospective outcome study. *Arthroscopy* 2002;18:469–482.

49. Segmuller HE, Alfred S, Zillion G, et al. Cutaneous nerve lesions of the shoulder and arm after arthroscopic shoulder surgery. *J Shoulder Elbow Surg* 1995;4:254–258.

50. Berjano P, Gonzalez BG, Olmedo JF, et al. Complications in arthroscopic shoulder surgery. *Arthroscopy* 1998;8:785–788.

51. Klein A, Fu F, Smith AE, et al. Measurement of brachial plexus strain in arthroscopy of the shoulder. *Arthroscopy* 1987;3:45–52.

52. Pitman MI, Nainzadeh N, Ergas E, et al. The use of somatosensory evoked potentials for detection of neuropraxia during shoulder arthroscopy. *Arthroscopy* 1988;4:250–255.

53. Pavlik A, Ang KC, Bell SN. Contralateral brachial plexus neuropathy after arthroscopic shoulder surgery. *Arthroscopy* 2002;6:305–309.

54. Bigliani LU, Dalsey RM, McCann PD, et al. An anatomical study of the suprascapular nerve. *Arthroscopy* 1990;6:301–305.

55. Goldberg BJ, Nirshl RP, McConnell JP, et al. Arthroscopic transglenoid suture capsulolabral repairs: Preliminary results. *Am J Sports Med* 1993;21:656–665.

56. Landsiedl F. Arthroscopic therapy of recurrent anterior luxation of the shoulder by capsular repair. *Arthroscopy* 1992;8:296–304.

57. Pearsall AW, Holovacs TF, Speer KP. The efficacy and safety of a low anterior portal established with an "outside-in" technique for arthroscopic shoulder surgery. Orlando, FL: Arthroscopy Association of North America, 17th Annual Meeting, May 1998.

58. Davidson PA, Tibone JE. Anterior inferior (5 o'clock" portal for shoulder arthroscopy. *Arthroscopy* 1995;5:519–525.

59. Pagnani MJ, Speer KP, Altcheck DW, et al. Arthroscopic fixation of superior labral lesions using biodegradable implant: A preliminary report. *Arthroscopy* 1995;11:194–198.

60. Samani JE, Marston SB, Buss DD. Arthroscopic stabilization of type II SLAP lesions using an absorbable tack. *Arthroscopy* 2001;17:19–24.

61. Dora C, Gerber C. Shoulder function after arthroscopic anterior stabilization of the glenohumeral joint using an absorbable tac. *J Shoulder Elbow Surg* 2000;9:106–110.

62. Speer KP, Warren RF, Pagnani M. An arthroscopic technique for anterior stabilization of the shoulder with a bioabsorbable tack. *J Bone Joint SurgAm* 1996;78:1801–1807.

63. Guyette TM, Bae H, Warren RF, et al. Results of arthroscopic subacromial decompression in patients with subacromial impingement and glenohumeral degenerative joint disease. *J Shoulder Elbow Surg* 2002;11:299–304.

64. Gartsman GM, Roddey TS, Hammerman SM. Arthroscopic treatment of anterior-inferior glenohumeral instability. Two to five-year follow-up. *J Bone Joint Surg Am* 2001;83:621–632.

65. Snyder SJ. Glenohumeral Instability. In: Snyder SJ, ed. *Shoulder Arthroscopy*, 2nd ed. Philadelphia: Lippincott Williams and Wilkins, 2003:97–108.

66. Burkhart SS, Wirth MA, Simonick, M, et al. Technical note: loop security as a determinant of tissue fixation security. *Arthroscopy* 1998;14:773–776.

67. Kim SH, Ha KI. The SMC knot–a new slipknot with locking mechanism. *Arthroscopy* 2000;16:563–565.

68. Snyder SJ. Technique of arthroscopic rotator cuff repair using implantable 4-mm Revo suture anchors, suture Shuttle relays, and no. 2 nonabsorbable mattress sutures. *Orthop Clin North Am* 1997;28:267–275.

69. Weston PV. A new cinch knot. *Obst Gynec* 1991;78:144–147.

Arthroscopy: Complications of Rotator Cuff Repair

13

Samer S. Hasan   *Gary M. Gartsman*

INTRODUCTION

All-arthroscopic rotator cuff repair is being performed by an ever-increasing number of orthopaedic surgeons. Although there is not as yet long-term follow-up, intermediate-term follow-up has demonstrated excellent results comparable to those attained following traditional open rotator cuff repair in terms of patient satisfaction, comfort, and function (1–7).

There are several advantages of an arthroscopic rotator cuff repair: it allows concurrent evaluation and treatment of intra-articular pathology, which is frequently present (8) and can affect outcome (3); it provides exceptional visualization of rotator cuff tear geometry, which may be superior to that afforded by open methods (9,10); and it facilitates precise soft-tissue releases to mobilize the rotator cuff and to allow for a tension-free repair (11,12). Furthermore, an arthroscopic repair avoids deltoid detachment and consequently the devastating complication of deltoid dehiscence (11). The mini-open repair, performed through a small deltoid split, also avoids deltoid detachment, but it has been associated with an increased incidence of postsurgical stiffness (13,14) that may relate to excessive deltoid retraction, which is avoided by an arthroscopic repair. Lastly, the small incisions are often more cosmetically acceptable to the patient, and the immediate postoperative pain is often considerably less than that experienced following open repair.

Many complications of arthroscopic rotator cuff repair are similar to those that follow open rotator cuff repair, such as postoperative stiffness and recurrent rotator cuff tear. However, the management and prevention of these problems is somewhat different when the surgery is performed arthroscopically. Other complications, such as those related to fluid extravasation or to the management of sutures within a cannula, are unique to arthroscopic techniques.

Complications of surgery are typically divided into those that arise from intraoperative errors and those that develop postoperatively. Intraoperative complications of arthroscopic rotator cuff repair include errors in assessment of tear geometry and reparability and in suture management. Postoperative complications include stiffness, retear, or infection. It is critical to note, however, that avoiding complications following arthroscopic rotator cuff repair begins prior to surgery.

PREOPERATIVE COMPLICATIONS

A careful history and physical examination are important in establishing the diagnosis of a rotator cuff tear and in excluding conditions, such as adhesive capsulitis, that may confound the diagnosis and impact treatment. Although it may be tempting to concurrently treat both adhesive capsulitis and rotator cuff tear, especially arthroscopically, it is generally best to treat the adhesive capsulitis and to delay the rotator cuff repair. Ancillary imaging, such as magnetic resonance imaging (MRI) or ultrasound, should be aimed at confirming, not establishing, the appropriate diagnosis. Plain radiographs and magnetic resonance imaging can also be used to gauge reparability. Upward migration of the humeral head on an anteroposterior radiograph with the arm internally rotated (15) and observations of fatty muscle changes by magnetic resonance imaging (16,17) are poor prognostic indicators of tendon reparability or of integrity following repair.

Another preoperative complication arises from the use of an arthroscopic repair by a surgeon uncomfortable with the technique. A durable repair is as dependent on the ability to perform an adequate bursectomy, evaluate tendon geometry, and assess reparability as it is on the ability to pass suture through tendon or tie knots arthroscopically. A less experienced surgeon can avoid those pitfalls and complications specific to arthroscopic repair by avoiding the technique altogether until sufficient experience has been gained.

Because an arthroscopic rotator cuff repair is characterized by a rather steep learning curve, a critical number of rotator cuff repairs is needed to justify the transition to arthroscopic repair and to gain mastery of the technique. Surgeons who do not perform an adequate number of shoulder procedures and who cannot justify undergoing the appropriate technical transition should continue to perform rotator cuff repair using the traditional open or mini-open techniques. It is useful to remember that although a number of shoulder surgeons currently repair all rotator cuff tears arthroscopically, many prefer to repair complete subscapularis tears, certain recurrent tears, or tears involving two or more tendons using open techniques.

The surgeon contemplating arthroscopic rotator cuff repair should be facile with shoulder arthroscopy, including subacromial bursoscopy, and be able to sequentially execute all the steps in the repair (3,9,10,18–21). There are no rules concerning who should perform an arthroscopic repair, but two useful guidelines for the surgeon contemplating the transition to arthroscopic rotator cuff repair are the ability to perform a diagnostic arthroscopy and subacromial decompression in 30 minutes or less and the surgical experience of 20 to 30 rotator cuff repairs annually (10).

The transition to arthroscopic rotator cuff repair is a gradual process that requires practice and demands patience. The steps in an arthroscopic repair should be mastered outside the operating room by practicing arthroscopic knot-tying on a knot-tying board and by gaining familiarity with the instruments needed to insert suture anchors and to pass suture. The shoulder arthroscopy model (Aptic Superbones, Vashon, WA) is a commercially available model of the shoulder that can aid in the transition (Fig. 13-1). The model consists of a felt rotator cuff and a plastic glenohumeral joint encased in a sturdy plastic shell that replicates shoulder surface anatomy. Courses specific to arthroscopic shoulder surgery are also an invaluable resource, especially for the surgeon who has had little formal training on arthroscopic rotator cuff repair. These courses, organized by the American Academy of Orthopaedic Surgeons and by various specialty societies, institutions, and vendors,

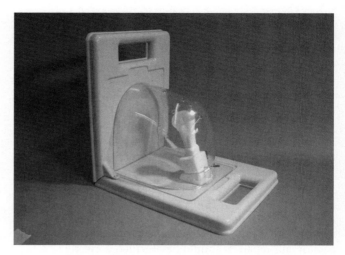

Figure 13-1 Shoulder arthroscopy model.

often provide an opportunity to perform repairs on cadaveric shoulders in a wet laboratory setting (10).

Ultimately, the transition to an all-arthroscopic rotator cuff repair is made incrementally, with the surgeon performing arthroscopically an increasing number of steps to a mini-open repair. Initially, the rotator cuff footprint can be decorticated and the suture anchors inserted arthroscopically. Later, some or all of the sutures can be passed, and the knots can be tied under direct visualization, until finally all that remains is an open inspection of the completed arthroscopic repair (10,13,22,23).

INTRAOPERATIVE COMPLICATIONS

If problems that are encountered during arthroscopic rotator cuff repair, especially during the transition to this technique, can be identified and corrected in the course of the operation, they do not affect the outcome; hence, they are not complications. However, failure to address them affects the ability to carry out the repair and adversely impacts the quality of the repair.

Subacromial Decompression

Complications related to arthroscopic subacromial decompression are reviewed elsewhere. However, it is important to point out that an inadequate subacromial bursectomy will interfere with tendon visualization and lead to difficulty in passive suturing and in tying knots. Although a complete bursectomy is not necessary, the bursectomy should be sufficient to enable clear visualization of all the steps of an arthroscopic rotator cuff repair from the various portals. Debridement of bursal tissue within the lateral gutter should not proceed beyond the bursal reflection (3 to 5 cm distally) to avoid axillary nerve injury (24,25).

An acromioplasty is not essential to arthroscopic rotator cuff repair, and neither author believes an acromioplasty is needed for visualization during rotator cuff repair (10). Moreover, the senior author has recently published a randomized study of arthroscopic rotator cuff repair with and without acromioplasty that showed that there was no difference in outcome at 1-year follow-up (26). Proper portal placement is more important than acromioplasty to optimize visualization and to facilitate the passage of sutures and instruments within the subacromial space (Fig. 13-2). The posterior portal used for viewing should be positioned somewhat superior and lateral to the traditional portal placement in the "soft spot" so that it affords "a room with a view" of the subacromial space (Fig. 13-3) (10).

If the surgeon elects to perform an acromioplasty with rotator cuff repair, it should be executed correctly (27,28), either before or following the rotator cuff repair. An inadequate or incorrectly performed acromioplasty may impair visualization and may also contribute to postoperative complications. A roughened, irregular undersurface may produce abrasion of the bursal surface of the rotator cuff, and excessive bleeding from the exposed cancellous bone may produce subacromial adhesions and stiffness postoperatively.

Tendon Releases

Adequate articular- and bursal-sided releases are essential for proper tendon mobilization and for affecting a tension-free repair. Scarring between the superior and posterior labrum and articular surface of the rotator cuff can be released bluntly or sharply using basket forceps or electrocautery (Fig. 13-4). Within the subacromial space, posterior adhesions are generally thin and amenable to blunt release, such as with a blunt trocar. Use of a motorized shaver is discouraged because bleeding posteromedially can be difficult to control (20). Anteriorly, the coracohumeral ligament is often thickened and scarred, which contributes to retraction of the distal supraspinatus (Fig. 13-5A) (29). Sharp

VIEW THROUGH ARTHROSCOPE

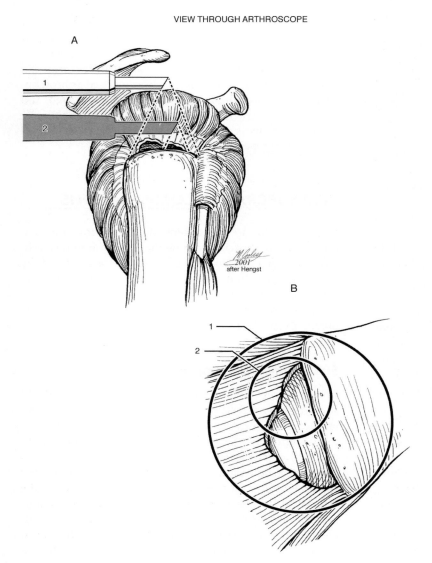

Figure 13-2 Placement of the arthroscope superiorly within the subacromial space **(A)** provides a "room with a view" **(B)**.

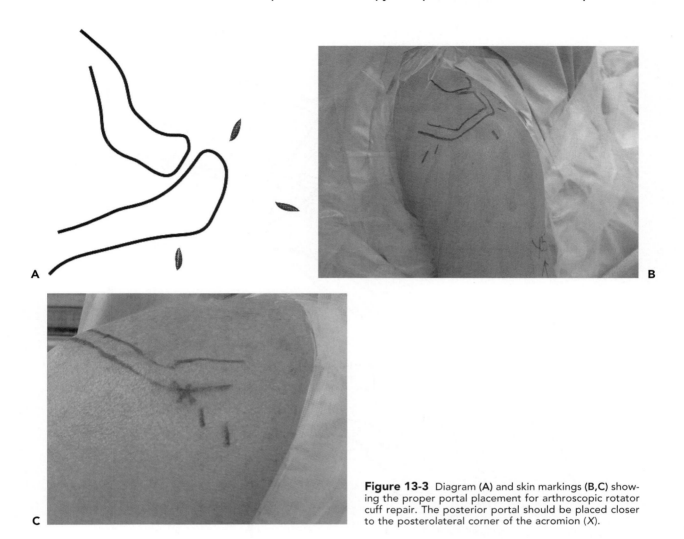

Figure 13-3 Diagram (**A**) and skin markings (**B,C**) showing the proper portal placement for arthroscopic rotator cuff repair. The posterior portal should be placed closer to the posterolateral corner of the acromion (*X*).

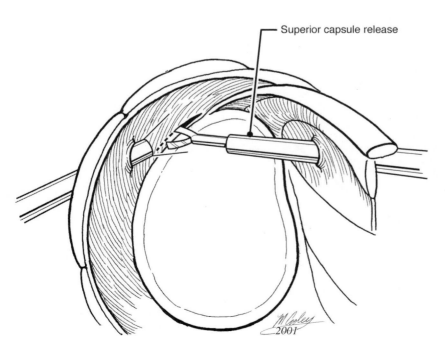

Superior capsule release

Figure 13-4 Release of the superior capsule and adhesions between labrum and rotator cuff.

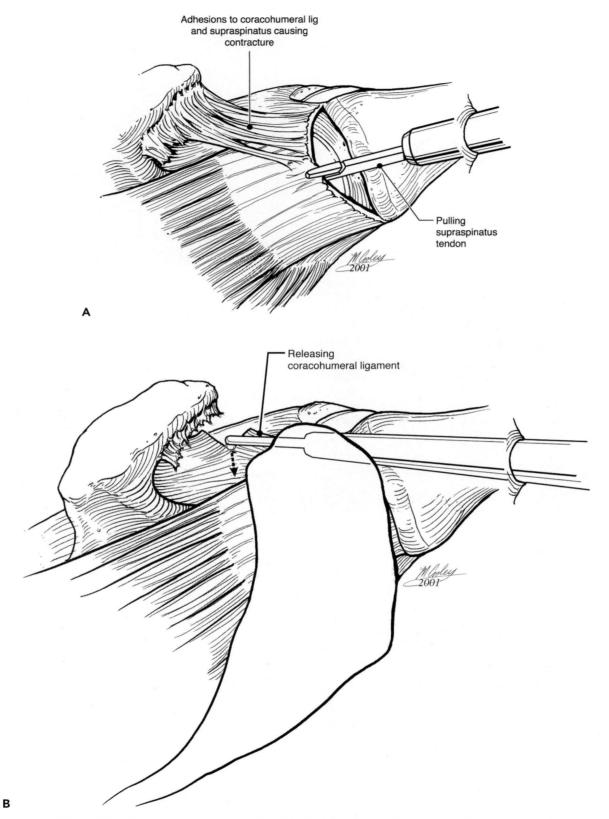

Figure 13-5 Coracohumeral adhesions (**A**) and their release (**B**) to mobilize a retracted supraspinatus tendon tear.

release of the coracohumeral ligament and related bursal adhesions using electrocautery or a shaver is often necessary to mobilize adequately the torn tendon (Fig. 13-5B).

For the most severely retracted large tears, a variety of interval releases and slides that aid in mobilizing the tendon have been described (Fig. 13-6) (30–33). However, it is important to recognize that the ability to repair the tendon, either to itself or to the tuberosity, does not guarantee a durable repair or outcome. Consequently, the use of these heroic releases for a contracted chronic rotator cuff tear needs to be weighed against overall tendon and muscle quality.

Assessment of Tear Morphology

Assessment of tear geometry is essential for successful rotator cuff repair. Arthroscopy has served to enhance this aspect of repair, especially for the largest, most retracted tears. For U-shaped tears with significant medial retraction, margin convergence as described by Burkhart (12,34–36) has been used to facilitate a tension-free repair (Fig. 13-7). The technique foregoes heroic attempts to repair the most retracted portions of the tendon directly to bone in favor of side-to-side repair of the medial extension of the tear followed by tendon to bone repair so that a tension-free repair can be obtained.

The arthroscope is also invaluable for evaluating smaller tears and for distinguishing between partial thickness and full thickness tears. With the arthroscope in the glenohumeral joint, an O-polydiaxanone (O-PDS) suture can be placed through a spinal needle inserted across an articular side tear that has already been debrided to help localize the cuff defect within the subacromial space (13,37–39).

In general, debrided tears that are less than 50% of the tendon thickness are not repaired (28), whereas higher-grade tears are repaired. Various techniques to repair a partial thickness tear either in situ (40,41) or by first completing the tear (38,39) have been described.

Assessment of tear reparability is important for rotator cuff repair and the arthroscope is ideally suited for this task (42). The two principal determinants of reparability are tendon excursion with the ability to obtain a tension-free repair and overall tendon quality. The former is established by thorough assessment of tear geometry and meticulous releases to mobilize the tendon. Tendon quality can be checked by placing braided no. 2 sutures across the tendon and applying the traction needed to advance the tendon to the repair site and slightly beyond. In tears that are delaminated or that have upper and lower leaves, the suture limb must be passed through both portions (13). Bone quality is also a determinant, and extremely osteopenic bone may preclude the placement of suture anchors. Although this problem is rarely encountered with currently available suture anchors, the security of each anchor should be tested immediately after it is inserted.

Bone Preparation

To improve tendon-to-bone healing, the rotator cuff insertion site or footprint must be prepared to accept the tendon. Traditional open techniques employ a trough prepared with a bur or osteotome (29) to facilitate the passage of sutures transosseously. The use of suture anchors obviates the need for a trough. Instead, the rotator cuff footprint is lightly abraded or decorticated to a depth of 1 to 2 mm

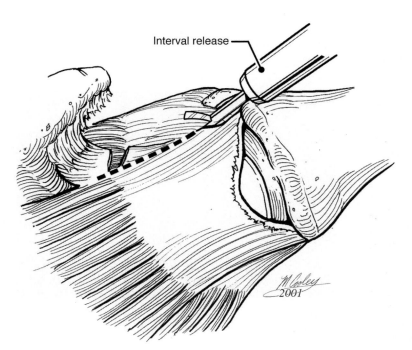

Figure 13-6 Rotator interval release.

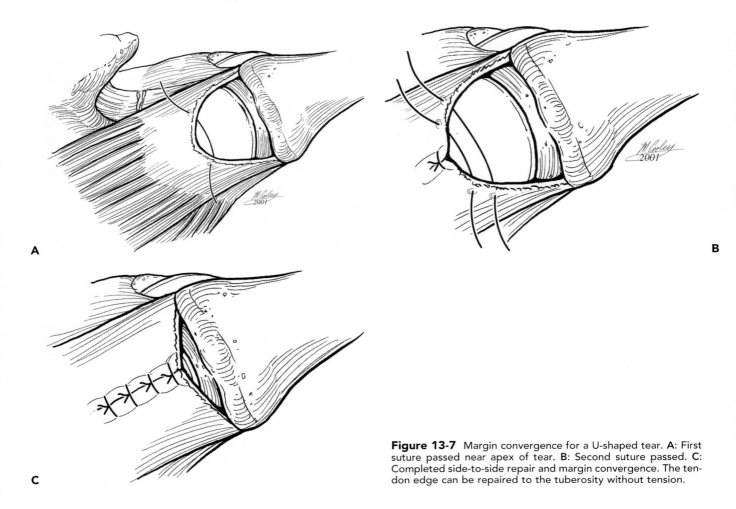

A

B

C

Figure 13-7 Margin convergence for a U-shaped tear. **A:** First suture passed near apex of tear. **B:** Second suture passed. **C:** Completed side-to-side repair and margin convergence. The tendon edge can be repaired to the tuberosity without tension.

and to a width of at least 1 cm starting just lateral to the articular surface (9,10,37,43).

Arthroscopic Instruments

Familiarity with various instruments for suture passage is essential during arthroscopic rotator cuff repair. In general, sutures are passed through rotator cuff tissue using either a direct or an indirect method. The direct method uses instruments that directly pass the suture through the tendon or instruments that first pierce the tendon and then retrieve the suture. Examples of these instruments are Cuff Stitch, Cuff Sew, and Arthropierce (Smith-Nephew Endoscopy, Andover, MA), Viper and Penetrator (Arthrex, Naples, FL), ExpressSew (U.S. Surgical), and Blitz (Linvatec, Largo, FL). The indirect method involves placing a passing suture or shuttle relay through the rotator cuff tissue and then using this transport suture to pull the repair suture through the tissue. The Caspari suture punch or Spectrum instruments are examples of instruments that employ an indirect method of suture transport (Fig. 13-8). The Caspari suture punch and Spectrum instruments can also be used to pass a suture directly (e.g., for side-to-side repair with a monofilament suture) (10). The Viper and the ExpressSew are su-

ture punches that allow direct passage of braided no. 2 suture.

The specific instrument used during tendon repair depends on multiple factors including tear geometry, location of the working portals, tissue thickness, and surgeon's pref-

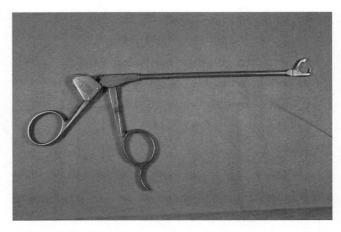

Figure 13-8 Caspari suture punch. (Reprinted with permission from Gartsman GM. *Shoulder Arthroscopy.* Philadelphia: WB Saunders, 2003.)

erence. Direct methods are often employed during side-to-side repair of a rotator interval rent or during margin convergence (10,35). A suture punch is often used to pass sutures from suture anchors through the lateral edge of a tear when visualizing from the posterior portal. Most instruments easily penetrate rotator cuff tissue, but occasionally the tendon edge is so thick that suture punches cannot penetrate the tendon. This may occur during the repair of acute traumatic tears in younger patients. The Caspari suture punch has been modified with a longer needle that is helpful in this situation (38).

The Spectrum instruments or the Caspari suture punch can be loaded with a shuttle wire, but this can abrade or damage tissue. An alternative is to use a 2-0 nylon suture folded in half so that the two free ends are passed into the suture punch and the loop end exits from the handle (Fig. 13-9) (10,20). Once the suture punch punctures the tendon and the two free ends are retrieved from the subacromial space through the anterior cannula, the suture punch is withdrawn from the lateral cannula, and one suture limb from the suture anchor is then retrieved from the lateral cannula. After placing a looping grasper around the nylon sutures to ensure they are not entangled with the suture limb from the anchor, the end of the suture limb is placed within the nylon loop. Finally, traction on the two ends of the nylon suture anteriorly is used to shuttle the suture limb from the lateral cannula into the subacromial space, through the tendon, and out through the anterior cannula (20).

Suture Anchors

Suture anchors represent a technical advance that has facilitated arthroscopic rotator cuff repair, but their use is not without risk. The senior author has put forth the following characteristics of the ideal suture anchor:

1. It should allow firm fixation in the greater tuberosity.
2. The surgeon should be able to select the type of suture loaded on the anchor.
3. The anchor should be inserted manually, without pre-drilling or power instruments.
4. The suture should slide easily in the anchor so that the eyelet orientation is irrelevant.
5. The anchor should be removable from bone if placed suboptimally or if the suture breaks.
6. The anchor must be fixed securely to the inserting device so that it does not dislodge within the subacromial space during insertion.
7. The anchor must be able to penetrate bone at an acute angle.
8. The anchor should be biodegradable (20).

No currently available suture anchor meets all these criteria, but many complications associated with the use of suture anchors can be minimized or avoided by knowing the specifics of the anchor being used. The surgeon should know whether the sutures are preloaded onto the anchor

or they must be loaded in the operating room; whether the suture anchor accommodates one or two sutures and the type of suture employed; and whether the sutures can be switched. When an anchor accommodates two sutures, the surgeon should know whether the sutures are stacked within the same eyelet or in two eyelets and whether the eyelet has sharp edges or is made from suture material. When two sutures are stacked within the same eyelet, the top suture should be tied first so that it does not bind the bottom suture (Fig. 13-10) (10). When an anchor is used that has an eyelet with a sharp edge, the final orientation of the anchor is important. In general, the anchor should be inserted so that the eyelet is parallel to the tendon edge instead of facing the edge (10), because in this orientation the sutures make a 90 degrees turn with respect to the eyelet in order to minimize suture abrasion (Fig. 13-11) (10). Most anchors are inserted with devices that clearly mark the location of the eyelet to facilitate proper orientation (Fig. 13-12).

Suture anchors are inserted lateral to the decorticated rotator cuff footprint so that they can be inserted into cortical bone and inserted at a 45-degree angle relative to the footprint or at deadman's angle (Fig. 13-13), which has been shown to optimize anchor pullout strength (35,44). Avoiding the footprint increases the area available for tendon-to-bone healing. The lateral anchor position permits an anatomic repair because the tendon is pulled laterally toward the tendon bed, and it also allows the sutures to be tied laterally to limit suture impingement, which is a frequent postoperative nuisance. A few recent studies have reported on the use of two rows of suture anchors to increase the contact area for rotator cuff healing (45–47). However, concerns have been raised over the consequences of placing additional anchors into the soft bone of the greater tuberosity (11), and there are no clinical studies demonstrating superior tendon healing or clinical outcome with this method.

When an anchor is chosen based on the above criteria, it is preferable to first practice anchor insertion on a model. This includes learning to prepare the bone with a drill or tap, determining the force needed for insertion, and learning to orient the eyelet properly so that the suture will slide easily. The authors favor screw-in anchors so that the purchase can be appreciated during screw insertion, but other anchors are also used commonly.

Regardless of the type of anchor employed, the insertion of each anchor to the appropriate depth and orientation and an adequate purchase in bone must be verified individually. After an anchor has been inserted and before withdrawing the inserter, the suture ends should be tugged firmly while viewing the insertion site arthroscopically. If the anchor pulls out, it should be inserted again at a different site, either more laterally, anteriorly, or posteriorly. Alternatively, a larger anchor, obtainable from some vendors, can be inserted at the same site in place of the loose anchor. Anchor pullout that occurs intraoperatively during inser-

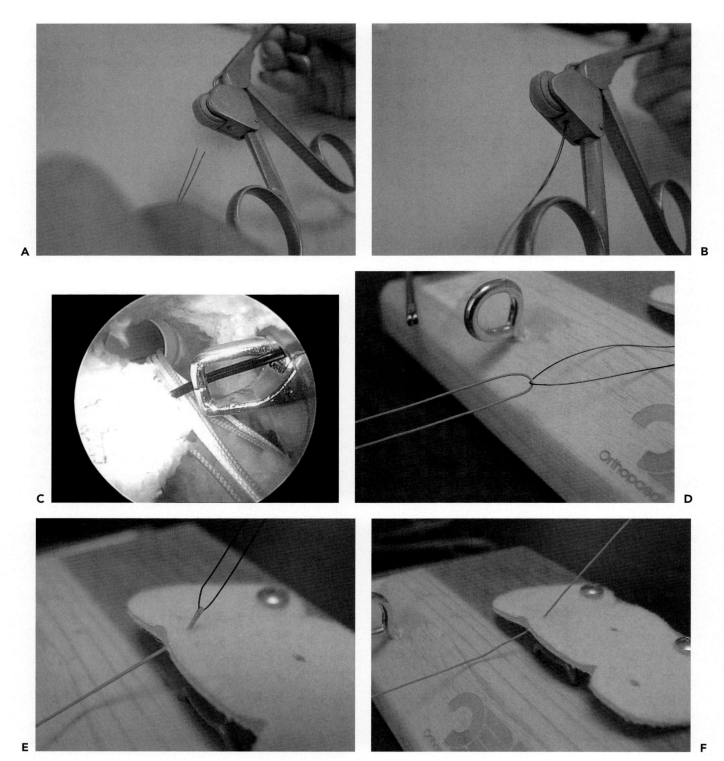

Figure 13-9 Use of the Caspari suture punch with nylon suture shuttle. **A,B:** Loading the folded 2-0 nylon suture. **C:** Retrieving the nylon suture ends using the looping grasper. **D:** Loading no. 2 braided suture onto suture shuttle loop. **E,F:** Suture shuttled through tendon.

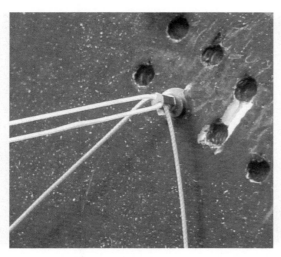

Figure 13-10 Close-up of suture anchor eyelet showing stacked arrangement of the two no. 2 sutures. (Reprinted with permission from Hasan SS, Gartsman GM. Pearls and pitfalls of arthroscopic rotator cuff repair. *Op Tech Orthop Surg* 2002;12:176–185.)

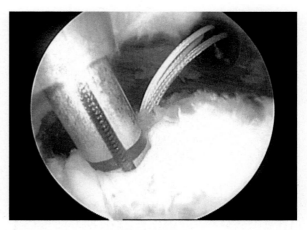

Figure 13-12 Arthroscopic view of suture anchor attached to insertion device. The vertical mark on the inserter identifies the orientation of the eyelet. (Reprinted with permission from Hasan SS, Gartsman GM. Pearls and pitfalls of arthroscopic rotator cuff repair. *Op Tech Orthop Surg* 2002;12:176–185.)

tion and testing can be corrected and is not a complication, but anchor loosening that occurs postoperatively is a potentially serious complication. Adherence to the above recommendations on anchor insertion will help to minimize the risk of anchor loosening.

Other problems related to the use of suture anchors can occur intraoperatively. If the anchor has been inserted but the location has been found to be less than optimal, the anchor position can be changed. For a screw-in anchor,

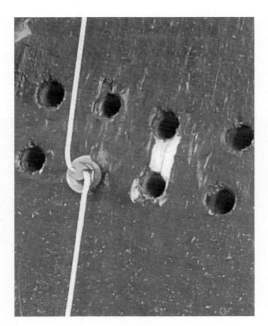

Figure 13-11 Close-up of suture anchor eyelet showing correct orientation to minimize suture abrasion against eyelet edge. (Reprinted with permission from Hasan SS, Gartsman GM: Pearls and pitfalls of arthroscopic rotator cuff repair. *Op Tech Orthop Surg* 2002;12:176–185.)

load the inserter and engage the anchor, pull the anchor out half way, use a grasper to grab the anchor, load the anchor onto the inserter, and finally reinsert the anchor.

If an anchor becomes dislodged and is free-floating within the subacomial space or in glenohumeral joint, it must be removed. This problem can be encountered intraoperatively (Fig. 13-14) or postoperatively (Fig. 13-15). A magnetized Wissinger rod or switching stick may help locate a metal anchor. Once the anchor is identified, use a large grasper through a large cannula to grab the anchor and then back the grasper out until the anchor is flush with the edge of the cannula. If the anchor is grasped in line with the anchor, then it can be retrieved through the cannula. If the anchor is not grasped in line with the anchor but it is just longer than the outer diameter of the cannula, then the cannula, grasper, and anchor can be carefully withdrawn together from the shoulder. Otherwise, it is best to use a second grasper from a different portal to retrieve the anchor from the first grasper by grasping in line with the anchor to facilitate removal.

Biodegradable suture anchors may be preferable, but currently the authors have no compelling arguments for or against current metallic or bioabsorbable anchors. Concerns have been raised over the damage caused by metallic anchors if they become dislodged (48), but metallic anchors are also easily imaged using plain radiographs. Bioabsorbable anchors produce less magnetic resonance imaging artifact, thereby allowing better rotator cuff visualization postoperatively (49). However, the anchors themselves are often visible by magnetic resonance imaging several years after surgery, suggesting at best incomplete degradation, and concerns have been raised regarding the potential for bioabsorbable anchors to fragment and to cause painful synovitic reactions (50). Neither author uses tacks for rotator cuff repair and neither can recommend this technique because of concerns over difficulties achieving a tension-free repair, repair failure by tearing around the tack,

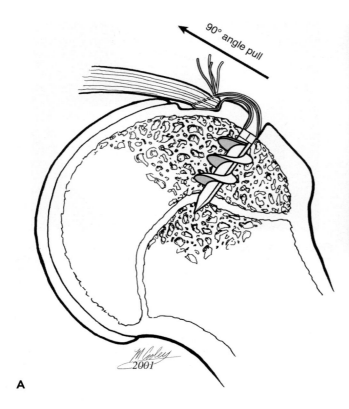

A

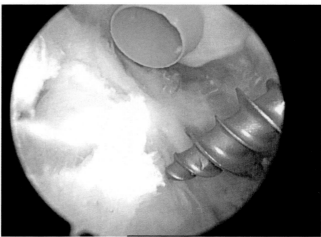

B

Figure 13-13 Schematic (**A**) and arthroscopic view (**B**) demonstrating lateral placement of a suture anchor inserted at deadman's angle. (Reprinted with permission from Hasan SS, Gartsman GM. Pearls and pitfalls of arthroscopic rotator cuff repair. *Op Tech Orthop Surg* 2002;12:176–185.)

prominent tack heads that may break (51,52), and the potential for tack-induced synovitis.

Suture Management and Passage through Tendon

Once the anchors have been inserted into the greater tuberosity, the remaining task becomes mainly one of suture management; that is, preventing entanglement as the sutures are passed through rotator cuff tissue and then tied. Strict adherence to a routine is essential to minimizing suture management problems. The authors prefer retrieving all sutures through the anterior cannula save for the suture being passed from anchor to tendon, which is placed in the lateral cannula.

Many anchors used for rotator cuff repair are loaded with two sutures so that additional points of rotator cuff fixation can be obtained without the need for additional anchors (35,37). When anchors loaded with two sutures

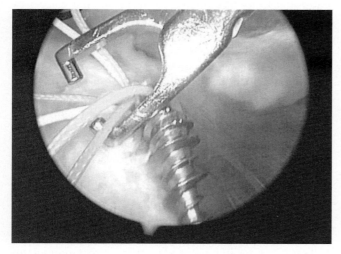

Figure 13-14 Retrieving an anchor that became loose intraoperatively. In this instance, a looping grasper was used for retrieval because one of the sutures had not been cut.

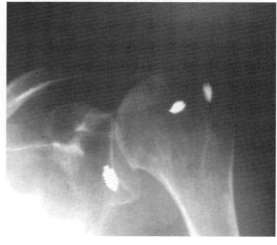

Figure 13-15 Radiograph of a shoulder with an irreparable tear showing a loose metallic anchor.

are used, it is helpful to use different colored suture (Fig. 13-10) (10,20), especially when suture-tying is performed after all the sutures have been passed through the tendon.

The authors use simple stitches for arthroscopic rotator cuff repair (9,10), but mattress repairs have also been described (1,5). Another stitch, the modified Mason-Allen stitch, is a locking stitch that has been shown to be superior in laboratory testing (15,53) but may be impractical for routine arthroscopic use (54). Recently, a novel stitch, termed the MaC stitch, has been described for arthroscopic use that appears to provide some of the advantages of the Mason-Allen stitch (55). However, biomechanical testing often ignores the fact that simple stitches can be placed close to one another to allow for a greater number of fixation points (35), and this is especially true when anchors loaded with two sutures are employed.

When two suture limbs (or one suture limb and a suture shuttle or shuttle relay) are located within a single cannula, it is imperative that the sutures not be entangled. This entanglement can occur when retrieving a suture limb prior to loading onto a suture shuttle and immediately before knot-tying when both suture ends are retrieved from the same cannula. A looping grasper can be inserted through the cannula and used to loop around one of the suture limbs (Fig. 13-16). As the grasper exits the cannula, it pulls the suture limb with it and untangles it from the other suture limb or from the shuttle suture.

All but the smallest rotator cuff tears require multiple suture anchors for repair. In general, sutures passed through tendon are spaced 5 mm apart so that a tear of 1 to 1.5 cm in length or smaller may require only one anchor with two sutures for repair, but a tear 3 cm or longer may require three or four suture anchors. First the anchors are inserted, then all the sutures are passed through the tendon before any of them are tied. As the anchors are inserted, the sutures are typically retrieved from the anterior cannula and clamped in pairs outside the cannula using hemostats. When using two or more suture anchors, retrieving the sutures percutaneously through an accessory portal created by an anterolateral stab incision can greatly facilitate suture management.

Suture anchors are inserted in the same sequence from anterior to posterior so that the anchors already in bone do not impair visualization when subsequent anchors are inserted (10). This order also minimizes the risk of suture entanglement because sutures that are retrieved from the first anchor through the anterior portal remain anterior to any subsequent anchor (10). Sutures are generally tied in sequence beginning with the most posterior one. Once the sutures have been passed through tendon, the two ends of the most posterior suture are retrieved through the same cannula, typically the lateral one, so that the sutures can be tied.

Arthroscopic Knot Tying

Before tying the knots, it is important to determine which one of the suture limbs is going to serve as the post. Typically, the most lateral limb, which is the one that has not been passed through the tendon, is used as the initial post. This enables the knots to lie flat (10) and as far laterally as possible, which prevents suture impingement against the undersurface of the acromion. A looping grasper placed through the lateral cannula is used around the post to identify it correctly and to ensure that the other strand is not wrapped around it. The subacromial space should be inspected as well for swollen bursal tissue that may become entrapped as the knots are tied. It is preferable to debride these bursal edges with a motorized shaver rather than after the knots have been tied because interposed tissue may affect knot security. Of course, the shaver blade should be directed away from sutures or knots.

Sutures are tied arthroscopically in the typical manner

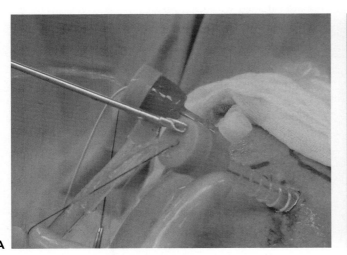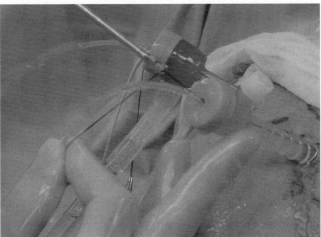

A   B

Figure 13-16 Use of the looping grasper to ensure that sutures are not tangled. **A:** Looping grasper. **B:** Verifying that no other sutures are entangled. (Reprinted with permission from Gartsman GM. *Shoulder Arthroscopy*. Philadelphia: WB Saunders, 2003.)

(9,10,38,39,56,57). There are many different stitches, each with its advocates, but the principles underlying proper knot-tying are the same. The strength of the knot is dependent on a number of factors including the characteristics of the suture employed, the knot security, and the loop security (57–60).

In general, it is important to master one sliding and one nonsliding knot and to know when to use each one. Sliding knots, such as the Duncan loop, are typically used for monofilament suture but can be used to tie braided suture so long as the suture slides freely. A nonsliding knot, such as the Revo knot, can be used for braided suture, but it is important to seat the knot squarely before locking it. A knot-pusher can be used to seat the knot securely before three or four additional half-hitches are placed to secure the knot (61,62). It is important to change the direction of the throw and post with consecutive half-hitches to improve pullout strength (61). This can be accomplished rather easily without physically changing posts by adjusting differential tension on the two limbs so that the throw changes at once from an underhand throw on one post to an overhand throw on the other post (63).

Other Intraoperative Pitfalls

Occasionally other problems occur that relate to suture anchors and the passage of sutures using specialized instruments. One such problem is suture pullout from the anchor. When this occurs, it is often best to continue the repair by using the remaining suture from that particular anchor. However, the anchor can also be backed out until its eyelet is visible and a wire-loop used to thread another suture through the eyelet. This technique can also been employed when sutures break inadvertently (for example, during knot-tying), although this problem is uncommon because the no. 2 braided suture typically used in rotator cuff repair does not break easily. When a suture breaks, it is often because the suture was already frayed from poor handling. This problem can be avoided by using looping graspers for suture manipulation instead of graspers with teeth, as well as by clamping sutures only at their tips when they are outside of the cannulas.

Occasionally, cannula-containing sutures will back out of the subacromial space. When this happens, retrieve the sutures using a looping grasper from an adjacent portal or cannula, reposition the cannula within the subacromial space, and then retrieve the sutures from the reinserted cannula. The authors favor the use of threaded cannulas because they do not back out as easily.

POSTOPERATIVE COMPLICATIONS

Postoperative complications include recurrent tears and stiffness, as well as medical complications, neurologic complications, and infection. The causes of recurrent tears and stiffness are multifactorial, but both complications are strongly influenced by postoperative rehabilitation. It is important to recognize that rehabilitation following arthroscopic repair is essentially identical to that following mini-open repair (10), because neither technique influences the biology of tendon healing (25). The initial rehabilitation differs from rehabilitation following traditional open repair only in that the deltoid does not need to be protected because it is not detached from its origin.

To protect the rotator cuff tendon during the early stages following repair, the patient should wear a simple sling at all times during the first 4 to 6 weeks, except when performing passive or gentle active-assisted exercise. The arm can hang comfortably at the side when an anatomic repair is carried out; hence, a large abduction pillow is not required to minimize tension across the repair. At the same time, passive or active-assisted motion is initiated early to prevent the formation of subdeltoid and subacromial adhesions that can limit movement. Specific postoperative complications are noted below.

Recurrent Tear

Factors that influence the durability of repair include conditions specific to the patient (for example, smoking and noncompliance), as well as conditions specific to the tear (for example, tendon retraction, scarring, and overall quality of tendon and bone). Other factors that influence the durability of the repair relate to technical aspects of the repair such as accurate assessment of the tear geometry, careful articular and bursal-sided release, the suture anchor and type of stitch employed, the anchor configuration employed, and the spacing of stitches across the repair.

Several studies have documented a high retear rate following open rotator cuff repair, especially following repair of large, chronic tears (15,17,64). However, revision surgery is rarely undertaken for a retear because most patients remain satisfied with their result (65). A retear can be suspected if there is trauma during the initial postoperative period leading to decreased mobility, comfort, or strength. Clinical examination may reveal increased crepitus, a palpable defect, and loss of strength on resistive strength testing. A loose metallic anchor on postoperative radiograph is confirmation that the tendon has retorn, but often the findings are considerably more subtle. Magnetic resonance imaging, even with contrast enhancement, is rather unreliable and may miss all but the largest retears.

The durability of arthroscopic rotator cuff repairs, especially those of large or massive tears, has been called into question. A recent study of 18 arthroscopic repairs of tears longer than 3 cm evaluated the repairs using ultrasound and found that 17 repairs had failed, nearly all retorn to their original size (66). Despite this complication, most patients remained pleased with their shoulders and no further intervention was needed. Another study recently compared the durability of arthroscopic and open rotator cuff repair performed by a single surgeon (67). Using magnetic resonance imaging at a minimum 1-year follow-up, the authors found that 69% of the open repairs and 53% of the arthroscopic repairs were intact. Of tears less than 3 cm in length, 74% of the open repairs and 84% of the arthroscopic repairs were intact. By contrast, of tears longer than 3 cm, only 24% in the arthroscopic group were intact. Despite these high retear rates following arthroscopic rotator cuff repair, patient satisfaction remained quite high and the clinical results appeared to be durable at intermediate follow-up. The majority of recurrent tears are asymptomatic or marginally symptomatic, so that very few patients go on to require revision repair. Most published series have documented revision rates between 0% and 4% (3,5,68–70).

Indications for revision rotator cuff repair are mainly symptom-based. An MRI or ultrasound should not be obtained to evaluate the rotator cuff for possibility of retear unless the patient is symptomatic (for example, persistent pain and weakness despite recovery of shoulder motion). Moreover, because of postsurgical artifacts from metallic debris, anchors, sutures, and scarring, MRI, even when contrast-enhanced, is often inaccurate in evaluating small recurrent tears and in distinguishing these from incomplete rotator cuff lesions. Ultrasound may offer an advantage over MRI in this setting, but again, the decision is typically driven by the patient's symptoms. An interesting dilemma is whether or not to recommend revision surgery when there is some persistent weakness but no pain following rotator cuff repair. When this unusual situation occurs, surgery can be recommended with caution if, and only if, the patient's expectations remain realistic and there is unequivocal evidence of a substantial recurrent rotator cuff tear by imaging and clinical testing.

There is no contraindication to performing revision rotator cuff repair arthroscopically, but if the failure relates to a technical consideration, such as improper assessment of tear geometry or anchor pullout, these factors must be corrected. At revision surgery, suture debris and exposed or loose anchors must be removed (Fig. 13-17). Careful release of subdeltoid and subacromial adhesions must be performed followed by typical rotator cuff mobilization, as described earlier. It may be best to begin the dissection medially at the apex of the tear rather than anteriorly or posteriorly where the rotator cuff margin may be scarred to the deltoid fascia (71). Finally, it is also important to recognize the tear that is irreparable or not worth repairing (Fig. 13-18) because of factors such as poor tendon quality or patient noncompliance, so that any technical errors may not be repeated.

Postoperative Stiffness

Stiffness is another postoperative complication that is by no means specific to arthroscopic repair, but rather is a complication of rotator cuff repair in general. In fact, stiff-

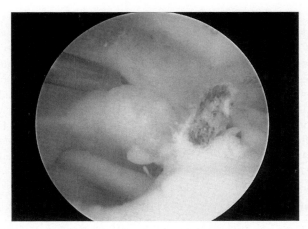

Figure 13-17 Suture and tendon debris following a failed rotator cuff repair.

ness from subdeltoid scarring may be more common following mini-open repair than following arthroscopic repair (14). A nonanatomic repair under tension and excessively cautious or delayed rehabilitation can produce a captured shoulder that is both painful and stiff (51,72). Consequently, neither repairs of marginal quality tissue nor repairs performed nonanatomically should be performed.

Rehabilitation following arthroscopic repair is identical to that following open repair, in that the tendon must be protected during the early stages of recovery. Moreover, passive or active-assisted motion should be initiated early to prevent the formation of subdeltoid and subacromial adhesions that can limit movement. Both authors use continuous passive motion as an adjunct to active-assisted exercises in forward elevation and external rotation to prevent stiffness. However, there are no objective data showing significant improvements in range of motion using continuous passive motion (73).

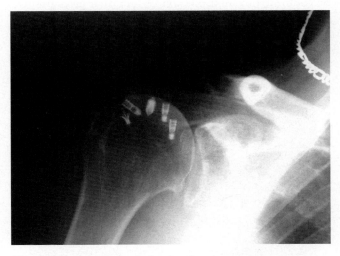

Figure 13-18 Radiograph showing three types of metallic anchors from three prior repairs, all of which failed. A fourth repair is unlikely to be successful.

When postoperative stiffness does occur, physical therapy and home exercises are important to improve the range of motion. Anti-inflammatory drugs and cortisone injections are discouraged because these may retard soft-tissue healing. When physical therapy has failed, arthroscopic contracture release and lysis of subacromial and subdeltoid adhesions (Fig. 13-19) followed by vigorous physical therapy is often helpful to restore movement. Manipulation is often performed serially as the contracture release is carried out, but manipulation alone may jeopardize the repair and should be avoided.

Infection

Infection is a devastating complication following any surgery, and rotator cuff repair is no exception. The keys to avoiding this complication are strict adherence to aseptic measures, efficient operative technique, and the use of perioperative antibiotics.

Fortunately, infection is rarely encountered after arthroscopic shoulder surgery. General reviews of complications following shoulder arthroscopy have documented overall infection rates between 0% and 3% (74–78), and one review of complications following arthroscopic rotator cuff repair noted an approximately 1% to 2% risk of infection (51). A total of three superficial infections of sinus tracts and no deep infections were documented in seven outcome studies, encompassing a total of 392 arthroscopic rotator cuff repairs (3,5,7,14,68,70,79). The superficial infections responded to oral antibiotics and did not require reoperation.

Superficial wound or skin infections are treated with local wound care in addition to antibiotics that cover *Staphylococcus* and *Streptococcus* organisms (51). Persistent or increasing pain and stiffness, warmth, redness, swelling, and drainage, as well as systemic symptoms such as fever, suggest a deep infection. In equivocal cases, the diagnosis can be confirmed by an aspiration of fluid that gives positive

cultures and an elevated cell count. Laboratory tests showing an elevated erythrocyte sedimentation rate, C-reactive protein, and white blood cell count may aid in establishing the diagnosis, but in most cases the diagnosis of an infected shoulder is established clinically. Treatment should not await the availability of laboratory test results.

Treatment of an infected shoulder consists of immediate irrigation and debridement including the removal of necrotic and nonviable tissue and debris. Antibiotics should be withheld until tissue and fluid samples for intraoperative Gram stain and culture have been obtained (51). Irrigation and debridement of an infected shoulder is readily accomplished arthroscopically using previously established portals, but grossly infected tissue located superficially should be debulked prior to arthroscopy and this may necessitate enlarging the portals to enable adequate debridement. Antibiotic-impregnated fluid should be irrigated into both glenohumeral joint and subacromial space because both regions may be involved. This also enables a thorough inspection of the repair to document its integrity. There is no consensus on the minimum volume of fluid needed to irrigate an infected shoulder, but 6 L of fluid is usually adequate. A motorized shaver can be used to remove any synovitis or debris, and a mucus suction trap or similar device can be attached to the shaver suction to collect tissue for culture. Drains can be inserted into both glenohumeral joint and subacromial space under arthroscopic guidance at the end of the procedure.

In situations where the infection develops acutely following repair, sutures and anchors can be retained when the repair is found to be intact, despite the fact that monofilament sutures may offer an advantage in treating infection compared with the braided suture used typically in repairs. If the infection is chronic, then eradicating it takes precedence over rotator cuff repair (51) and the removal of all suture material and retained anchors becomes necessary. In either case, intravenous and oral antibiotics are an integral part of treating a postoperative infection.

If the repair has failed or if removal of foreign material becomes necessary in the course of treating an infection, then revision repair can be performed at the time of final washout. The repair can be performed open using transosseous sutures or arthroscopically using anchors if bone purchase is adequate. Monofilament suture may be advantageous because of concerns that braided suture may readily harbor bacteria. If the infection is particularly difficult to eradicate, then revision repair may have to be attempted at a later date (i.e., once the infection has been successfully treated). Additionally, if eradication of the infection requires arthrotomy because of the magnitude of the infection or for any other reasons, then (whenever possible) that incision should be used for repair.

NEUROLOGICAL COMPLICATIONS

Direct nerve injury during arthroscopic rotator cuff repair is extremely rare (74,78) because proper portal placement

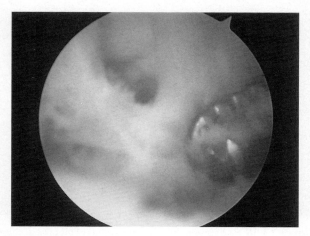

Figure 13-19 Dense subacromial adhesions in a patient with stiffness following rotator cuff repair.

does not put any of the peripheral nerves at risk. However, posterior or posterior-inferior portal malposition may place the axillary and suprascapular nerves at risk, and lateral or anterior portal malposition may place the axillary or musculocutaneous nerves at risk, respectively (51). Care should be exercised during the use of motorized instruments or electrocautery during coracohumeral ligament release, owing to the proximity of the musculocutaneous and axillary nerves. The suprascapular nerve is vulnerable to injury during intra-articular releases for contracted posterior rotator cuff tears. Surgeons considering arthroscopic subscapularis repair should be aware of the relationship of both the axillary and radial nerves to the subscapularis tendon, especially if the tear is retracted and chronic.

Other neurologic complications relate to the use of interscalene block for intraoperative and immediate postoperative analgesia (80–82). Most injuries are neuropraxias that resolve completely within a few weeks, but a few may persist for a year or longer (82).

Ipsilateral nerve injury can occur following arthroscopic shoulder surgery in the decubitus position (77,83). These injuries are usually neuropraxias that can be avoided by positioning the arm in approximately 70 degrees of abduction and 15 degrees of flexion (39) and by using the minimum weight (<7 kg) needed for distraction (84,85). Traction should always be released whenever it is not needed, and the wrist and forearm sleeve that connects to the traction apparatus should be adequately padded (75,85). Neuropraxia relating to excessive traction is more easily avoided when surgery is performed in the beach chair position (75,83,86) but it is not eliminated (87,88). Neuropraxia may also result from direct compression by excessive fluid extravasation (84,85). Lastly, both contralateral and lower-extremity neuropraxias can also occur following arthroscopic shoulder surgery in both the beach chair and lateral decubitus positions. These are generally attributed to improper patient positioning, inadequate padding around vulnerable sites, or excessively long surgery.

SYSTEMIC COMPLICATIONS

Fluid overload resulting from excessive fluid extravasation during arthroscopy can cause cardiac and respiratory failure (77,88). Vigilance is the key to preventing this complication. The surgeon should remain mindful of the duration of the procedure, operate at the minimum fluid pressure necessary for adequate visualization and hemostasis, and turn off the flow whenever there is an interruption (for example, while waiting for an anchor, a replacement cannula, or an instrument). In addition, fluid extravasation can be minimized by ensuring that the cannulas remain within the subacromial space and by promptly reinserting them whenever they back out. The shoulder should always be examined periodically for signs of excessive soft tissue swelling (85).

Epinephrine is frequently added to the lactated Ringer's solution used in arthroscopy, but it may be best to avoid it altogether (38). Epinephrine may introduce unnecessary risks and probably does little to improve visualization. If the surgeon finds epinephrine helpful, it can be added only to every other bag of Ringer's solution or to the first two bags of fluid when a longer surgery is anticipated.

Systemic complications, including pneumothorax and complications relating to inadvertent vascular injection, have been attributed to interscalene blocks (82), but an experienced regional anesthesia team can significantly minimize these risks. Interscalene block often produces diaphragmatic paralysis, which may last for several hours. Although this is a transient and frequently benign phenomenon, it can lead to respiratory failure, especially in a patient with poor pulmonary reserve.

COMPLICATION RATES AND CONCLUSIONS

Published series of arthroscopic rotator cuff repair have documented good to excellent results using shoulder-specific outcomes instruments in approximately 90% of patients (3,5,7,68,89), and this result is comparable to those following traditional open repair (90) or mini-open repair (91,92). These series have also documented very low rates of intraoperative and immediate postoperative complications. The senior author initially described the results of arthroscopic rotator cuff repair in a series of 73 patients published in 1998 (3) that showed, at a minimum 2-year follow-up, 84% of the results were rated as good or excellent and various outcome measures documented significant improvements over preoperative function and comfort. No complications such as infection, stiffness, neural injury, or those stemming from suture anchors were reported.

We recognize that the low complication rates for arthroscopic repairs in published series by experienced high-volume surgeons may not always be applicable to other providers, including those making the transition to arthroscopic repair. However, one should remember that any difficulty encountered during an arthroscopic repair should be addressed intraoperatively by prompt conversion to a mini-open repair. The incidence of postoperative complications, such as stiffness and infection, remains low and probably lower than that following mini-open or conventional open repair. Hopefully, careful adherence to the principles outlined above during the transition to an arthroscopic repair and afterwards will minimize these problems.

REFERENCES

1. Gazielly DF, Gleyze P, Montgagnon C, et al. Arthroscopic repair of distal supraspinatus tears with Revo Screw and permanent mat-

tress sutures. A preliminary report. Amelia Island, FL: 13th Annual Meeting of the American Shoulder and Elbow Surgeons, 1996.

2. Snyder SJ. Technique of arthroscopic rotator cuff repair using implantable 4-mm Revo suture anchors, suture Shuttle Relays, and no. 2 nonabsorbable mattress sutures. *Orthop Clin North Am* 1997; 28:267–275.

3. Gartsman GM, Khan M, Hammerman SM. Arthroscopic repair of full-thickness tears of the rotator cuff. *J Bone Joint Surg Am* 1998; 80:832–840.

4. Gartsman GM, Brinker MR, Khan M. Early effectiveness of arthroscopic repair for full-thickness tears of the rotator cuff—an outcome analysis. *J Bone Joint Surg* 1998;80A:33–40.

5. Tauro JC. Arthroscopic rotator cuff repair: analysis of technique and results at 2- and 3-year follow-up. *Arthroscopy* 1998;14:45–51.

6. Burkhart SS. Arthroscopic treatment of massive rotator cuff tears. *Clin Orthop* 2001;390:107–118.

7. Wolf EM, Pennington WT, Agrawal V. Arthroscopic rotator cuff repair: 4- to 10-year results. *Arthroscopy* 2004;20:5–12.

8. Miller C, Savoie FH. Glenohumeral abnormalities associated with full-thickness tears of the rotator cuff. *Orthop Rev* 1994;23: 159–162.

9. Gartsman GM, Hammerman SM. Arthroscopic rotator cuff repair. *Op Tech Shoulder Elbow Surg* 1999;1:2–8.

10. Hasan SS, Gartsman GM. Pearls and pitfalls of arthroscopic rotator cuff repair. *Op Tech Orthop Surg* 2002;12:176–185.

11. Ahmad CS, Levine WN, Bigliani LU. Arthroscopic rotator cuff repair. *Orthopedics* 2004;27:570–574.

12. Burkhart SS, Danaceau SM, Pearce CE Jr. Arthroscopic rotator cuff repair: Analysis of results by tear size and by repair technique-margin convergence versus direct tendon-to-bone repair. *Arthroscopy* 2001;17:905–912.

13. Norberg FB, Field LD, Savoie FH 3rd. Repair of the rotator cuff. Mini-open and arthroscopic repairs. *Clin Sports Med* 2000;19: 77–99.

14. Severud EL, Ruotolo C, Abbott DD, et al. All-arthroscopic versus mini-open rotator cuff repair: a long-term retrospective outcome comparison. *Arthroscopy* 2003;19:234–238.

15. Gerber C. Massive rotator cuff tears. In: Iannotti JP, Williams GR, eds. *Disorders of the Shoulder: Diagnosis and Management.* Philadelphia: Lippincott Williams & Wilkins, 1999: 57–92.

16. Fuchs B, Weishaupt D, Zanetti M, et al. Fatty degeneration of the muscles of the rotator cuff: assessment by computed tomography versus magnetic resonance imaging. *J Shoulder Elbow Surg* 1999; 8:599–605.

17. Jost B, Pfirrmann CW, Gerber C, et al. Clinical outcome after structural failure of rotator cuff repairs. *J Bone Joint Surg Am* 2000; 82:304–314.

18. Gartsman GM, Hammerman SM. Full-thickness tear: arthroscopic repair. *Orth Clin North Am* 1997;28:83–98.

19. Gartsman GM, Hammerman SM. Arthroscopic repair of full-thickness rotator cuff tears. *Op Tech Orth* 1998;8:226–235.

20. Gartsman GM. Arthroscopic rotator cuff repair. *Clin Orthop* 2001; 390:95–106.

21. Gartsman GM. All arthroscopic rotator cuff repairs. *Orthop Clin North Am* 2001;32:501–510.

22. Yamaguchi K, Ball CM, Galatz LM. Arthroscopic rotator cuff repair: transition from mini-open to all-arthroscopic. *Clin Orthop* 2001;390:83–94.

23. Yamaguchi K, Levine WN, Marra G, et al. Transitioning to arthroscopic rotator cuff repair: the pros and cons. *Instr Course Lect* 2003; 52:81–92.

24. Beals TC, Harryman DT 2nd, Lazarus MD. Useful boundaries of the subacromial bursa. *Arthroscopy* 1998;14:465–470.

25. Mazzoca AD, Cole BJ, Romeo AA. Arthroscopic repair of full-thickness rotator cuff tears: surgical technique. *Op Tech Orthop Surg* 2002;12:167–175.

26. Gartsman GM, O'Connor DP. Arthroscopic rotator cuff repair with and without arthroscopic subacromial decompression: a prospective, randomized study of one-year outcomes. *J Shoulder Elbow Surg* 2004;13:424–426.

27. Gartsman GM. Arthroscopic acromioplasty for lesions of the rotator cuff. *J Bone Joint Surg* 1990;72A:169–180.

28. Gartsman GM. Arthoscopic management of rotator cuff disease. *J Am Acad Orthop Surg* 1998;6:259–266.

29. Matsen FA III, Arntz CT, Lippitt SB. Rotator cuff. In: Rockwood CA Jr, Matsen FA III, eds. *The Shoulder.* 2nd ed. Philadelphia: WB Saunders, 1998;755–839.

30. Tauro JC. Arthroscopic "interval slide" in the repair of large rotator cuff tears. *Arthroscopy* 1999;15:527–530.

31. Lo IK, Burkhart SS. Arthroscopic repair of massive, contracted, immobile rotator cuff tears using single and double interval slides: technique and preliminary results. *Arthroscopy* 2004;20: 22–33.

32. Lo IK, Burkhart SS. The interval slide in continuity: a method of mobilizing the anterosuperior rotator cuff without disrupting the tear margins. *Arthroscopy* 2004;20:435–441.

33. Tauro JC. Arthroscopic repair of large rotator cuff tears using the interval slide technique. *Arthroscopy* 2004;20:13–21.

34. Burkhart SS, Athanasiou KA, Wirth MA. Margin convergence: a method of reducing strain in massive rotator cuff tears. *Arthroscopy* 1996;12:335–338.

35. Burkhart SS. A stepwise approach to arthroscopic rotator cuff repair based on biomechanical principles. *Arthroscopy* 2000;16: 82–90.

36. Lo IK, Burkhart SS. Current concepts in arthroscopic rotator cuff repair. *Am J Sports Med* 2003;31:308–324.

37. Millstein ES, Snyder SJ. Arthroscopic management of partial, full-thickness, and complex rotator cuff tears: indications, techniques, and complications. *Arthroscopy* 2003;19(Suppl 1):189–199.

38. Gartsman GM. *Shoulder Arthroscopy.* Philadelphia: WB Saunders, 2003.

39. Snyder SJ. *Shoulder Arthroscopy,* 2nd ed. Philadelphia: Lippincott Williams & Wilkins, 2003.

40. Lo IK, Burkhart SS. Transtendon arthroscopic repair of partial-thickness, articular surface tears of the rotator cuff. *Arthroscopy* 2004;20:214–220.

41. Fox JA, Romeo AA. PASTA lesion: trans-tendon technique for repair. *Op Tech Orthop* 2002;12:191–196.

42. Gartsman GM. Arthroscopic assessment of rotator cuff tear reparability. *Arthroscopy* 1996;12:546–549.

43. Stollsteimer GT, Savoie FH 3rd. Arthroscopic rotator cuff repair: current indications, limitations, techniques, and results. *Instr Course Lect* 1998;47:59–65.

44. Burkhart SS. The deadman theory of suture anchors: observations along a south Texas fence line. *Arthroscopy* 1995;11:119–123.

45. Apreleva M, Ozbaydar M, Fitzgibbons PG, et al. Rotator cuff tears: the effect of the reconstruction method on three-dimensional repair site area. *Arthroscopy* 2002;18:519–526.

46. Lo IK, Burkhart SS. Double-row arthroscopic rotator cuff repair: re-establishing the footprint of the rotator cuff. *Arthroscopy* 2003; 19:1035–1042.

47. Meier SW, Meier JD, Levy AS. Rotator cuff repair: the effect of double row versus single row fixation on the three-dimensional area of repair site. 71st Annual Meeting Proceedings, American Academy of Orthopaedic Surgeons, 2004:533–534.

48. Kaar TK, Schenck RC Jr, Wirth MA, et al. Complications of metallic suture anchors in shoulder surgery: a report of 8 cases. *Arthroscopy* 2001;17:31–37.

49. Magee T, Shapiro M, Hewell G, et al. Complications of rotator cuff surgery in which bioabsorbable anchors are used. *AJR Am J Roentgenol* 2003;181:1227–1231.

50. Freehill MQ, Harms DJ, Huber SM, et al. Poly-L-lactic acid tack synovitis after arthroscopic stabilization of the shoulder. *Am J Sports Med* 2003;31:643–647.

51. Cohen BS, Hatzidakis AM, Romeo AA. Complications of rotator cuff surgery. In: *Orthopaedic Knowledge Update: Shoulder and Elbow 2.* Rosemont, IL: American Academy of Orthopaedic Surgeons, 2002: 181–189.

52. Cummins CA, Strickland S, Appleyard RC, et al. Rotator cuff repair with bioabsorbable screws: an in vivo and ex vivo investigation. *Arthroscopy* 2003;19:239–248.

53. Gerber C, Schneeberger AG, Beck M, et al. Mechanical strength of repairs of the rotator cuff. *J Bone Joint Surg* 1994;76B:371–380.

54. Schneeberger AG, von Roll A, Kalberer F, et al. Mechanical strength of arthroscopic rotator cuff repair techniques: an in vitro study. *J Bone Joint Surg Am* 2002;84:2152–2160.

55. MacGillivray JD, Ma CB. An arthroscopic stitch for massive rotator cuff tears: the Mac stitch. *Arthroscopy* 2004;20:669–671.

56. Nottage WM, Lieurance RK. Arthroscopic knot typing techniques. *Arthroscopy* 1999;15:515–521.
57. Kim SH, Yoo JC. Arthroscopic knot tying. *Tech Shoulder Elbow Surg* 2003;4:35–43.
58. Burkhart SS, Wirth MA, Simonick M, et al. Loop security as a determinant of tissue fixation security. *Arthroscopy* 1998;14:773–776.
59. Burkhart SS, Wirth MA, Simonich M, et al. Knot security in simple sliding knots and its relationship to rotator cuff repair: how secure must the knot be? *Arthroscopy* 2000;16:202–207.
60. Lo IK, Burkhart SS, Chan KC, et al. Arthroscopic knots: determining the optimal balance of loop security and knot security. *Arthroscopy* 2004;20:489–502.
61. Loutzenheiser TD, Harryman DT II, Yung SW, et al. Optimizing arthroscopic knots. *Arthroscopy* 1995;11:199–206.
62. Loutzenheiser TD, Harryman DT II, Ziegler DW, et al. Optimizing arthroscopic knots using braided or monofilament suture. *Arthroscopy* 1998;14:57–65.
63. Chan KC, Burkhart SS. How to switch posts without rethreading when tying half-hitches. *Arthroscopy* 1999;15:444–450.
64. Harryman DT II, Mack LA, Wang KY, et al. Repairs of the rotator cuff: correlation of functional results with integrity of the cuff. *J Bone Joint Surg* 1991;73A:982–989.
65. Zanetti M, Jost B, Hodler J, et al. MR imaging after rotator cuff repair: full-thickness defects and bursitis-like subacromial abnormalities in asymptomatic subjects. *Skeletal Radiol* 2000;29:314–319.
66. Galatz LM, Ball CM, Teefey SA, et al. The outcome and repair integrity of completely arthroscopically repaired large and massive rotator cuff tears. *J Bone Joint Surg* 2004;86A:219–224.
67. Bishop J, Lo IK, Klepps S, et al. Cuff integrity following arthroscopic versus open rotator cuff repair: a prospective study. San Francisco, CA: 20th Open Meeting of the American Shoulder and Elbow Surgeons, 2004.
68. Murray TF, Latjai G, Mileski RM, et al. Arthroscopic repair of medium to large full-thickness rotator cuff tears: outcome at 2- to 6-year follow-up. *J Shoulder Elbow Surg* 2002;11:19–24.
69. Kim SH, Ha KI, Park JH, et al. Arthroscopic versus mini-open salvage repair of the rotator cuff tear: outcome analysis at 2 to 6 years' follow-up. *Arthroscopy* 2003;19:746–754.
70. Bennett WF. Arthroscopic repair of full-thickness supraspinatus tears (small-to-medium): a prospective study with 2- to 4-year follow-up. *Arthroscopy* 2003;19:249–256.
71. Lo IK, Burkhart SS. Arthroscopic revision of failed rotator cuff repairs: technique and results. *Arthroscopy* 2004;20:250–267.
72. Mormino MA, Gross RM, McCarthy JA. Captured shoulder. A complication of rotator cuff surgery. *Arthroscopy* 1996;12:457–461.
73. Lastayo PC, Wright T, Jaffe R, et al. Continuous passive motion after repair of the rotator cuff. A prospective outcome study. *J Bone Joint Surg Am* 1998;80:1002–1011.
74. Gill TJ, Warren RF, Rockwood CA Jr, et al. Complications of shoulder surgery. *Instr Course Lect* 1999;48:359–374.
75. Weber SC, Abrams JS, Nottage WM. Complications associated with arthroscopic shoulder surgery. *Arthroscopy* 2002;18(2 Suppl 1):88–95.
76. Bigliani LU, Flatow EL, Deliz ED. Complications of shoulder arthroscopy. *Orthop Rev* 1991;20:743–751.
77. McFarland EG, O'Neill OR, Hsu CY. Complications of shoulder arthroscopy. *J South Orthop Assoc* 1997;6:190–196.
78. Small NC. Complications in arthroscopic surgery performed by experienced arthroscopists. *Arthroscopy* 1988;4:215–221.
79. Jones CK, Savoie FH 3rd. Arthroscopic repair of large and massive rotator cuff tears. *Arthroscopy* 2003;19:564–571.
80. Conn RA, Cofield RH, Byer DE. Interscalene block anesthesia for shoulder surgery. *Clin Orthop* 1987;216:94–98.
81. Tetzlaff JE, Yoon HJ, Brems J. Interscalene brachial plexus block for shoulder surgery. *Reg Anesth* 1994;19:339–343.
82. Brown AR. Anesthesia for shoulder surgery. In: Iannotti JP, Williams GR, eds. *Disorders of the Shoulder: Diagnosis and Management*. Philadelphia: Lippincott Williams & Wilkins, 1999:1075–1102.
83. Skyhar MJ, Altchek DW, Warren RF, et al. Shoulder arthroscopy with the patient in the beach-chair position. *Arthroscopy* 1988;4:256–259.
84. Ogilvie-Harris DJ, D'Angelo G. Arthroscopic surgery of the shoulder. *Sports Med* 1990;9:120–128.
85. Stanish WD, Peterson DC. Shoulder arthroscopy and nerve injury: pitfalls and prevention. *Arthroscopy* 1995;11:458–466.
86. Ogilvie-Harris DJ, Wiley AM. Arthroscopic surgery of the shoulder. *J Bone Joint Surg* 1986;68:201–207.
87. Mullins RC, Drez D Jr, Cooper J. Hypoglossal nerve palsy after arthroscopy of the shoulder in the beach chair position. *J Bone Joint Surg* 1992;74A:137–139.
88. Berjano P, González BG, Olmedo JF, et al. Complications in arthroscopic shoulder surgery. *Arthroscopy* 1998;14:785–788.
89. Wilson F, Hinov V, Adams G. Arthroscopic repair of full-thickness tears of the rotator cuff: 2- to 14-year follow-up. *Arthroscopy* 2002;18:136–144.
90. Cofield RH, Parvizi J, Hoffmeyer PJ, et al. Surgical repair of chronic rotator cuff tears. A prospective long-term study. *J Bone Joint Surg Am* 2001;83:71–77.
91. Liu SH, Baker CL. Arthroscopically assisted rotator cuff repair: correlation of functional results with integrity of the cuff. *Arthroscopy* 1994;10:54–60.
92. Youm T, Murray DS, Rokito AS, et al. Outcome and patient satisfaction of arthroscopic rotator cuff repair versus mini-open rotator cuff repair: medium term follow-up. San Francisco, CA: 20th open meeting of the American Shoulder and Elbow Surgeons, 2004.

Complications of Arthroscopic Subacromial Decompression and Acromioclavicular Joint Resection

14

Ilya Voloshin   Kevin J. Setter
Sean F. Bak   Louis U. Bigliani

In the past decade, we have seen an exponential increase in arthroscopic surgery of the shoulder. Consequently, complications related to these arthroscopic procedures have also increased. These complications can be divided into two categories: complications related to the arthroscopic techniques in general and those to specific arthroscopic procedures. The goal of this chapter is to discuss the complications specific to arthroscopic subacromial decompression (ASD) and acromioclavicular (AC) joint resection, as well as to provide clinical advice for prevention and treatment of these complications.

OVERVIEW OF ARTHROSCOPIC SUBACROMIAL DECOMPRESSION

In 1972, Neer described subacromial impingement syndrome (IS) of the shoulder (1). The principles of open subacromial decompression include resection of the acromial spur, coracoacromial ligament, inflamed hypertrophic bursa, and when indicated, the distal clavicle. In 1987, Ellman described the technique for arthroscopic subacromial decompression while maintaining the treatment principles set forth by Dr. Neer (2). ASD has proven to be a reliable procedure with success rates being equivalent to open subacromial decompression (80% to 90%) (2–7). The advantages of the arthroscopic approach include preservation of the origin of the deltoid muscle, a more rapid rehabilitation, and more pleasing results cosmetically. According to most reports, the complication rate of ASD has been the lowest with respect to arthroscopic procedures of the shoulder, ranging between 0.7% to 2% (8,9). However, the reported success rate of 80% to 90% points to a "failure" rate of 10% to 20%. The failure of a procedure may be a consequence of complications of treatment, which can be the result of preoperative diagnostic errors or intraoperative technical errors. However, the failure may also be the result of the intrinsic physiologic response of the patient and factors beyond the control of the surgeon and unrelated to diagnostic or technical errors, including worker's compensation (4,10).

COMPLICATIONS AND FAILURE OF ASD

Diagnostic Errors

The failure of ASD can be multifactorial and a systematic approach is important in deciphering the factors responsible for failures. The definition of a failed ASD would include at least one of the following: persistent pain, motion loss, weakness, and inability to return to an active lifestyle enjoyed prior to the onset of symptoms. Several investigators have attributed nearly 50% of acromioplasty failures to incorrect or missed diagnosis (4,10,11). It is important to differentiate IS from other conditions that may cause similar symptoms in the shoulder, such as glenohumeral instability, os acromiale, AC arthritis, cervical radiculitis, calcific tendonitis, adhesive capsulitis, and nerve compression.

Glenohumeral instability is common in younger patients, and especially in athletes involved in overhead activity sports (12). Ogilvie-Harris et al. (4) found that 25% of all diagnostic errors in their study were due to instability of the shoulder. The diagnosis of IS in this patient population should be thoroughly scrutinized. Patients with instability may have symptoms and signs of IS, most likely secondary to nonphysiologic kinematics of the shoulder and secondary bursitis. Internal impingement is also possible source of pain in these patients (13). Even though ASD would remove potential associated bursitis in these patients, it would also further destabilize the shoulder unless the capsular laxity and labral pathology are addressed at the same time.

Presence of os acromiale should certainly be sought when considering ASD (Fig. 14-1). Point tenderness over the midacromion is the most reliable sign of a symptomatic os. Currently, the treatment of os acromiale is controversial with some reports showing successful results following arthroscopic excision or near-total excision of mesoacromion without residual sequalae. This approach must be used with caution, realizing that there is no good solution to pain secondary to the loss of the deltoid origin and biomechani-

cal force-couple responsible for shoulder function. The authors' preferred treatment is coracoacromial ligament release and acromioplasty, which effectively decreases contact pressure between the greater tuberosity and acromion. We have consistently achieved satisfactory results with this method. Other authors have reported success using internal fixation supplemented by bone graft (14,15).

Degenerative symptomatic AC joint not only can contribute to IS (1), but also can be the cause of persistent pain after subacromial decompression unless addressed at the time of surgery (16). However, the resection of the distal clavicle should not be performed routinely for all patients who have IS, rather only in patients who are symptomatic in the region of the AC joint. For the failed ASD secondary to the AC joint symptoms, subsequent removal of the diseased AC joint offers a reasonable chance of success.

ASD is inappropriate for other potential diagnoses, such as cervical radiculitis, calcific tendonitis, adhesive capsulitis and nerve compression that can be confused with IS and will lead to persistent or exacerbated symptoms.

IS has become an increasingly common diagnosis for patients with painful shoulder. The authors recommend that each patient is approached thoroughly without expeditious attribution of their pain to IS. Complete history and a detailed physical examination must be performed specifically looking for other potential sources of symptoms in patients complaining of the anterosuperior shoulder pain, weakness, and difficulty with overhead activities. Appropriate radiographic workup as well as diagnostic injections are also important to differentiate potential other diagnoses. If the preoperative diagnosis was wrong or missed, ASD is bound to fail. It has been our experience that the most common entity misdiagnosed as IS is AC arthritis. In

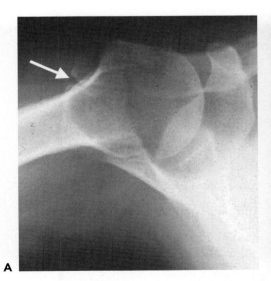
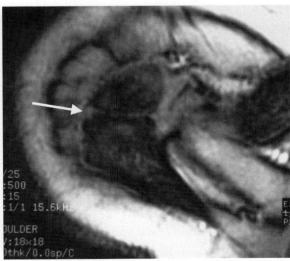

Figure 14-1 **A:** Axillary projection is typically the best radiographic view for demonstration of os acromiale (*arrow*). **B:** Axial magnetic resonance imaging in same patient.

younger patients, subtle instability can be missed. Differentiation of these processes can be simplified using selective injection of the subacromial space, AC joint, and glenohumeral joint. A positive impingement test (relief of pain during the Neer impingement maneuver after subacromial injection) is particularly useful in confirming the diagnosis of IS. It is essential that a systematic and thorough evaluation for other diagnoses is performed in the patient who has previously failed ASD.

Technical Errors

Perhaps one of the most common technical errors in ASD is the inadequate acromial resection (17). Poor visualization due to bleeding is probably the most crucial factor responsible for this complication. Visualization can be improved with good arthroscopic techniques, hypotensive anesthesia (18), and epinephrine in the irrigation fluid (19). Complete bursectomy is also very important for adequate visualization. The senior author successfully employed the "preemptive strike" technique where the electrocautery is passed just anterior to the coracoacromial ligament with the goal of cauterizing the acromial branch of the thoracoacromial trunk prior to the ligament detachment (Fig. 14-2). After this maneuver is performed, the ligament is taken directly off the anterior acromion without any major bleeding. A release rather than a resection of the coracoacromial ligament is performed, allowing for eventual healing of the ligament back to the bone in an elongated fashion. In the event of a massive rotator cuff tear, the ligament is left intact.

With the exception of younger patients with purely functional impingement and bursitis, we do a bony acromioplasty on the majority of patients with IS. To ensure adequate bone removal, the authors start the acromioplasty at the anterolateral corner of the acromion and set the resection level as a reference for the rest of the acromion. Removal of the spur along with 2 to 4 mm of additional bone anteriorly "raises the roof" of the acromion. Inadequate bone removal responsible for persistent IS usually can be successfully treated with revision ASD.

Although inadequate decompression is one of the most common technical errors, fracture of the acromion secondary to excessive bone removal has also been reported (20,21). Obtaining good quality preoperative radiographs, especially the outlet view, allows the surgeon to plan the appropriate amount of bone resection. The shape of the acromion can also be assessed, focusing on the curvature and the presence of the anterior spur. Again, starting the acromioplasty at the anterolateral corner of the acromion and setting the resection level is a useful technique to prevent this complication. These fractures can usually be treated with tension band fixation (21) or excision of the anterior fragment depending on its size.

Detachment of the anterior deltoid origin has been reported in literature (3,22) and can be a devastating complication causing anterosuperior subluxation of the humeral head and dysfunctional shoulder. Extreme care must be utilized to prevent this complication because there is no reliable treatment for anterosuperior humeral head subluxation. If diagnosed intraoperatively, the deltoid must be securely reattached to the anterior acromion to prevent chronic detachment and retraction, which is difficult to treat (22). The authors resect the anterior acromion just to the inferior attachment of the deltoid muscle (Fig. 14-3). Excessive anterior acromionectomy can also cause deltoid origin detachment. Chronic deltoid detachment is best treated with an attempt at soft tissue repair if an adequate cuff remains on the acromion. In the absence of a good soft-tissue stump, the deltoid is reattached via heavy non-

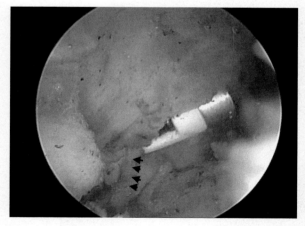

Figure 14-2 Arthroscopic view from posterior portal of right shoulder. The electrocautery device is used to come anterior to the coracoacromial ligament to coagulate the acromial branch (*arrows*) of the thoracoacromial trunk which lies within the ligament.

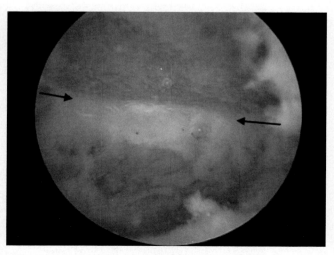

Figure 14-3 Arthroscopic view from posterior portal of left shoulder. The periosteal attachment of the deltoid (*arrows*) is left intact following thorough anterior subacromial decompression.

absorbable suture through bone tunnels in the anteriolateral acromion. It is important to perform a complete subcutaneous and bursal sided mobilization of the deltoid prior to repair to ensure high-tissue quality.

Inadequate bursectomy can potentially be the cause of persistent bursitis and pain in patients after ASD. Not only is complete bursectomy important for visualization, but it is also important for removal of the inflammatory mediators, which play a role in the catabolic processes and continued degeneration in patients with IS (23). The study at our institution demonstrated increased levels of the inflammatory mediators in the bursae of patients with IS compared to controls (23). Gotoh et al. (24) identified increased levels of neuromediators responsible for pain generation in the bursae of patients with IS. Based on these studies, the authors believe that complete bursectomy is an important part of ASD.

Biceps tendon pathology must be addressed at the time of ASD. Our preference is to pull the biceps into the joint and look laterally down the biceps groove to visualize as much of the tendon as possible. This should be a part of the routine diagnostic glenohumeral arthroscopy. In general, where severe inflammation or greater than 50% fraying exists, the biceps is tenodesed. Less extensive disease is treated with debridement. The presence of biceps pathology can often be noted preoperatively on axial magnetic resonance imaging (MRI).

There seems to be a controversy in literature regarding the address of the osteophytes on the distal clavicle (Fig. 14-4). Many reports advocate partial resection or coplaning of the AC joint if necessary to adequately decompress the subacromial space (25–29). On the other hand, Fischer et al. (30) reported on postoperative AC joint symptoms secondary to the violation of the AC joint during acromioplasty. The authors of this paper advocated an "all-or-none" approach to the AC joint and recommended distal

clavicle resection any time the inferior capsule or the inferior osteophytes were removed. The senior author has addressed the inferior osteophytes of the distal clavicle impinging on the rotator cuff by using the coplaning technique. There has not been an increase in postoperative complications related to the AC joint when using this technique (Fig. 14-5). Kuster et al. (31) demonstrated that removal of inferior impinging osteophytes from the distal clavicle in asymptomatic AC joints exhibiting arthrosis did not result in any instability or pain postoperatively; however, routine violation of the inferior capsule of the AC joints with no arthrosis resulted in mild instability and tenderness in 9 out of 12 patients. We remove the impinging osteophytes and do not excise the entire distal clavicle in an otherwise asymptomatic AC joint; however, we try not to violate the AC joint if no impinging osteophytes are present. Percutaneous placement of a needle through the AC joint is an excellent guide during ASD for the location of the AC joint viewed from the subacromial space.

Failure to address potential rotator cuff pathology can be the reason for an unsatisfactory result. Careful inspection of the rotator cuff is important and complete repairable tears must be addressed at the time of ASD. The patient should be informed about this possibility and prepared for it. The treatment of partial tears is controversial (32–34). The senior author repair the tears involving greater than 50% of the footprint of the rotator cuff tendon, especially in a younger patient population.

Physiologic Factors

The reformation of the anterior spur and the reattachment of the coracoacromial ligament can be responsible for re-

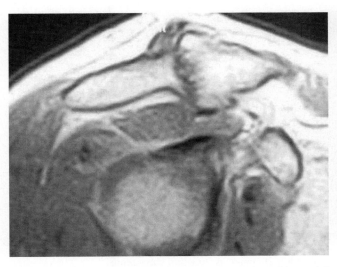

Figure 14-4 Coronal magnetic resonance imaging of large AC osteophytes (*top*).

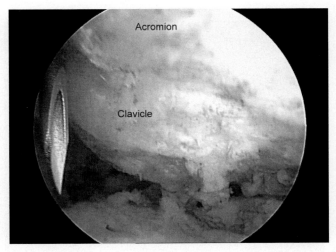

Figure 14-5 Arthroscopic view from lateral portal of left shoulder. A needle has been inserted into the AC joint anteriorly and prominent osteophytes off the undersurface of the distal clavicle are seen after anterior subacromial decompression.

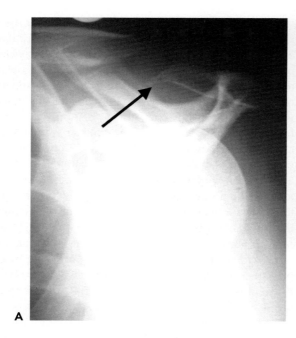

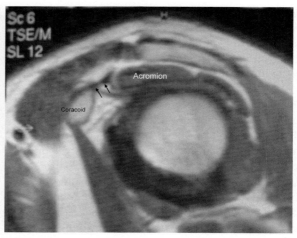

Figure 14-6 **A:** Outlet view of patient several years after arthroscopic subacromial decompression demonstrating reformation of spur. **B:** Sagittal magnetic resonance imaging of same patient with visible coracoacromial ligament (*arrows*).

current IS (Figs. 14-6 and 14-7) (35–37). Despite adequate decompression and complete bursectomy, some patients reform the removed bone and the coracoacromial ligament. The factors responsible for this phenomenon are unknown. The authors routinely perform a radial cut in the midsubstance of the coracoacromial ligament after detachment from the anterior acromion (Fig. 14-8). We feel that even if the ligament heals back to the anterior acromion, it would be lengthened by the radial cut and exhibit less pressure on the underlying rotator cuff. We have no proof that this is actually what happens; however, we have not seen this phenomenon on our revision cases since the implementation of this technique.

Severe heterotopic ossification (HO) has been reported

(38), as well as mild HO, which did not affect the outcome of the ASD (35). The authors of these reports did not know what caused the formation of the HO, but speculated that it could be related to slow rehabilitation and prolonged immobilization.

Another complication most likely related to the postoperative rehabilitation is "captured shoulder" or arthrofibrosis resulting in stiffness (39). Some patients seem to be predisposed to this complication and must be aggressively rehabilitated in the postoperative period. If the nonoperative treatment fails, arthroscopic release has been shown to be effective and does not cause glenohumeral instability (39,40). In our institution, patients are encouraged to start motion on the first postoperative day after the ASD and

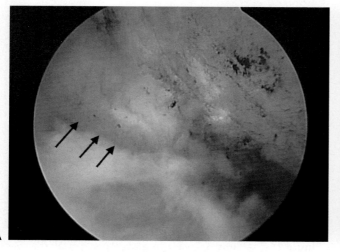

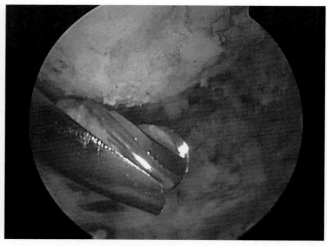

Figure 14-7 Arthroscopic view from posterior portal of left shoulder. **A:** Revision subacromial decompression revealing reformation of a stout CA ligament (*arrows*). A partial resection medially of the ligament has already been performed. **B:** Significant spur reformation in the same patient.

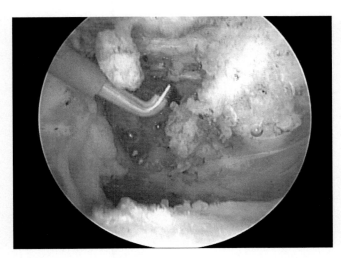

Figure 14-8 Arthroscopic view from posterior portal of right shoulder. After peeling the CA ligament off the anterior acromion, cautery is then used to radially cut the remaining ligament, disrupting any residual continuity it may have should it heal back to the acromion.

undergo a course of physical therapy stressing stretching and strengthening of the rotator cuff musculature.

Patients Receiving Worker's Compensation Benefit

Several reports have indicated that the patients receiving worker's compensation did significantly worse after ASD compared to patients receiving no such benefit (4,41). Often no diagnostic and/or technical errors can be found despite continued symptoms after ASD. We find it impossible to predict which patients will benefit from ASD in this patient population. Ogilvie-Harris et al. (42) reported only a 43% success rate after acromioplasty in patients receiving worker's compensation. A clear discussion must occur preoperatively with these patients regarding the expectations from ASD.

OVERVIEW OF ARTHROSCOPIC DISTAL CLAVICLE RESECTION

Arthroscopic distal clavicle resection has been well documented in literature (43–46). Johnson et al. (47) described a direct superior approach to the AC joint for resection of the distal clavicle in patients with isolated AC symptoms. The clinical success of this procedure has been well documented (43,44,48,49). Ellman (2) and Esch et al. (50) first described the arthroscopic subacromial approach to the distal clavicle resection. This approach is used for patients who have a concomitant subacromial IS and AC joint arthritis or patients who have impinging inferior osteophytes on the distal clavicle (51). This procedure was reported to be successful by several authors (45,46,52). Martin et al.

(53) reported excellent results with arthroscopic distal clavicle resection and concomitant ASD. Few complications have been reported following either the isolated arthroscopic distal clavicle resection or in conjunction with ASD. As with ASD, careful patient selection for the arthroscopic AC resection, as well as precise surgical technique, are important to achieve satisfactory results.

COMPLICATIONS AND FAILURE OF THE ARTHROSCOPIC AC RESECTION

Patient Selection

Several studies from our institution pointed out to the inferior results of arthroscopic distal clavicle resection in patients with subtle AC instability and previous history of trauma (44,54,55). In addition to palpation, the AC joint should be routinely tested not only for superoinferior instability but also for anteroposterior instability, using the contralateral shoulder for comparison. Biomechanical studies have shown that the acromioclavicular capsule and ligaments represent 90% of the restraint to posterior translation of the clavicle at both small and large displacements (56,57). These structures are damaged in grade II AC injuries and are probably the cause of failure of the arthroscopic AC joint resections in patients with AC instability. Flatow et al. (44) reported a 42% failure rate in patients with AC instability after arthroscopic distal clavicle resection. The authors recommended an AC stabilization procedure in combination with the distal clavicle resection as a treatment of choice in this group of patients. Capsular and ligamentous laxity in these patients probably results in posterior abutment that has been described after open distal clavicle resection (58).

As mentioned above, in the section on complications of ASD, there is controversy about the appropriate management of the inferior osteophytes of the distal clavicle causing impingement. Some authors advocate an "all-or-none" approach by recommending complete distal clavicle excision if the AC joint is violated (59). Their argument is that subtle instability related to the disruption of the inferior capsular restraints causes AC joint symptoms in the long-term. Others, including the senior author, have not noted any complications following coplaning of the distal clavicle to remove impinging osteophytes (25–29).

Technical Errors

Technical errors in the arthroscopic AC resection are mostly related to an imprecise resection level of the distal clavicle. This resection has to be complete, yet not extensive, to prevent the instability of the distal clavicle. Inadequate bone removal most commonly occurs at the posterosuperior cor-

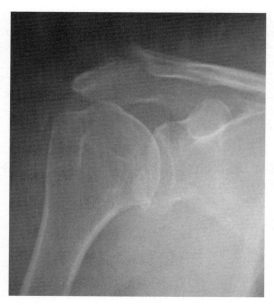

Figure 14-9 AP view of patient with residual AC symptoms over one year after distal clavicle resection which was superiorly incomplete.

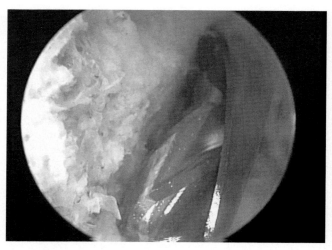

Figure 14-11 Arthroscopic view of right shoulder from the posterior portal using the direct approach demonstrates the excellent visualization and access given by this method.

ner of the AC joint (Fig. 14-9). This occurs most commonly with the subacromial approach, which provides challenging visualization of that part of the AC joint. Placement of the arthroscope through the anterior portal provides excellent views and allows verification of the accomplished resection (Fig. 14-10). Also, a 70-degree arthroscope is useful during the subacromial approach. It allows the visualization of the posterior part of the AC joint without the need to move the arthroscope to the anterior portal. Recently the authors have been placing the 30-degree arthroscope

in the lateral portal and have been resecting the distal clavicle with a burr from the anterior portal. Keeping the 30-degree arthroscope in the lateral portal allows visualization of the entire AC joint when the camera is directed from the anterior side of the joint in a posterior direction. This technique obviates the need to switch viewing portals or to use a 70-degree arthroscope to confirm complete resection. The direct approach described by Johnson (47) provides better visualization of all parts of the AC joint and can be utilized in patients with isolated AC symptoms (Fig. 14-11).

Extensive resection of the distal clavicle compromises the capsular restraints of the AC joint and has been reported

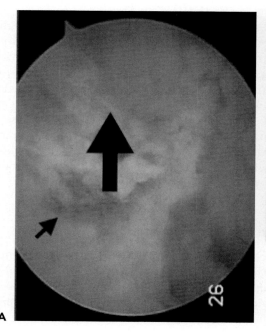

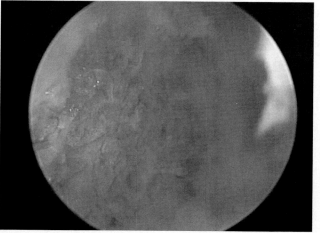

Figure 14-10 **A:** Arthroscopic view of a left shoulder from the anterior portal reveals residual superior clavicle (*large arrow*) after resection from the posterior viewing portal. The resected portion of distal clavicle is marked by the smaller arrow. **B:** Anterior viewing portal, left shoulder of another patient. The anterior view has confirmed circumferential resection of the distal clavicle.

to be associated with symptomatic AC instability (60). The clavicle positions the scapular during motion of the upper extremity. Transmission of forces are generated by the attached muscles through the coracoclavicular and acromioclavicular ligaments (61). The loss of these ligaments is likely to cause abnormal motion and increase the demand on the surrounding musculature that coordinates scapular motion and stabilization. Symptoms of myalgia, decreased stability leading to drooping shoulder, weakness, and irritation of the brachial plexus may ensue (60). Most authors have recommended excision of up to 2 or even 2.5 cm of the distal clavicle (2,45,50,56), suggesting that less resection will cause the abutment of the distal clavicle against the acromion with arm motion (62). Rockwood (62) and Kennedy and Cameron (63) have shown that only minimal relative motion of the clavicle in relation to the scapula exists in normal shoulders. Flatow et al. (44) demonstrated that as little as 5-mm resection of the distal clavicle was enough to achieve successful results. The posterior abutment is most likely related to the disruption of the ligamentous restraints caused by excessive resection or preexisting AC instability (Fig. 14-12).

Recently, Renfree et al. (64) described the anatomic ligamentous insertions around the AC joint. The study demonstrated that the superior AC ligament disruption can occur with as little as 5.2 mm of resection of the distal clavicle in women and 7.6 mm in men, and resection of as little as 4.7 mm of the medial acromion in women and 8.0 mm in men. Based on these findings, we have been removing a few millimeters from the medial acromion and from the distal clavicle, achieving a complete resection and clearance of at least 5 mm between the acromion and the distal clavicle without compromising outcomes (Fig. 14-13).

Treatment of extensive distal clavicle resections, espe-

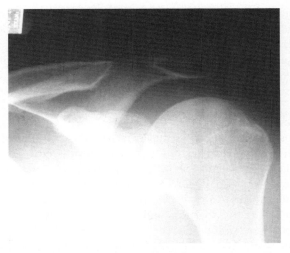

Figure 14-13 AP radiograph of patient two years after arthroscopic distal clavicle resection who had continued pain localizing to the AC joint as well as symptomatic anteroposterior AC instability. This patient underwent a revision distal clavicle resection with coracoacromial ligament transfer with excellent relief of pain.

cially with compromised integrity of the coracoclavicular ligaments, is challenging. The treatment is similar to that of AC instability and involves the transfer of the coracoacromial ligament, if it is available, to the distal clavicle. This construct can be reinforced with nonabsorbable sutures wrapped around the coracoid and the distal clavicle or suture anchors placed in the coracoid base with sutures tied over the clavicle. If the coracoacromial ligament is not available due to the previous acromioplasty, various autograft and allograft tissues (such as hamstring tendons) can be used for reconstruction of the coracoclavicular ligaments. Recently, Murthi and Moinfar (65) performed an

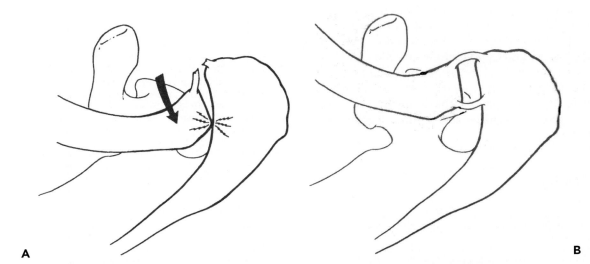

A   **B**

Figure 14-12 **A:** An AC joint with disruption of the superior capsule allows posterior translation and abutment against the acromial base. **B:** Preservation of the superior ligaments maintaining AC stability and preventing abutment. (Reproduced with permission from American Academy of Orthopaedic Surgeons; Flatow EL: The biomechanics of the acromioclavicular, sternoclavicular, and scapulothoracic joints. *Instr Course Lect* 1993;42:237–45.)

anatomical study describing the use of the pectoralis minor tendon for reconstruction of the coracoclavicular ligaments. This could potentially obviate the need for allograft tissue or distant autograft tissue to stabilize the distal clavicle.

Physiologic Factors

Reossification and even fusion across the AC joint after arthroscopic distal clavicle resection have been reported (66,67). The factors that influence partial or complete reossification of the AC joint are probably multifactorial and related to the extent of the resection, the leftover boney debris after the resection, and most importantly, the postoperative rehabilitation. The partial reossification of the AC joint is not necessarily symptomatic (46). Kay et al. (46) demonstrated that 25% of the patients showed partial or even complete reformation of the distal clavicle without any symptoms at an average of a 6 year follow-up. Tytherleigh-Strong et al. (66) described a case report of a complete fusion of the AC joint following the arthroscopic distal clavicle resection, resulting in limited range of motion. We believe that an aggressive rehabilitation program stressing range-of-motion exercises is extremely important to prevent symptomatic reformation of bone at the end of the distal clavicle following arthroscopic resection.

CONCLUSION

Arthroscopic subacromial decompression and the AC joint resection are successful and safe procedures. Most of the complications of these procedures are related to diagnostic or technical errors. Strict patient selection and precise and sound surgical technique will prevent most of the complications. Postoperative rehabilitation stressing range-of-motion exercises is also extremely important to achieve successful results. The authors have discussed their personal clinical approach and techniques to help avoid complications. A systematic approach to address the failures of ASD and distal clavicle resection is crucial and has to be directed at identifying the cause of failure. The treatment of the complications is often challenging and at times there are no good solutions.

REFERENCES

1. Neer CS 2nd. Anterior acromioplasty for the chronic impingement syndrome in the shoulder: a preliminary report. *J Bone Joint Surg Am* 1972;54:41–50.
2. Ellman H. Arthroscopic subacromial decompression: analysis of one- to three-year results. *Arthroscopy* 1987;3:173–181.
3. Stephens SR, Warren RF, Payne LZ, et al. Arthroscopic acromioplasty: a 6- to 10-year follow-up. *Arthroscopy* 1998;14:382–388.
4. Ogilvie-Harris DJ, Wiley AM, Sattarian J. Failed acromioplasty for impingement syndrome. *J Bone Joint Surg Br* 1990;72:1070–1072.
5. Tibone JE, Jobe FW, Kerlan RK, et al. Shoulder impingement syndrome in athletes treated by an anterior acromioplasty. *Clin Orthop* 1985;198:134–140.
6. Altchek DW, Warren RF, Wickiewicz TL, et al. Arthroscopic acromioplasty. Technique and results. *J Bone Joint Surg Am* 1990;72: 1198–1207.
7. Norlin R. Arthroscopic subacromial decompression versus open acromioplasty. *Arthroscopy* 1989;5:321–323.
8. Muller D. Arthroscopy of the shoulder joint: a minimal invasive and harmless procedure? *Arthroscopy* 2000;16:425.
9. Small N. Complications in arthroscopy: the knee and other joints. *Arthroscopy* 1986;2:253–258.
10. Hawkins RJ, Chris T, Bokor D, et al. Failed anterior acromioplasty. A review of 51 cases. *Clin Orthop* 1989;243:106–111.
11. Rockwood CA, Lyons FR. Shoulder impingement syndrome: diagnosis, radiographic evaluation, and treatment with a modified Neer acromioplasty. *J Bone Joint Surg Am* 1993;75:409–424.
12. Jobe FW, Kvitne RS, Giangarra CE. Shoulder pain in the overhand or throwing athlete. The relationship of anterior instability and rotator cuff impingement. *Orthop Rev* 1989;18:963–975.
13. Paley KJ, Jobe FW, Pink MM, et al. Arthroscopic findings in the overhand throwing athlete: evidence for posterior internal impingement of the rotator cuff. *Arthroscopy* 2000;16:35–40.
14. Ryu RK, Fan RS, Dunbar WHT. The treatment of symptomatic os acromiale. *Orthopedics* 1999;22:325–328.
15. Warner JJ, Beim GM, Higgins L. The treatment of symptomatic os acromiale. *J Bone Joint Surg Am* 1998;80:1320–1326.
16. Penny JN, Welsh RP. Shoulder impingement syndromes in athletes and their surgical management. *Am J Sports Med* 1981;9: 11–15.
17. Matthews LS, Blue JM. Arthroscopic subacromial decompression: avoidance of complications and enhancement of results. *Instr Course Lect* 1998;47:29–33.
18. Morrison DS, Jackson DW. Correlation of acromial morphology and results of arthroscopic subacromial decompression. *Orthop Trans* 1988;12:731–732.
19. Jensen KH, Werther K, Stryger V, et al. Arthroscopic shoulder surgery with epinephrine saline irrigation. *Arthroscopy* 2001;17: 578–581.
20. Matthews LS, Blue JM. Arthroscopic subacromial decompression—avoidance of complications and enhancement of results. *Instr Course Lect* 1998;47:29–33.
21. Rupp S, Seil R, Muller B, et al. Complications after subacromial decompression. *Arthroscopy* 1998;14:445.
22. Bonnel S. Detached deltoid during arthroscopic subacromial decompression. *Arthroscopy* 2000;16:745–748.
23. Voloshin I, Gelinas J, Maloney MD, et al. The rotator cuff disease is associated with inflammatory mediators in the subacromial bursa. San Diego, CA: AOSSM Annual Meeting, 2003.
24. Gotoh M, Hamada K, Yamakawa H, et al. Increased substance P in subacromial bursa and shoulder pain in rotator cuff diseases. *J Orthop Res* 1998;16:618–621.
25. Caspari RB, Thal R. A technique for arthroscopic subacromial decompression. *Arthroscopy* 1992;8:23–30.
26. Burns TP, Turba JE. Arthroscopic treatment of shoulder impingement in athletes. *Am J Sports Med* 1992;20:13–16.
27. Levy HJ, Gardner RD, Lemak LJ. Arthroscopic subacromial decompression in the treatment of full-thickness rotator cuff tears. *Arthroscopy* 1991;7:8–13.
28. Olsewski JM, Depew AD. Arthroscopic subacromial decompression and rotator cuff debridement for stage II and stage III impingement. *Arthroscopy* 1994;10:61–68.
29. Barber FA. Coplaning of the acromioclavicular joint. *Arthroscopy* 2001;17:913–917.
30. Fischer BW, Gross RM, McCarthy JA, et al. Incidence of acromioclavicular joint complications after arthroscopic subacromial decompression. *Arthroscopy* 1999;15:241–248.
31. Kuster MS, Hales PF, Davis SJ. The effects of arthroscopic acromioplasty on the acromioclavicular joint. *J Shoulder Elbow Surg* 1998; 7:140–143.
32. Weber SC. Arthroscopic debridement and acromioplasty versus mini-open repair in the management of significant partial-thickness tears of the rotator cuff. *Orthop Clin North Am* 1997;28: 79–82.

33. Ogilvie-Harris DJ, Wiley AM. Arthroscopic surgery of the shoulder. A general appraisal. *J Bone Joint Surg Br* 1986;68:201–207.

34. Ellman H. Diagnosis and treatment of incomplete rotator cuff tears. *Clin Orthop* 1990;254:64–74.

35. Berg EE, Ciullo JV, Oglesby JW. Failure of arthroscopic decompression by subacromial heterotopic ossification causing recurrent impingement. *Arthroscopy* 1994;10:158–161.

36. Anderson K, Bowen MK. Spur reformation after arthroscopic acromioplasty. *Arthroscopy* 1999;15:788–791.

37. Levy O, Copeland SA. Regeneration of the coracoacromial ligament after acromioplasty and arthroscopic subacromial decompression. *J Shoulder Elbow Surg* 2001;10:317–320.

38. Boynton MD, Enders TJ. Severe heterotopic ossification after arthroscopic acromioplasty: A case report. *JSES* 1999;8:495–497.

39. Mormino MA, Gross RM, McCarthy JA. Captured shoulder: A complication of rotator cuff surgery. *Arthroscopy* 1996;12:457–461.

40. Warner JJ, Allen AA, Marks PH, et al. Arthroscopic release of postoperative capsular contracture of the shoulder. *J Bone Joint Surg Am* 1997;79:1151–1158.

41. Ryu RK. Arthroscopic subacromial decompression: a clinical review. *Arthroscopy* 1992;8:141–147.

42. Ogilvie-Harris DJ, D'Angelo G. Arthroscopic surgery of the shoulder. *Sports Med* 1990;9:120–128.

43. Bigliani LU, Nicholson GP, Flatow EL. Arthroscopic resection of the distal clavicle. *Orthop Clin North Am* 1993;24:133–141.

44. Flatow EL, Duralde XA, Nicholson GP, et al. Arthroscopic resection of the distal clavicle with a superior approach. *J Shoulder Elbow Surg* 1995;4(1 Pt 1):41–50.

45. Gartsman GM. Arthroscopic resection of the acromioclavicular joint. *Am J Sports Med* 1993;21:71–77.

46. Kay SP, Dragoo JL, Lee R. Long-term results of arthroscopic resection of the distal clavicle with concomitant subacromial decompression. *Arthroscopy* 2003;19:805–809.

47. Johnson LL. *Diagnostic and Surgical Arthroscopy.* St. Louis: CV Mosby, 1981.

48. Flatow EL, Cordasco FA, Bigliani LU. Arthroscopic resection of the outer end of the clavicle from a superior approach: a critical, quantitative, radiographic assessment of bone removal. *Arthroscopy* 1992;8:55–64.

49. Novak PJ, Bach BR Jr, Romeo AA, et al. Surgical resection of the distal clavicle. *J Shoulder Elbow Surg* 1995;4(1 Pt 1):35–40.

50. Esch JC, Ozerkis LR, Halgager JA, et al. Arthroscopic subacromial decompression: results according the degree of rotator cuff tear. *Arthroscopy* 1988;4:241–249.

51. Petersson CJ, Gentz CF: Ruptures of the supraspinatus tendon. The significance of distally pointing acromioclavicular osteophytes. *Clin Orthop* 1983;174:143–148.

52. Tolin BS, Snyder SJ. Our technique for the arthroscopic Mumford procedure. *Orthop Clin North Am* 1993;24:143–151.

53. Martin SD, Baumgarten TE, Andrews JR. Arthroscopic resection of the distal aspect of the clavicle with concomitant subacromial decompression. *J Bone Joint Surg Am* 2001;83A:328–335.

54. Levine WN, Barron OA, Yamaguchi K, et al. Arthroscopic distal clavicle resection from a bursal approach. *Arthroscopy* 1998;14:52–56.

55. Zawadsky M, Marra G, Wiater JM, et al. Osteolysis of the distal clavicle: long-term results of arthroscopic resection. *Arthroscopy* 2000;16:600–605.

56. Fukuda K, Craig EV, An KN, et al. Biomechanical study of the ligamentous system of the acromioclavicular joint. *J Bone Joint Surg Am* 1986;68:434–440.

57. Salter EG Jr, Nasca RJ, Shelley BS. Anatomical observations on the acromioclavicular joint and supporting ligaments. *Am J Sports Med* 1987;15:199–206.

58. Flatow EL. The biomechanics of the acromioclavicular, sternoclavicular, and scapulothoracic joints. *Instr Course Lect* 1993;42:237–245.

59. Fischer BW, Gross RM, McCarthy JA, et al. Incidence of acromioclavicular joint complications after arthroscopic subacromial decompression. *Arthroscopy* 1999;15:241–248.

60. Adolfsson L, Lysholm J, Nettelblad H. Adverse effects of extensive clavicular resections and a suggested method of reconstruction. *J Shoulder Elbow Surg* 1999;8:361–364.

61. Abbott LC, Lucas DB. The function of the clavicle: its surgical significance. *Ann Surg* 1954;140:583–599.

62. Rockwood CAJ, Young DC. Disorders of the acromioclavicular joint. In: Rockwood CAJ, Matsen FA, eds. *The Shoulder.* Philadelphia: WB Saunders, 1990:413–476.

63. Kennedy JC, Cameron H. Complete dislocation of the acromioclavicular joint. *J Bone Joint Surg Br* 1954;36B:202–208.

64. Renfree KJ, Riley MK, Wheeler D, et al. Ligamentous anatomy of the distal clavicle. *J Shoulder Elbow Surg* 2003;12:355–359.

65. Murthi AM, Moinfar A. Anatomy of the pectoralis minor tendon and its use in acromioclavicular joint reconstruction. Washington, DC: 9th International Congress on Surgery of the Shoulder and Elbow, 2004.

66. Tytherleigh–Strong G, Gill J, Sforza G, et al. Reossification and fusion across the acromioclavicular joint after arthroscopic acromioplasty and distal clavicle resection. *Arthroscopy* 2001;17:E36.

67. Berg EE, Ciullo JV. Heterotopic ossification after acromioplasty and distal clavicle resection. *J Shoulder Elbow Surg* 1995;4:188–193.

Complications of Thermal Capsulorrhaphy

15

Charles L. Getz   *Matthew L. Ramsey*
David Glaser   *Gerald R. Williams Jr.*

INTRODUCTION

Thermal energy has been used in the management of gleno-humeral instability to modify the structure of collagen. Applying the energy with a small probe makes thermal capsulorrhaphy a relatively easy technique to add to a shoulder arthroscopist's repertoire. In part, the ease of thermal capsulorrhaphy has resulted in its widespread use. However, application of heat in shoulder surgery has raised concerns about the potential complications that may occur. Risk to the axillary nerve, stiffness, capsular necrosis, and chondral injury have been reported as the major complications of thermal capsulorrhaphy. The following chapter will review the basic science of thermal modification of tissue, the indications and results for its use in shoulder surgery, and the major complications associated with thermal capsulorrhaphy.

BASIC SCIENCE

The most common structural protein contained within ligaments is type I collagen. Type I collagen is comprised of a triple-helix tropocollagen molecule composed of three polypeptide chains, each with unique repeating triple amino acid sequences (1,2). The individual polypeptide chains that combine to form the triple helix are bound together by crosslinking. Additional crosslinks between separate triple-helix tropocollagen molecules also occur. The crosslinking within and between the tropocollagen molecules is responsible for the tensile properties of collagen and maintains the highly organized structure.

When tissue containing type I collagen is heated to a temperatures above 65°C, the crosslinked bonds that stabilize the structures are dissolved (Fig. 15-1) (1,2). The "melting" of collagen transforms the previously organized structure into a gel by both uncoiling the triple helices and disrupting the crosslinks between the tropocollagen molecules. As the tissue cools, the individual chains are free to form new crosslinks, resulting in a less organized, smaller protein. Over time, the tissue is remodeled to a more normal state.

The ability to shrink collagen fibers has allowed thermal energy to be used as a possible tool to decrease the overall length of the individual capsular regions and the overall volume of the glenohumeral joint. Luke et al. were able to show that thermal energy, when applied to cadeveric specimens, reduced capsular volume but not to the same extent that can be achieved by open shift techniques (3). In a series of articles, Tibone, Lee, and colleagues demonstrated reduced glenohumeral translation in cadaveric shoulders following thermal shrinkage (4–9).

Thermal modification of type I collagen not only results in physical changes, but also in mechanical and biologic changes as well. The mechanical properties of strength and stiffness are both decreased as a result of thermal capsulor-

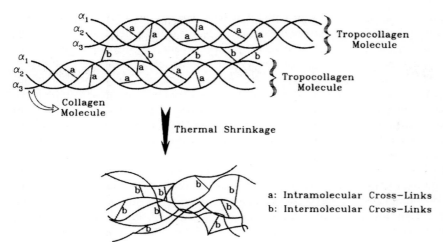

Figure 15-1 The structure of type I collagen is a highly organized triple-helix with a repeating amino-acid sequence. The structure is stabilized by polar bonds between the amino acid chains, as well as cross-linking within and between triple-helix units. When temperatures of 65°C are reached within polar bonds, crosslinking is broken. The previously highly organized structure reforms bonds in a random pattern with a smaller volume. (Reprinted from Arnoczky SP, Aksan A. Thermal modification of connective tissues: basic science considerations and clinical implications. *J Am Acad Orthop Surg* 2000;8:305–313, with permission.)

rhaphy. The decreases in strength and stiffness are directly proportional to the length change that has occurred during heat application (10–12). Following the thermal injury, the treated tissue must then undergo protracted tissue remodeling, requiring up to 3 months (in a rabbit model) before normal mechanical characteristics return (13). The biologic impact of thermal injury is primarily related to the effect of heat on cells within the capsular tissue. Cell death has been reported to occur at temperatures of greater than 45°C (14,15). Therefore, in tissue that has been thermally modified (heated to at least 65°C), cell death has certainly occurred and probably extends to a zone of injury adjacent to but not directly under the heat probe.

INDICATIONS AND RESULTS

Traumatic Unidirectional

Instability can be defined as increased rotational or translational motion associated with pain and disability. A common type of glenohumeral instability is unidirectional anterior instability. This instability pattern often results following a frank anterior dislocation of the shoulder and is secondary to an avulsion of the anterior glenoid rim (bony Bankart lesion), labrum (classic Bankart lesion), or humeral insertion of the anterior-inferior glenohumeral ligament (HAGL). Intracapsular stretch injury also contributes to traumatic unidirectional instability in patients who have had multiple dislocations or who have sustained an anterior dislocation in the presence of pre-existing multidirectional laxity. Therefore, surgery to address unidirectional anterior instability is aimed at restoring the premorbid anatomy (i.e., reattaching the capsule or labrum and addressing any pathologic capsular laxity). Open repair of the injured anterior shoulder restraints has a long proven track record with recurrence rates of less then 10% (16–19). Arthroscopic repair of the same structures has continued to

improve and results are now approaching those obtained in open reconstruction, especially when capsular stretch and capsular avulsion have been addressed. Gartsman has reported excellent results (92% success rate) for 53 patients with anterior instability arthroscopically treated with thermal capsulorrhaphy added to arthroscopic labral repair if increased translation exists after the labrum is repaired (20).

Atraumatic and Microtraumatic Instability

Atraumatic and microtraumatic instability may develop with repetitive use of the arm over months to years, not in a single event. Various regions of the joint capsule become attenuated and allow increased motion of the glenohumeral joint. The labrum, glenoid, and ligamentous insertions are typically normal. Neer (21) described an inferior capsular shift procedure that reduced the over all volume of the shoulder in patients with multidirectional instability patterns; his results were greater then 90% successful. Arthroscopic plication of the capsule to address capsular redundancy has also been described (22). All of these surgical techniques aim to restore normal function to the shoulder by reducing the length of the ligaments of the shoulder and therefore reducing the overall capsular volume.

Arthroscopic thermal modification of the collagen-rich glenohumeral capsule has also been described as a method of shortening capsular ligaments and reducing capsular volume (3). The ability to watch the tissues as they shorten provides the surgeon tactile feedback to assess the overall amount of volume contraction that is taking place. The procedure has been applied to a wide range of instability patterns with varied success.

Anterior Atraumatic Instability

Jobe (23) described an open anterior capsular reconstruction for primarily overhead athletes with anterior, microtraumatic instability in 1991. An open subcapularis sparing approach with plication of the anterior inferior glenohumeral ligament returned 17 of 25 overhand athletes to a high level of play (mainly professional baseball players) and resulted in 92% good or excellent results. In a similar group of patients, Levitz et al. (24) reported on the use of thermal capsulorrhaphy in 2001. Surgery was performed using arthroscopy with and without thermal capsulorrhaphy in this group of throwing athletes with presumed recurrent anterior microtraumatic subluxation. Patients with partial rotator cuff tears and/or superior labral tears were treated with arthroscopic debridement of the partial rotator cuff tear and debridement or repair of superior labral pathology. At an average of 30 months follow-up, a significant difference was noted between those patients who underwent thermal treatment and those who did not. In all, 90% of patients treated by thermal capsulorrhaphy were still throwing at follow-up as compared to 60% in the nonthermally treated group.

Enad et al. (25,26) have recently reported less favorable results for overhand athletes treated with selective thermal shrinkage. In one series, only 10 of 20 patients returned to their previous level of play (25). In the second series, 17% of patients required an open stabilization procedure following thermal capsulorrhaphy for continued instability (26).

Multidirectional Instability

As previously noted, Neer (21) has reported considerable success with an open shift to address multidirectional instability. Other surgeons have also noted success with open capsular shift techniques (27,28). Success with thermal capsulorrhaphy in the management of multidirectional instability has been quite variable. Reports by Fanton, Thabit, and Savoie have been favorable (29–31). Gartsman combined thermal capsulorrhaphy with other techniques to successfully treat patients with bidirectional instability (32). However, the literature also has reports of less favorable results from Anderson, Fitzgerald, Levy, Frostick, Noonan, Miniaci, and D'Alessandro (33–39).

In an attempt to define patients that may be more likely to have early recurrent instability after undergoing thermal capsulorrhaphy, Anderson et al. (40) reviewed the results of 106 patients all with at least 6 months of follow-up. The study found a significantly higher failure rate among patients with a history of more than two dislocations or prior surgery. Other factors reviewed such as contact sports, multidirectional instability, and other procedures performed concurrent with the thermal capsulorrhaphy did not result in significantly higher rates of failure.

COMPLICATIONS

Axillary Nerve Injury

Several authors have reported injury to the axillary nerve after thermal shrinkage. Greis (41) reported a case series of four patients with axillary nerve injury. Two had pure sensory disturbances, whereas the others were mixed injuries. Miniaci (38) reported four patients with transient sensory disturbances in a series of 19 patients. One of the patients also had deltoid weakness. The neurologic symptoms were completely resolved by 9 months in all patients. D'allessandro (39) reported 12 patients (out of 84) who experienced temporary axillary nerve dysesthesias. Fortunately, all symptoms related to nerve irritation resolved by 3 months.

In an attempt to gauge the rate and variety of axillary nerve injuries, Wong and Williams (42) surveyed 379 surgeons who had performed 14,277 thermal capsulorrhaphy procedures over a 5-year period. Response to the survey found 196 cases of axillary nerve injury (1.4%) (Fig. 15-2).

Gryler (44) evaluated the temperatures along the axillary nerve in a cadaver model during thermal capsulorrhaphy. In two of nine specimens, axillary nerve temperature exceeded 65°C, and in seven specimens the temperature was above 45°C. McCarty (45) reported similar results and was unable to decrease temperatures along the nerve with arm abduction during heat application.

Several techniques have been proposed to reduce the risk of nerve injury. These include avoiding the axillary pouch completely, reducing the power on the heat probe in the axillary pouch, and reducing the application pressure and time at the tip of the probe. Avoiding the pouch would prevent treatment of patients with pathologic laxity of the axillary pouch. Reducing the power setting is a reasonable thought. However, whether or not that reduction would result in fewer nerve injuries is unknown. Moreover, the effect on efficiency of shrinkage is also unknown. Finally decreasing the application pressure or time of application, although logical, may also decrease the efficiency of shrinkage (29).

Nerve monitoring during thermal capsulorrhaphy can provide real time feedback on the function of the nerve and may be able to detect irritation of the nerve prior to frank injury (46). Nerve monitoring does require advance planning, additional setup time, availability of qualified neurophysiologists, changes in anesthesia technique (no blocks or inhaled agents), and additional cost. These factors have limited nerve monitoring from becoming more widely accepted.

Author's Preferred Treatment of Axillary Nerve Injuries

Nerve injury following thermal capsulorrhaphy may present in one of four scenarios or types. Type I is a sensory disturbance that produces dysasthesias about the shoulder. Type II is a mixed sensory and motor disturbance with partial retention of deltoid function. Type III injury is complete motor and sensory loss. Type IV is a nerve injury induced

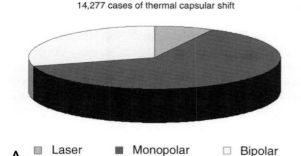

14,277 cases of thermal capsular shift

A ▣ Laser ■ Monopolar ☐ Bipolar

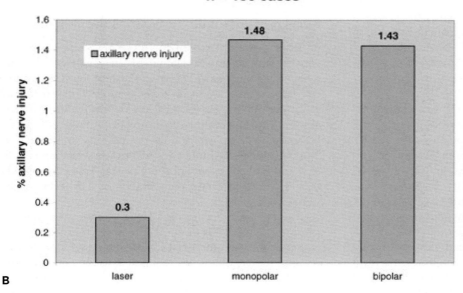

**Percentage of patients with axillary neuropathy
n = 196 cases**

B

Figure 15-2 A: The breakdown by type of heat application used to perform thermal capsulorrhaphy for 14,273 procedures. **B:** The rate of axillary nerve injury as reported for monopolar, bipolar, and laser procedures. The average length of recovery of axillary nerve injury reported by type of nerve injury. (Reprinted from Wong KL, Williams GR. Complications of thermal capsulorrhaphy of the shoulder. *J Bone Joint Surg Am* 2001;83(Suppl 2 Pt 2):151–155, with permission.)

complex regional pain syndrome (i.e., reflex sympathetic dystrophy) (Table 15-1).

Type I nerve injuries manifest mild to moderate pain about the shoulder. Cutaneous sensation over the lateral deltoid is abnormal, with patients commonly describing a tingling sensation when lightly touched. They will also describe burning pain similar to the pain felt with sunburn. Type II nerve injuries have similar sensory disturbances with the addition of deltoid weakness. The use of an electromyelogram (EMG) can confirm the diagnosis of axillary nerve injury and will serve as a baseline for comparison during recovery. The treatment of patients with Type I and

TABLE 15-1

CLASSIFICATION OF THERMAL CAPSULLORRHAPHY NERVE INJURY

Type	Clinical Features	Management	Prognosis
I	Sensory disturbance	Observation with or without gabapentin or amitriptyline	Good
II	Sensory disturbance with partial motor loss	Observation with or without gabapetin or amitriptyline; EMG at 6 weeks postop to confirm diagnosis	Variable
III	Complete sensory and motor deficit	EMG, if no recovery at 3 months consider exploration and nerve grafting	Poor
IV	Reflex sympathetic dystrophy	Multidisciplinary approach—physical therapy, medications, injection	Poor

II nerve injuries is mainly expectant. Occasionally, the use of gabapentin or amitriptyline may be required to manage nerve-related pain.

Type III nerve injuries represent a profound change in nerve physiology. A flaccid deltoid that does not have motor function is the hallmark finding. Sensory disturbance is variable because of overlap of cutaneous innervation about the lateral deltoid. Pain is nearly always moderate to severe in the first few weeks to months following surgery. An initial EMG is performed within 6 weeks of surgery to characterize the extent of injury. A repeat EMG at 3 months postoperatively will hopefully show signs of early reinnervation. If signs of reinervation are present, then the treatment is the same as type I and II injuries. An EMG that has no signs of reinnervation at 3 months is worrisome. At this point, discussion with the patient concerning possible nerve grafting is warranted. If no clinical or EMG evidence of nerve recovery is noted by 4 to 6 months postoperatively, referral to a surgeon specializing in nerve-grafting procedures is requested.

Type IV nerve injuries present as a complex regional pain syndrome (i.e., reflex sympathetic dystrophy). Any of the other types of nerve injuries may degenerate into a type IV injury. Patients' initial complaints of intense shoulder pain may spread to the rest of the upper extremity and, rarely, other extremities. Cutaneous sensitivity is markedly increased and the skin may appear mottled. Complaints of temperature changes in the hand and hyperhydrosis signal vasomotor instability. Examination is limited because of the pain. Treatment of complex regional pain syndromes is very difficult and is carried out in conjunction with a multidisciplinary team potentially consisting of pain management specialists, psychiatrists, psychologists, specialized physical and occupation therapists, and practitioners of alternative medicine techniques such as acupuncture. Physical therapy, desensitization techniques, medications

such as gabapentin and amitriptyline, and stellate ganglion blocks may be used alone or in combination.

The best treatment of axillary nerve injury is prevention. Although avoiding the axillary pouch, turning down the application power, and minimizing application pressure and time may be helpful, their efficacy is unknown. Intraoperative nerve monitoring has been shown to identify the course of the axillary nerve and prevent injury (46). The technique involves placement of cutaneous brachial plexus leads on the neck and peripheral leads into the deltoid (Fig. 15-3). Continuous transspinal motor evoked potentials and electromyography can then be monitored for disturbance in their normal activity.

Recurrent Instability and Capsular Necrosis

Recurrent instability following thermal capsulorrhaphy is variable and diagnosis-dependent. In general, the recurrence rates in more subtle forms of instability, such as anterior subluxation, are lower than in more global forms of instability. The causes for recurrent instability are also variable and include reinjury, incomplete correction of capsular laxity, recurrent capsular laxity, and capsular deficiency. The pathology encountered at revision may be amenable to traditional open and arthroscopic stabilization methods or may require capsular augmentation or substitution techniques.

The incidence of capsular deficiency following thermal capsulorraphy (43) is unknown. However, several authors have documented the need for capsular augmentation in revision surgery. Rath (47) reported a case of a catastrophic capsular disruption following thermal capsulorrhaphy for posterior instability. Not only were the treated tissues necrosed, but extensive damage of surrounding tissue was also found. Jensen (48) presented the findings of 11 patients who underwent open revision following thermal capsulor-

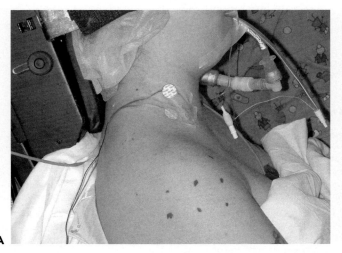
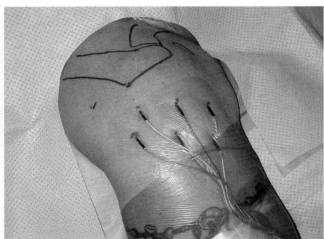

A   **B**

Figure 15-3 Nerve monitoring setup includes placement of transcutaneous pads used to stimulate the brachial plexus **(A)** and peripheral leads used to record axillary nerve function **(B)**.

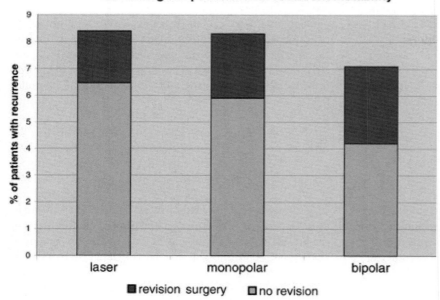

Figure 15-4 Recurrent instability rates for patients undergoing 14,273 thermal capsulorrhaphy procedures broken down into type of heat application. (Reprinted from Wong KL, Williams GR. Complications of thermal capsulorrhaphy of the shoulder. *J Bone Joint Surg Am* 2001; 83(Suppl 2 Pt 2):151–155, with permission.)

rhaphy. Two patients had frank necrosis of the capsule and six others had thin friable tissue for the capsule. Wong and Williams (42) surveyed surgeons with an aggregate total of 14,273 thermal capsulorrhaphy procedures. Ultimately, 363 patients underwent revision surgery for recurrent instability (Fig. 15-4). At the time of revision surgery, capsular attenuation was found in 33%, 18%, and 20% of patients who had previously undergone laser, monopolar, and bipolar shrinkage, respectively. Seven patients required tissue augmentation.

Application of heat in a striped pattern may spare cells in untreated areas to facilitate remodeling and prevent frank necrosis (Fig. 15-5). However, adjacent tissues can some-

times reach temperatures high enough to result in cell death despite not undergoing direct heat application. The concept of capsular striping has been advocated as a means of reducing the risk of capsular necrosis, but to date no studies have examined this technique's effectiveness. Despite lacking supporting data, striping techniques seem to be logical alternatives to decrease the overall cell death and prevent capsular necrosis.

Author's Preferred Treatment for Recurrent Instability

Evaluation of patients with recurrent instability following thermal capsulorrhaphy is really no different from evaluation of other patients with instability. The primary evaluation tools are history and physical examination, which are supplemented with plain radiography and magnetic resonance arthrography. The primary difference between patients with recurrent instability following prior thermal treatment and those who have not had any thermal modification is the possibility of capsular insufficiency. It is not always possible to identify the presence of capsular deficiency preoperatively. However, with careful evaluation, significant capsular deficiency can be suspected.

Important historical features to identify include presence or absence of a traumatic event or documented dislocation, any change in frequency or severity of instability episodes since the thermal treatment, the nature of the current complaints (i.e., pain or instability), and the types of concomitant procedures performed at the time of thermal treatment. If a significant traumatic event or recurrent dislocation requiring reduction is identified, it is possible that a labral avulsion is present. It is unlikely that the labrum could have been avulsed with severe capsular deficiency.

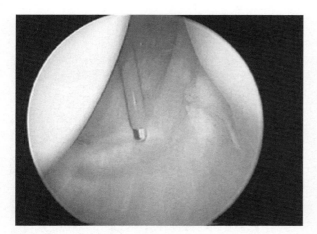

Figure 15-5 Capsular striping technique leaves areas of the capsule untreated to provide cells to repopulate the heat-treated areas of the capsule. Striping technique may lessen the chance of capsular necrosis from developing. (Reprinted from D'Alessandro DF, Bradley JP, Fleischli JE, et al. Prospective evaluation of thermal capsulorrhaphy for shoulder instability: indications and results, two- to five-year follow-up. *Am J Sports Med* 2004;32:21–33, with permission.)

Therefore, under these circumstances, standard open or arthroscopic techniques may be used. Conversely, if the patient has recognized recurrent instability episodes with little or no trauma, especially if the frequency and severity of these episodes is greater than before the thermal treatment, capsular deficiency is more likely.

A myriad of physical findings has been described for the diagnosis of glenohumeral instability. A complete discussion of all of these physical findings and diagnostic techniques is beyond the scope of this chapter. However, certain findings may suggest the presence of capsular deficiency and deserve emphasis. Changes in humeral head translation in the awake patient with recurrent instability can be difficult to quantify. However, changes in passive rotation in specific arm positions can be a proxy for increased length or deficiency of various capsular regions. For example, increased passive external rotation with the arm at the side (in the presence of a negative abdominal compression test) is indicative of rotator interval capsular laxity, increased passive external rotation with the arm at 90 degrees of scapular plane elevation is indicative of laxity or deficiency of the anterior portion of the inferior glenohumeral ligament, and increased passive internal rotation with the arm at 90 degrees of scapular plane elevation is indicative of deficiency or laxity of the posterior portion of the inferior glenohumeral ligament. When increased passive rotation is identified, the possibility of capsular deficiency should at least be entertained.

Plain radiography is primarily helpful in determining whether bone deficiencies exist that might affect the results of revision instability surgery. The presence of large humeral (2 cm) or glenoid (1 cm) defects may indicate the need for bone grafts. Although the amount of bone deficiency requiring grafting has not yet been determined, the indications are no different in patients who have failed

thermal procedures than in those who have failed other stabilization procedures.

Magnetic resonance arthrography can be a helpful diagnostic tool in the evaluation of recurrent instability following thermal capsulorrhaphy, especially when capsular deficiency is suspected. It is critical that gadolinium is injected directly into the joint and not extra-articularly. If, under these circumstances, dye is visualized outside the glenohumeral joint capsule, capsular deficiency is a virtual certainty. Even in the absence of a frank defect in the capsule, the presence of dye in the joint may allow the identification of very thin areas of the capsule and some estimation of the quality of the remaining capsule (Fig. 15-6).

When a decision has been made to perform revision surgery for recurrent instability following prior thermal treatment, several principles may help to guide treatment. First, diagnostic arthroscopy may provide a better assessment of the degree and location of capsular deficiency than open visualization. Second, minor amounts of capsular deficiency may be addressed arthroscopically through capsular plication techniques. Third, when major capsular deficiency exists, capsular substitution or replacement techniques are required.

Examination under anesthesia is used to confirm any differences in translation and rotation between the operative side and the normal side. Diagnostic arthroscopy is performed in either the beach chair or lateral decubitus position. In our practice, the beach chair position is preferred, especially in this situation because open capsular reconstruction may be required. If small localized areas of capsular deficiency are identified, they are repaired using arthroscopic suture plication techniques. This technique is especially good if the area of capsular deficiency is close enough to the glenoid so that the intact capsule can be anchored to the labrum or the glenoid rim (Fig. 15-7). If

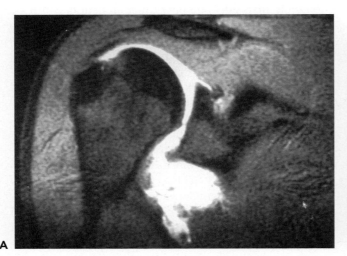
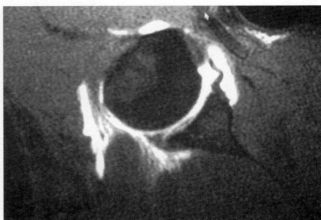

A   **B**

Figure 15-6 A: An magnetic resonance arthrogram of a patient with recurrent instability after thermal capsulorrhaphy displays excessive pooling of contrast below the glenoid on the sagital views. B: The thinned attenuated capsule on axial cuts.

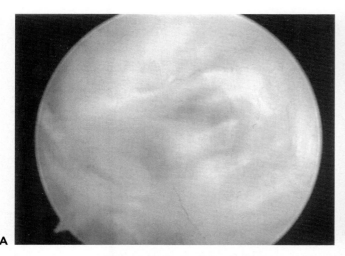
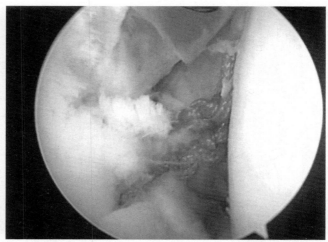

A   B

Figure 15-7 **A:** Arthroscopic pictures obtained in a patient with capsular deficiency following arthroscopic thermal capsulorrhaphy. **B:** The area was able to be plicated and anchored to the labrum to close the defect.

the capsular deficiency is too extensive to address arthroscopically, open reconstruction is indicated. The decision to convert to an open procedure should be made as early as possible in the arthroscopic portion of the procedure, so as not to compromise the open procedure because of massive amounts of soft-tissue swelling.

An anterior axillary incision is made and the subscapularis is exposed through a standard deltopectoral approach. Because of the potential need for a capsular allograft and the probability that at least some portion of the axillary pouch will be involved, the capsule is exposed by reflecting the upper two-thirds of the subscapularis rather than by splitting it. Once the upper two-thirds of the subscapularis has been reflected, any capsular deficiency will be obvious. If possible, the capsule can be incised in such a way as to incorporate areas of deficiency. During subsequent closure, the intact capsular layers can be closed, thereby excluding the areas of deficiency. Alternatively, if the capsular deficiency is so extensive that this type of plication would cause too much motion loss, allograft capsular reconstruction will be required.

Although many types of allograft reconstruction are possible, we prefer an iliotibial band allograft (49). With care, the remaining native capsule can be identified. This usually consists of at least the midportion of the axillary recess and the rotator interval capsule. In order to reconstruct the deficient portion of the capsule, a 6 × 15 cm iliotibial band allograft is folded on itself twice along the long axis. This creates a three-ply layer of iliotibial band that is approximately 2 cm in width and 15 cm in length. How much of the graft is used depends on how much of the capsule is deficient. In most cases, the capsule requires reconstruction from the anterior edge of the rotator interval capsule or supraspinatus to some portion of the axillary recess.

The graft is first attached to the glenoid rim at the ante-

rior edge of the biceps origin with two suture anchors. It is then brought over to the humerus and fixed to the upper portion of the anterior edge of the bicipital groove using two suture anchors (Fig. 15-8). The lateral sutures are tied with the arm in 5 to 10 degrees of abduction and neutral rotation. If the biceps was dislocated and can be reduced, it can be preserved if there is no tendency toward redislocation and it is structurally sound. Otherwise a biceps tenodesis is performed.

The graft is then folded back on itself and secured to the anterior glenoid rim with two suture anchors. The location of this second glenoid attachment site is inferior to the first so that the inferior edge of the superior portion of the graft approximates the superior border of the inferior portion of the graft. The second portion of the graft should be secured to the glenoid with the arm in slightly more abduction (20 to 30 degrees) and slightly more external rotation (10 to 15 degrees). If the remaining portion of the inferior native capsule is close enough to the inferior edge of the graft, the two structures should be sewn together and the excess graft excised. If, however, there is still a significant gap between the native capsule and the graft, the graft should be folded on itself again and attached to the humerus with suture anchors. This provides a Z-shaped graft. The edges of the graft should be sewn together, as should the most inferior portion of the graft and the remaining inferior native capsule (Fig. 15-9). Fortunately, in these cases, the subscapularis is normal and can be anatomically repaired without difficulty.

Postoperative rehabilitation is slower than in primary cases, regardless of whether or not an open capsular reconstruction has been required. A sling is maintained for 10 days to 2 weeks. The shoulder is examined at that point. If external rotation is greater than 30 degrees with the arm at the side, pendulum exercises only are started. Passive

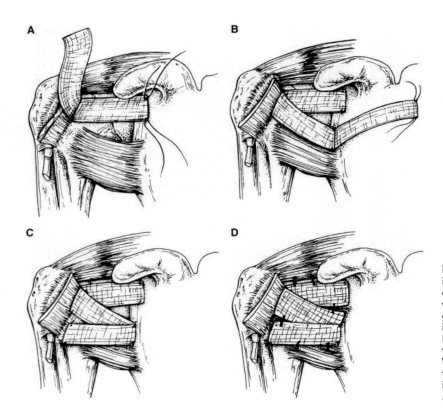

Figure 15-8 A: The graft is sewn into the glenoid in a superior location and attached the the medial edge of the bicepital groove. **B:** The graft is then weaved back and secured more inferiorly onto the glenoid with two more suture anchors. **C:** The graft is folded over to form a Z-shaped reconstruction. **D:** Remaining capsule is sutured to the graft to reinforce the repair. (Reprinted from Iannotti JP, Antoniou J, Williams GR, et al. Iliotibial band reconstruction for treatment of glenohumeral instability associated with irreparable capsular deficiency. *J Shoulder Elbow Surg* 2002;11:618–623, with permission.)

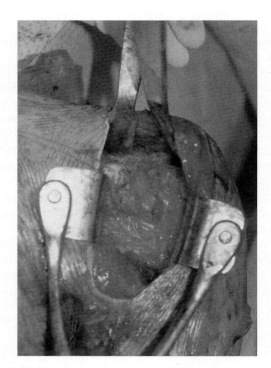

Figure 15-9 The Z-shaped reconstruction of the anterior capsule recreates the deficient anterior ligamentous structures. (Reprinted from Iannotti JP, Antoniou J, Williams GR, et al. Iliotibial band reconstruction for treatment of glenohumeral instability associated with irreparable capsular deficiency. *J Shoulder Elbow Surg* 2002;11: 618–623, with permission.)

external rotation and flexion are added at 4 to 6 weeks postoperatively. If, at 10 days to 2 weeks postoperatively, external rotation is 30 degrees or less, passive flexion to 130 degrees and passive external rotation to not more than 45 degrees are instituted. Full passive motion, within the limits of pain, is started at 6 weeks postoperatively. Strengthening is instituted at 8 to 10 weeks postoperatively.

Stiffness

Several surgeons have reported the development of postoperative stiffness following thermal capsulorrhaphy. Miniaci (38) reported a 10% rate of occurrence, whereas Fanton (27) reported one incidence out of 54 patients. Wong and Williams (42) found 41 cases developing in 14,277 thermal shoulder procedures.

Stiffness can be the result of the procedure itself or the amount of postoperative immobilization. Care should be taken to shrink only those areas of the capsule associated with symptoms. In addition, thermally treated tissue can take several months to obtain the normal tissue strengths. Therefore, some immobilization and protection are required. Serial examinations of joint range of motion should occur in the early postoperative period to identify those patients developing stiffness. The amount of passive mobilization can then be adjusted accordingly.

Author's Preferred Treatment of Stiffness

The patient who develops stiffness postoperatively typically has a painful synovitis in the weeks following surgery.

Gently externally rotating the arm while at the side of the body should produce minimal pain after the first postoperative week. Patients who develop synovitis will find the end range-of-motion extremely painful.

Synovitis in the first month following surgery is often greatly relieved with an intra-articular steroid injection. However, infection can also look very similar to aseptic synovitis. Therefore, infection should be excluded prior to considering an injection. The timing of passive stretching exercises can be difficult. Because of the known tendency of thermally treated tissues to stretch out in the early postoperative period, it is often delayed until 6 weeks postoperatively. However, if passive external rotation is less than 30 degrees at 3 weeks postoperatively, passive stretching exercises are instituted at that time.

Consideration for manipulation under anesthesia or arthroscopic capsular release is not considered until at least 3 months postoperatively. We prefer controlled arthroscopic release over manipulation under anesthesia alone. This is performed at 3 months postoperatively in only the most severe cases (i.e., external rotation of 0 degrees and flexion less than 90 degrees), otherwise it is reserved until 6 months postoperatively. The technique of arthroscopic release is no different than what has been described elsewhere (50,51), except that additional care must be taken to protect the axillary nerve. Because of the prior thermal trauma and scarring in the axillary recess, the nerve may be tethered to the inferior capsule.

Chondral Injury

The potential for chondral injuries exists either by directly applying heat to the articular surface or through heating of the fluid within the joint. Petty et al. (52) reported a case series of three patients who developed chodrolysis after shoulder arthroscopy. One patient had undergone a thermal capsulorrhaphy and another an extensive synovectomy utilizing heat within the joint. Burkhead et al. (53) recently reported severe chondrolysis in five shoulders of patients who had undergone an arthroscopic procedure that included thermal treatment and hypothesized that increased temperature of the arthroscopic fluid or direct thermal energy may have propagated through the capsule to the joint surface and resulted in cell death. The authors reviewed video of the surgeries in an attempt to identify another source for the joint injury but could not identify one. Avoidance of direct application of heat to the articular surface as well as assessing the temperature of the arthroscopy fluid as it exits through portals could potentially reduce the risk of chondrolysis. It should be noted, however, that no conclusive evidence linking the use of thermal capsular shrinkage to progressive chondrolysis has been established.

Author's Preferred Treatment of Chondral Injuries

The treatment options for chondolysis are limited. If joint stiffness has occurred in conjunction with the cartilage injury, then arthroscopic capsular release may result in improved motion, decreased joint contact forces, and improved pain. If the chondral damage is localized, arthroscopic debridement and microfracture arthroplasty may provide symptom improvement. The use of cartilage transplantation—either autologous or allograft—has been sparsely used in the shoulder. However, this patient population is typically young and not well suited for joint replacement. Therefore, an attempt at cartilage transplantation in localized defects may be warranted. Interpositional arthroplasty using the anterior capsule or an allograft substitute in cases of capsular deficiency is another potential joint sparing technique in these young, unfortunate patients.

When the chondral damage is extensive, especially when it involves both sides of the joint, joint sparing techniques may not be possible. Under these circumstances, traditional total shoulder arthroplasty, hemiarthroplasty, hemiarthroplasty combined with soft-tissue interposition, and arthrodesis are considered.

CONCLUSION

Thermal capsulorrhaphy is one method of reducing pathologic capsular laxity and decreasing capsular volume. Its ease of application and potential for low morbidity are its greatest draw. However, the real potential for axillary nerve injury, reported high recurrence rates in some series of multidirectional patients, and the development and refinement of arthroscopic suture plication techniques have led to the apparent decrease in popularity of thermal capsulorraphy. Intraoperative nerve monitoring is a successful method for decreasing the risk of nerve injury to very low levels. Unfortunately, it remains expensive and only available in a few centers. Further work is necessary to determine safe and effective practices for thermal capsulorraphy if it is to remain a viable treatment for glenohumeral instability—alone or in combination with other treatment methods.

REFERENCES

1. Arnoczky SP, Aksan A. Thermal modification of connective tissues: basic science considerations and clinical implications. *J Am Acad Orthop Surg* 2000;8:305–313.
2. Arnoczky SP, Aksan A. Thermal modification of connective tissues: basic science considerations and clinical implications. *Instr Course Lect* 2001;50:3–11.
3. Luke TA, Rovner AD, Karas SG, et al. Volumetric change in the shoulder capsule after open inferior capsular shift versus arthroscopic thermal capsular shrinkage: a cadaveric model. *J Shoulder Elbow Surg* 2004;13:146–149.
4. Tibone JE, McMahon PJ, Shrader TA, et al. Glenohumeral joint translation after arthroscopic, nonablative, thermal capsuloplasty with a laser. *Am J Sports Med* 1998;26:495–498.
5. Tibone JE, Lee TQ, Black AD, et al. Glenohumeral translation after arthroscopic thermal capsuloplasty with a radiofrequency probe. *J Shoulder Elbow Surg* 2000;9:514–518.

6. Tibone JE, Lee TQ, Csintalan RP, et al. Quantitative assessment of glenohumeral translation. *Clin Orthop* 2002:93–97.

7. Selecky MT, Vangsness CT Jr, Liao WL, et al. The effects of laser-induced collagen shortening on the biomechanical properties of the inferior glenohumeral ligament complex. *Am J Sports Med* 1999;27:168–172.

8. Selecky MT, Tibone JE, Yang BY, et al. Glenohumeral joint translation after arthroscopic thermal capsuloplasty of the posterior capsule. *J Shoulder Elbow Surg* 2003;12:242–246.

9. Selecky MT, Tibone JE, Yang BY, et al. Glenohumeral joint translation after arthroscopic thermal capsuloplasty of the rotator interval. *J Shoulder Elbow Surg* 2003;12:139–143.

10. Hayashi K, Massa KL, Thabit G 3rd, et al. Histologic evaluation of the glenohumeral joint capsule after the laser-assisted capsular shift procedure for glenohumeral instability. *Am J Sports Med* 1999;27:162–167.

11. Vangsness CT Jr, Mitchell W 3rd, Nimni M, et al. Collagen shortening. An experimental approach with heat. *Clin Orthop* 1997;337:267–271.

12. Schaefer SL, Ciarelli MJ, Arnoczky SP, et al. Tissue shrinkage with the holmium:yttrium aluminum garnet laser. A postoperative assessment of tissue length, stiffness, and structure. *Am J Sports Med* 1997;25:841–848.

13. Sandusky MD, Schultz MM, McMahon PJ, et al. The effects of laser on joint capsular tissue: an in vivo rabbit study. *Trans Orthop Res Soc* 1999;24:366.

14. Peacock EE, Van Winkle W. *Wound Repair*, 2nd ed. Philadelphia: WB Saunders, 1976.

15. Boykin JV Jr, Molnar JA. Burn scar and skin equivalants. In: Cohen IK, Diegelmann RF, Lindblad WJ, eds. *Wound Healing: Biochemical and Clinical Aspects*. Philadelphia: WB Saunders, 1992:523–540.

16. Rowe CR, Patel D, Southmayd WW. The Bankart procedure: a long-term end-result study. *J Bone Joint Surg Am* 1978;60:1–16.

17. Magnusson L, Kartus J, Ejerhed L, et al. Revisiting the open Bankart experience: a four- to nine-year follow-up. *Am J Sports Med* 2002;30:778–782.

18. Pagnani MJ, Dome DC. Surgical treatment of traumatic anterior shoulder instability in american football players. *J Bone Joint Surg Am* 2002;84:711–715.

19. Wirth MA, Blatter G, Rockwood CA Jr. The capsular imbrication procedure for recurrent anterior instability of the shoulder. *J Bone Joint Surg Am* 1996;78:246–259.

20. Gartsman GM, Roddey TS, Hammerman SM. Arthroscopic treatment of anterior-inferior glenohumeral instability. Two to five-year follow-up. *J Bone Joint Surg Am* 2000;82:991–1003.

21. Neer CS 2nd, Foster CR. Inferior capsular shift for involuntary inferior and multidirectional instability of the shoulder. A preliminary report. *J Bone Joint Surg Am* 1980;62:897–908.

22. Duncan R, Savoie FH 3rd. Arthroscopic inferior capsular shift for multidirectional instability of the shoulder: a preliminary report. *Arthroscopy* 1993;9:24–27.

23. Jobe FW, Giangarra CE, Kvitne RS, et al. Anterior capsulolabral reconstruction of the shoulder in athletes in overhand sports. *Am J Sports Med* 1991;19:428–434.

24. Levitz CL, Dugas J, Andrews JR. The use of arthroscopic thermal capsulorrhaphy to treat internal impingement in baseball players. *Arthroscopy* 2001;17:573–577.

25. Enad JG, ElAttrache NS, Tibone JE, et al. Isolated electrothermal capsulorrhaphy in overhand athletes. *J Shoulder Elbow Surg* 2004;13:133–137.

26. Enad JG, Kharrazi FD, ElAttrache NS, et al. Electrothermal capsulorrhaphy in glenohumeral instability without Bankart tear. *Arthroscopy* 2003;19:740–745.

27. Cooper RA, Brems JJ. The inferior capsular-shift procedure for multidirectional instability of the shoulder. *J Bone Joint Surg Am* 1992;74:1516–1521.

28. Altchek DW, Warren RF, Skyhar MJ, et al. T-plasty modification of the Bankart procedure for multidirectional instability of the anterior and inferior types. *J Bone Joint Surg Am* 1991;73:105–112.

29. Fanton GS. Arthroscopic electrothermal surgery of the shoulder. *Oper Tech in Sports Med* 1998;6:139–146.

30. Thabit G 3rd. The arthroscopically assisted holmium: YAG laser surgery in the shoulder. *Oper Tech in Sports Med* 1998;6:131–138.

31. Savoie FH 3rd, Field LD. Thermal versus suture treatment of symptomatic capsular laxity. *Clin Sports Med* 2000;19:63–75.

32. Gartsman GM, Roddey TS, Hammerman SM. Arthroscopic treatment of bidirectional glenohumeral instability: two- to five-year follow-up. *J Shoulder Elbow Surg* 2001;10:28–36.

33. Anderson SP, McCarty EC, Warren RF. Thermal capsulorrhaphy: where are we now? *Sports Med Arthr Rev* 1999;7:117–127.

34. Fitzgerald BT, Watson BT, Lapoint JM. The use of thermal capsulorrhaphy in the treatment of multidirectional instability. *J Shoulder Elbow Surg* 2002;11:108–113.

35. Levy O, Wilson M, Williams H, et al. Thermal capsular shrinkage for shoulder instability. Mid-term longitudinal outcome study. *J Bone Joint Surg Br* 2001;83:640–645.

36. Frostick SP, Sinopidis C, Al Maskari S, et al. Arthroscopic capsular shrinkage of the shoulder for the treatment of patients with multidirectional instability: minimum 2-year follow-up. *Arthroscopy* 2003;19:227–233.

37. Noonan TJ, Tokish JM, Briggs KK, et al. Laser-assisted thermal capsulorrhaphy. *Arthroscopy* 2003;19:815–819.

38. Miniaci A, McBirnie J. Thermal capsular shrinkage for treatment of multidirectional instability of the shoulder. *J Bone Joint Surg Am* 2003;85:2283–2287.

39. D'Alessandro DF, Bradley JP, Fleischli JE, et al. Prospective evaluation of thermal capsulorrhaphy for shoulder instability: indications and results, two- to five-year follow-up. *Am J Sports Med* 2004;32:21–33.

40. Anderson K, Warren RF, Altchek DW, et al. Risk factors for early failure after thermal capsulorrhaphy. *Am J Sports Med* 2002;30:103–107.

41. Greis PE, Burks RT, Schickendantz MS, et al. Axillary nerve injury after thermal capsular shrinkage of the shoulder. *J Shoulder Elbow Surg* 2001;10:231–235.

42. Wong KL, Williams GR. Complications of thermal capsulorrhaphy of the shoulder. *J Bone Joint Surg Am* 2001;83(Suppl 2 Pt 2):151–155.

43. Lephart SM, Myers JB, Bradley JP, et al. Shoulder proprioception and function following thermal capsulorraphy. *Arthroscopy* 2002;18:770–778.

44. Gryler EC, Greis PE, Burks RT, et al. Axillary nerve temperatures during radiofrequency capsulorrhaphy of the shoulder. *Arthroscopy* 2001;17:567–572.

45. McCarty EC, Warren RF, Deng XH, et al. Temperature along the axillary nerve during radiofrequency-induced thermal capsular shrinkage. *Am J Sports Med* 2004;32:909–914.

46. Esmail A, DeLong WG, Ramsey ML. Axillary nerve monitoring during monopolar radiofrequency thermal capsulorrhaphy of the shoulder. Washington, DC: Arthroscopy Association of North America, 2002.

47. Rath E, Richmond JC. Capsular disruption as a complication of thermal alteration of the glenohumeral capsule. *Arthroscopy* 2001;17(3):E10.

48. Jensen K. Management of complications associated with thermal capsulorrhaphy. Orlando, FL: ASES Open Meeting, 2000.

49. Iannotti JP, Antoniou J, Williams GR, et al. Iliotibial band reconstruction for treatment of glenohumeral instability associated with irreparable capsular deficiency. *J Shoulder Elbow Surg* 2002;11:618–623.

50. Holloway GB, Schenk T, Williams GR, et al. Arthroscopic capsular release for the treatment of refractory postoperative or post-fracture shoulder stiffness. *J Bone Joint Surg Am* 2001;83:1682–1687.

51. Warner JJ, Allen A, Marks PH, et al. Arthroscopic release for chronic, refractory adhesive capsulitis of the shoulder. *J Bone Joint Surg Am* 1996;78:1808–1816.

52. Petty DH, Jazrawi LM, Estrada LS, et al. Glenohumeral chondrolysis after shoulder arthroscopy: case reports and review of the literature. *Am J Sports Med* 2004;32:509–515.

53. Burkhead WZ, Krishnan SG, Ruark D. Focal osteonecrosis and severe chondrolysis following thermal capsulorrhaphy. San Francisco: AOSSM Specialty Day, 2004.

Index

A

AC joint. *See* Acromioclavicular joint
Acromial fracture, rotator cuff repair
    with, 39–40
Acromioclavicular joint (AC joint), 77
Acromioclavicular joint resection, 162,
    167–170, *168, 169*
  patient selection for, 167
  physiologic factors complicating, 170
  technical errors with, 167–170, *168,*
    169
Acromioclavicular joint surgery, 77–81
  anatomy for, 77
  complications of, 77–80, *78–80*
  pathology with, 77
  Rockwood's classification with, *78, 78*
  treatment with, 77
Adhesive capsulitis, 163
Adult Self-Expression Scale (ASES), 31
Allograft reconstruction, 179
ALPSA lesion. *See* Anterior labrum
    periosteal sleeve avulsion lesion
American Shoulder and Elbow Surgeons
    (ASES), 95
Anesthesia
  arthroscopic shoulder surgery, 126
  manipulation of frozen shoulder
    under, 100–103
Anterior-inferior labral tears, 3
Anterior labrum periosteal sleeve
    avulsion lesion (ALPSA lesion),
    133
Anterior shoulder instability, 3–12
  illustrative cases of, *8,* 8–12, *10, 11*
    arthrosis as, *8,* 8–9, *10*
    hardware-related, 11–12
    neurologic injury as, 11
    subscapularis tendon rupture as,
      9–11, *11*
  imaging of, 5, *5*
  neurologic injury with, 88
  nonanatomic repairs of, 4
  principles of, 3–4
  prior surgery failure with, 3
  recurrent, 4–5, *5*
  rehabilitation of, 12
  surgical options for, 5–7, *6, 7*
  surgical technique for, 51–52, *51–53*
  total shoulder arthroplasty with,
    50–52, *50–53*
Arthritis, 43, 80
Arthrofibrosis, 165
Arthrography, frozen shoulder in, 99
Arthroplasty. *See* Total shoulder
    arthroplasty

Arthroscopic capsular release, 106*t,* 107*t*
Arthroscopic distal clavicle resection,
    167
Arthroscopic shoulder surgery, 125–131,
    126–129
  AC joint resection using, 162,
    167–170, *168, 169*
    patient selection for, 167
    physiologic factors complicating,
      170
    technical errors with, 167–170, *168,*
      169
  anatomic structures at risk during, *128,*
    128–130, *129*
    axillary nerve as, *128,* 128–129
    musculocutaneous nerve as, 129,
      129
    suprascapular nerve as, 129
    variants in, 129–130
  anesthesia concerns for, 126
  draping for, 128
  extravasation with, 130
  implants/devices complications in,
    130
  infection with, 130
  patient positioning for, *126,* 126–128,
    127
    beach chair position in, 126, *126*
    hips/knees flexion in, 126, *127,*
      128
    lateral decubitus position in, 127,
      127
    neutral cervical spine position in,
      126, *127,* 128
  patient selection for, 125–126
  postoperative pain from, 130–131
  rotator cuff repair complications with,
    144–159, *145–150, 152–155,*
    157, 158
    intraoperative, 145–156, *146–150,*
      152–155
    neurological, 158–159
    postoperative, 156–158, *157, 158*
    preoperative, 144–145, *145*
    rates of, 159
    systemic, 159
Arthroscopic subacromial decompression
    (ASD), 162–167, *163–167,* 170
  diagnostic errors with, *163,* 163–164
  glenohumeral instability v., 163
  heterotopic ossification with, 165
  overview of, 162
  physiologic factors complicating,
    165–167, *166, 167*

technical errors with, *164,* 164–165,
    165
  worker's compensation benefit
    following, 167
Arthroscopy, 132–142
  arthrosis following, 136, 140–141
  frozen shoulder treatment with,
    103–105, *104, 105,* 106*t,* 107*t*
    postoperative treatment following,
      105
    results/complications from, 105,
      105, 106*t,* 107*t*
    technique of, 103–105, *104*
  hardware/implant-related
    complications following,
    136–138, 136–139, 141
  loss of motion without arthrosis
    following, 135–136, 140
  neurovascular injury following,
    139–140, 141
  recurrent instability following,
    132–135, *133–135,* 140
  repair revision following, 139
Arthrosis
  anterior shoulder instability with, *8,*
    8–9, *10*
  arthroscopy with, 136, 140–141
  posterior/multidirectional
    postoperative complications of,
    24–26, *25*
ASD. *See* Arthroscopic subacromial
    decompression
ASES. *See* Adult Self-Expression Scale;
    American Shoulder and Elbow
    Surgeons
Avascular necrosis, proximal humeral
    fracture with, 74
Axillary nerve injury
  arthroscopic shoulder surgery with,
    128, 128–129
  EMG for, 175, 175*t*
  preferred treatment of, 174–176, 175*t,*
    176
  prognosis for, 175*t*
  thermal capsulorrhaphy with,
    174–176, *175,* 175*t, 176*
Axonotmesis, 89, 90

B

Band-aid surgery, 125
Bankart lesion, 5, *7*
Bankart procedure, 3, 9
Beach chair position, arthroscopic
    shoulder surgery in, 126, *126*
Belly press test, 9, *11*
Bone grafting, 115, 163
Bone regrowth, 81

Bone scanning, frozen shoulder in, 99
Bony procedures, posterior/
    multidirectional instability treated
    with, 22–24, *23, 24,* 27–28
Brachial plexus, 91, *91*
Brisement. *See* Capsular distention
Bristow-Helfet procedure, 5
Bristow procedure, 4

C

Calcific tendonitis, 163
Capsular distention, frozen shoulder
    treatment with, 100–103
Capsular necrosis, thermal
    capsulorrhaphy with, 176–177,
    177
Capsular striping technique, *177*
Capsulotomy, 21, *21*
Captured shoulder, 165
Cervical radiculitis, 163
Cervical spine pathology, 18
Chondral injury, thermal capsulorrhaphy
    with, 181
Clavicle fracture management, *75,*
    75–76
Component loosening
    glenoid, *44,* 44–45, *45*
    humeral, 45, *45*
    surgical technique for, 46–48, *46–49*
Computed tomography (CT)
    anterior shoulder instability in, 5
    posterior/multidirectional instability,
    17–18, *18*
Controlled manipulation, frozen
    shoulder treatment with,
    103–105, *104, 105,* 106t, 107t
CT. *See* Computed tomography
Cybex testing, 81

D

DCR. *See* Distal clavicle resection
Deltoid injury
    rotator cuff repair with, *35,* 35–36
    total shoulder arthroplasty with, 66,
    66
Deltopectoral approach, 92
Diagnosis
    imaging in, 17–18, *18*
    laxity in, 17, *17*
    patient history in, 15
    physical exam in, 16
    posterior/multidirectional instability,
    15–19, *16–18*
    voluntary subluxation in, 16, *16*
Diphtheroids, 37
Distal clavicle resection (DCR), *80,*
    80–81, *81*
Distention arthrography. *See* Capsular
    distention
Donor nerve grafts, 92

E

Electromyelogram (EMG)
    anterior shoulder instability in, 5
    axillary nerve injury in, 175, 175t
    deltoid injury in, 36
    neurologic injury in, 85, 88, 90

EMG. *See* Electromyelogram
Extravasation, arthroscopic shoulder
    surgery with, 130

F

Fracture management, 70–76
    clavicle, *75,* 75–76
    hardware complications with, 73
    heterotopic ossification with, 73, *73*
    infection with, 70–71, *71*
    neurovascular injuries with, 71–72
    proximal humeral, *73,* 73–75, *74*
        avascular necrosis with, 74
        four-part, 74–75
        instability with, 75
        prosthesis-associated complications
        with, 75
        three-part, 73–74, *74*
        tuberosity failure with, 74–75
        two-part, *73,* 73
    stiffness with, *72,* 72–73
    wire breakage with, 73
Fractures, glenohumeral arthrodesis with,
    114
Frozen shoulder, 95–110
    classification of, 95, *96*
    clinical presentation of, 99
    defined, 95
    development of, 95, *96*
    epidemiology of, 95–96
    imaging of, 99
    laboratory studies on, 99
    natural history of, 99–100
    pathogenesis of, 96–97, 97t
    pathology of, 97–98
    patient history with, 99
    physical examination for, 99
    postsurgical stiffness as, 99
    secondary, 98
    staging of, 98
    treatment of, 100–110, *101, 102, 104,*
    105, 106t, 107t, *108, 109*
        arthroscopy in, 103–105, *104, 105,*
        106t, 107t
        capsular distention as, 100–103
        controlled manipulation as,
        103–105, *104, 105,* 106t, 107t
        management of complications with,
        108–109
        manipulation under anesthesia as,
        100–103
        open release as, 105–108, *108, 109*
        pain management as, 100
        physical therapy as, 100, *101*
        preferred approach to, 109–110

G

Glenohumeral arthrodesis, 113–119,
    115, 116
    complications with, 113–114
    fractures with, 114
    infection with, 114
    malposition with, 114–115
    nonunion with, 114
Glenohumeral instability, 163

Glenoid component instability, total
    shoulder arthroplasty with,
    48–50, *50*
Glenoid component loosening, total
    shoulder arthroplasty with, *44,*
    44–45, *45*
Gunslinger brace, 119, *119,* 120

H

HAGL. *See* Humeral avulsion of
    glenohumeral ligament
Heterotopic ossification (HO)
    arthroscopic subacromial
    decompression with, 165
    fracture management with, 73, *73*
    rotator cuff repair with, 37–38
Hill-Sachs lesion, 5, *5,* 6, 125
HO. *See* Heterotopic ossification
Horner's syndrome, 126
Humeral avulsion of glenohumeral
    ligament (HAGL), 133
Humeral component loosening, total
    shoulder arthroplasty with, 45, *45*
Humeroscapular arthrodesis, 113. *See also*
    Glenohumeral arthrodesis

I

Iatrogenic chondral damage, 129
Iliotibial band allograft, 179
Imaging. *See also* Magnetic resonance
    imaging (MRI)
    anterior shoulder instability in, 5, *5*
    diagnosis using, 17–18, *18*
    failed rotator cuff repair in, 33, 34
    frozen shoulder, 99
Impingement syndrome (IS), 162
Implants
    complications following arthroscopy
    with, *136–138,* 136–139, 141
    complications from, 130
    failure/dissociation, 65–66
    polydioxanone, 136
    polyglycolic acid, 130, 136
    polylactic acid, 130, 136
    total shoulder arthroplasty with, 46,
    65–66
Infection
    arthroscopic shoulder surgery with, 130
    arthroscopy rotator cuff repair with,
    158
    fracture management with, 70–71, *71*
    glenohumeral arthrodesis with, 114
    rotator cuff repair with, 36–37
    total shoulder arthroplasty with,
    63–65, *64*
    treatment technique for, *64,* 64–65
Inferior instability
    surgical technique for, 58–60, *59, 60*
    total shoulder arthroplasty with,
    57–60, *58–60*
Instability. *See also* Specific instability
    defined, 17, *17*
Intraoperative errors
    bony procedures in, 22–24, *23, 24*
    defined, 15
    patient positioning with, 19, 22
    posterior approach in, 19–22, *20, 21*

posterior/multidirectional instability, 19–24, *20, 21, 23, 24*
rotator cuff repair, 145–156, *146–150, 152–155*
  arthroscopic instruments with, *150,* 150–151, *152*
  arthroscopic knot tying with, 155–156
  bone preparation with, 149–150
  passage through tendon with, 154–155, *155*
  subacromial decompression with, 145–146, *146, 147*
  suture anchors with, 151–154, *153, 154*
  suture management with, 154–155, *155*
  tear morphology assessment with, 149, *150*
  tendon releases with, 146–149, *147–149*
Intraoperative fractures
  surgical technique for, 61
  total shoulder arthroplasty with, 60–61, *61*
IS. *See* Impingement syndrome

L
Labral tears, 3
Lateral decubitus position, arthroscopic shoulder surgery in, 127, *127*
Latarjet procedure, 5, 125
Laxity, 17, *17*

M
Magnetic resonance imaging (MRI)
  ALPSA lesion in, 133
  anterior shoulder instability in, 5
  arthroscopic subacromial decompression with, 165
  deltoid injury in, 36
  failed rotator cuff repair in, 33
  frozen shoulder in, 99
  neurologic injury in, 85
  posterior/multidirectional instability, 17
Magnuson-Stack procedure, 3, 4, 9
Malposition, glenohumeral arthrodesis with, 114–115
Manipulation under anesthesia, frozen shoulder treatment with, 100–103
MDI. *See* Multidirectional instability
MRI. *See* Magnetic resonance imaging
Multidirectional instability (MDI), 14–29
  arthroscopic techniques for, 15
  diagnosis of, 15–19, *16–18,* 28
  intraoperative errors with, 19–24, *20, 21, 23, 24*
    bony procedures in, 22–24, *23, 24*
    posterior approach in, 19–22, *20, 21*
  patient evaluation following failed repair of, 28
  postoperative complications with, 24–28, *25*
    arthrosis as, 24–26, *25*
    bony procedures, 27–28

coracoid impingement syndrome as, 27
  loss of motion as, 24–26, *25*
  new anterior instability as, 26–27
  recurrent instability as, 26–27
  preoperative errors with, 15–19, *16–18*
    incorrect diagnosis as, 15–19, *16–18*
    patient expectations in, 19
Musculocutaneous nerve, arthroscopic shoulder surgery with, 129, *129*

N
Nerve transfer (Neurotization), 92
Neurologic injury, 85–93, 163. *See also* Axillary nerve injury
  anterior shoulder instability from, 11, 88
  arthroscopic rotator cuff repair with, 158–159
  axonotmesis, 89, 90
  classification of, 89–90
  electrodiagnostic studies on, 90
  incidence of, 88–89
  musculocutaneous nerve and, 87, *87*
  neurapraxia, 89
  neurotmesis, 89
  operation safe zones for, 86
  overview of, 85–88, *86, 87*
  preoperative assessment of, 85
  prosthetic shoulder arthroplasty with, 89
  rotator cuff repair with, 88–89
  scapulothoracic arthrodesis complications as, 120–121
  Seddon and Sunderland classification of, 89
  suprascapular nerve and, *86,* 86–87, *87*
  surgical techniques for, 90–93, *91*
    brachial plexus in, 91, *91*
    clavicular osteotomy as, 92
    deltopectoral approach in, 92
    donor nerve grafts as, 92
    neurotization as, 92
    recovery from, 93
    shoulder fusion as, 92–93
  total shoulder arthroplasty with, 65, *65*
  treatment technique for, 65
  Wallerian degeneration, 90
Neurapraxia, 89
Neurotmesis, 89
Neurovascular injuries
  arthroscopy with, 139–140, *141*
  fracture management with, 71–72, 76
Nonanatomic repairs, anterior shoulder instability with, 4
Nonunion, glenohumeral arthrodesis with, 114

O
Open reduction and internal fixation (ORIF), 70, 80
Open release, frozen shoulder treatment with, 105–108, *108, 109*
Ophthalmoplegia, 126
ORIF. *See* Open reduction and internal fixation

Osteolysis, clavicle, 80, *80*
Osteotomy
  clavicular, 92
  humeral, 114–115
  humeral shaft, 46, *46*

P
Pain management, frozen shoulder treatment with, 100
Pancapsular arthroscopic capsular release, frozen shoulder treatment with, 107*t*
PDS implants. *See* Polydioxanone implants
Peel-back maneuver, 129
Peptostreptococcus magnus, 37
Periprosthetic fractures
  postoperative, *62,* 62–63, *63*
  surgical technique for, 62–63, *63*
  total shoulder arthroplasty with, 60, *62,* 62–63, *63*
PGA implants. *See* Polyglycolic acid implants
Physical therapy, frozen shoulder treatment with, 100, *101*
PLA implants. *See* Polylactic acid implants
Pneumomediastinum, 126
Pneumothorax, 120
Polydioxanone implants (PDS implants), 136
Polyglycolic acid implants (PGA implants), 130, 136
Polylactic acid implants (PLA implants), 130, 136
Posterior glenoid labral tears, 3
Posterior instability, 14–29
  arthroscopic techniques for, 15
  classification of, 14
  diagnosis of, 15–19, *16–18,* 28
  intraoperative errors with, 19–24, *20, 21, 23, 24*
    bony procedures in, 22–24, *23, 24*
    posterior approach in, 19–22, *20, 21*
  patient evaluation following failed repair of, 28
  postoperative complications with, 24–28, *25*
    arthrosis as, 24–26, *25*
    bony procedures, 27–28
    coracoid impingement syndrome as, 27
    loss of motion as, 24–26, *25*
    new anterior instability as, 26–27
    recurrent instability as, 26–27
  preoperative errors with, 15–19, *16–18*
    incorrect diagnosis as, 15–19, *16–18*
    patient expectations in, 19
  surgical technique for, *56,* 56–57, *57*
  total shoulder arthroplasty with, 55–57, *56, 57*
Preoperative errors
  defined, 15
  incorrect diagnosis as, 15–19, *16–18*
  patient expectations in, 19
  posterior/multidirectional instability, 15–19, *16–18*
  rotator cuff repair, 144–145, *145*

Propionibacter, 37
Prosthetic loosening, total shoulder
    arthroplasty with, 44, *44*
Prosthetic shoulder arthroplasty,
    neurologic injury with, 89
Proximal humeral fracture management,
    73, 73–75, *74*
  avascular necrosis with, 74
  four-part, 74–75
  instability with, 75
  prosthesis-associated complications
    with, 75
  three-part, 73–74, *74*
  tuberosity failure with, 74–75
  two-part, 73, *73*
Pseudomonas aeruginosa, 63
Pulmonary complications,
    scapulothoracic arthrodesis with,
    120
Putti-Platt procedure, 3, 4, 9

R
Recurrent instability
  allograft reconstruction for, 179
  postoperative rehabilitation for,
    179–180
  preferred treatment for, 177–180,
    178–180
  rates for, *177*
  thermal capsulorrhaphy with,
    176–180, *177–180*
Reflex sympathetic dystrophy, 175,
    175*t*
Refractory disorders, scapulothoracic
    articulation, 118
Reverse humeral avulsion of
    glenohumeral ligaments (RHAGL)
    lesions, 133
Rockwood's classification of AC joint
    dislocations, 78, *78*
Rotator cuff repair, 31–41
  acromial fracture following, 39–40
  anterior superior humeral head
    subluxation following, 40–41
  arthroscopy complications with,
    144–159, *145–150, 152–155,
    157, 158*
    arthroscopic instruments, *150,*
      150–151, *152*
    arthroscopic knot tying, 155–156
    bone preparation, 149–150
    infection as, 158
    intraoperative, 145–156, *146–150,
      152–155*
    neurological, 158–159
    passage through tendon, 154–155,
      155
    postoperative, 156–158, *157, 158*
    postoperative stiffness as, 157–158,
      158
    preoperative, 144–145, *145*
    rates of, 159
    recurrent tear as, 156–157, *157*
    subacromial decompression,
      145–146, *146, 147*
    suture anchors, 151–154, *153, 154*
    suture management, 154–155, *155*

systemic, 159
  tear morphology assessment, 149,
    150
  tendon releases, 146–149, *147–149*
deltoid injury following, 35, *35–36*
failed, 31–35
  clinical evaluation of, 32–33, *34*
  etiology of, 31–32
  fixation technique effects with, 32
  imaging of, 33, *34*
  revision results for, 33–34
heterotopic ossification following,
    37–38
infection following, 36–37
neurologic injury with, 88–89
persistent OS acromiale following,
    39–40
persistent subacromial impingement
    following, 36
postoperative stiffness following,
    38–39
Rotator cuff tears, 3
  surgical technique for, 60
  total shoulder arthroplasty with, 60
Rotator interval (RI), 21

S
SC joint. *See* Sternoclavicular joint
Scapulohumeral periarthritis. *See* Frozen
    shoulder
Scapulothoracic arthrodesis, 118–121,
    119
  hardware complications with, 120
  neurologic complications with,
    120–121
  preferred surgical technique for,
    118–120, *119*
  pulmonary complications with, 120
  wound complications with, 121
Seddon and Sunderland classification, 89
Shoulder arthrodesis. *See*
    Humeroscapular arthrodesis
Shoulder fusion, 92–93
Staphylococcus, 37, 158
Sternoclavicular joint (SC joint), 77, 81
Sternoclavicular joint surgery, 77, 81–83,
    82, 83
  anatomy for, 81
  pathology with, 81–82, *82*
  reducing complications with, 82–83,
    83
Stiffness. *See also* Frozen shoulder
  fracture management with, 72, *72–73*
  glenohumeral, 83
  postoperative arthroscopy rotator cuff
    repair, 157–158, *158*
  thermal capsulorrhaphy with, 180–181
Streptococcus, 63, 158
Stryker notch, 5
Subacromial decompression, 145–146,
    146, 147
Subacromial impingement, rotator cuff
    repair with, 36
Subscapularis tendon rupture
  anterior shoulder instability from,
    9–11, *11*
  belly press test for, 9, *11*

Sulcus sign, 21, *21*
Superior instability
  surgical technique for, 53–55, *54, 55*
  total shoulder arthroplasty with,
    52–55, *54, 55*
Suprascapular nerve, arthroscopic
    shoulder surgery with, 129
Surgical techniques
  neurologic injury, 90–93, *91*
    brachial plexus in, 91, *91*
    clavicular osteotomy as, 92
    deltopectoral approach in, 92
    donor nerve grafts as, 92
    neurotization as, 92
    recovery from, 93
    shoulder fusion as, 92–93
  TSA anterior instability, 51–52, *51–53*
  TSA component loosening, 46–48,
    46–49
  TSA inferior instability, 58–60, *59, 60*
  TSA intraoperative fractures, 61
  TSA periprosthetic fractures, 62–63, *63*
  TSA posterior instability, *56,* 56–57,
    57
  TSA rotator cuff tears, 60
  TSA superior instability, 53–55, *54, 55*

T
Thermal capsulorrhaphy, 172–181, *173,
    175–180,* 175*t*
  axillary nerve injury following,
    174–176, *175,* 175*t, 176*
  basic science with, 172–173, *173*
  capsular necrosis following, 176–177,
    177
  chondral injury following, 181
  complications from, 174–181,
    175–180, 175*t*
  indications for, 173–174
    atraumatic instability as, 173–174
    multidirectional instability as, 174
    traumatic instability as, 173
  introduction to, 172
  recurrent instability following,
    176–180, *177–180*
  results with, 173–174
  stiffness following, 180–181
Total shoulder arthroplasty (TSA), 43–66
  anterior instability with, 50–52, *50–53*
    surgical technique for, 51–52, *51–53*
  deltoid dysfunction with, 66, *66*
  glenoid component instability with,
    48–50, *50*
  glenoid component loosening with,
    44, 44–45, *45*
  humeral component loosening with,
    45, *45*
  implant failure/dissociation with,
    65–66
  implant wear with, 46
  infection with, 63–65, *64*
    treatment technique for, *64,* 64–65
  inferior instability with, 57–60, *58–60*
    surgical technique for, 58–60, *59, 60*
  intraoperative fractures with, 60–61,
    61
    surgical technique for, 61

nerve injuries with, 65, *65*
    treatment technique for, 65
periprosthetic fractures with, 60, *62,*
        62–63, 63
    postoperative, *62, 62–63, 63*
    surgical technique for, 62–63, *63*
posterior instability with, 55–57, *56,*
        57
    surgical technique for, *56, 56–57, 57*

prosthetic loosening with, 44, *44*
rotator cuff tears with, 60
    surgical technique for, 60
superior instability with, 52–55, *54, 55*
    surgical technique for, 53–55, *54, 55*
technique for component loosening
        with, 46–48, *46–49*
Tracheal compression, 126
TSA. *See* Total shoulder arthroplasty

Tuberosity failure, proximal humeral
        fracture with, 74–75

U
Ultrasound, failed rotator cuff repair in,
        33

W
Wallerian degeneration, 90
Weaver-Dunn procedure, 78